Download Your
Ebook Tod

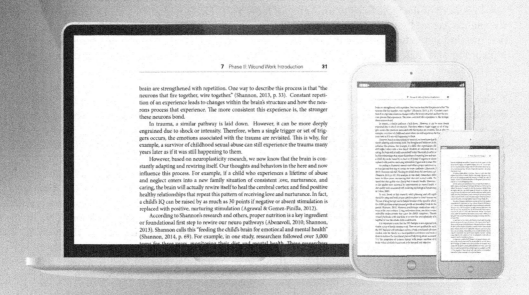
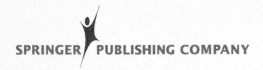

SPRINGER PUBLISHING COMPANY

SPC

Janna C. Heyman, PhD, LMSW, is Professor and Endowed Chair of the Henry C. Ravazzin Center on Aging and Intergenerational Studies at Fordham University Graduate School of Social Service. She is also Director of the Children & Families Institute at Fordham University. She has written numerous articles on health care, aging, palliative care, and social work education. Dr. Heyman is a Fellow at the New York Academy of Medicine and at the Gerontological Society of America. She was President of the State Society on Aging of New York. Dr. Heyman was awarded an Academic Excellence Award by the American Public Human Service Association for outstanding education and training in the field of human services. Prior to entering academia, she was a researcher and a planning and policy analyst, and served as Deputy Director of a large federal and state health care planning agency.

Elaine P. Congress, DSW, LCSW, is Associate Dean and Professor at Fordham University Graduate School of Social Service in New York City. Dr. Congress has published nine books including *Teaching Social Work Values and Ethics: A Curriculum Resource* (second edition in 2009), *Multicultural Perspectives in Social Work Practice With Families* (third edition in 2013), *Social Work With Immigrants and Refugees* (second edition in 2016), and *Nonprofit Management: A Social Justice Approach* (2017), as well as over 50 professional journal articles and book chapters. Dr. Congress is a Fellow at the New York Academy of Medicine, represents social work on the Governing Council of the American Public Health Association (APHA), and at Fordham coordinates the MSW/MPH program with the Icahn School of Medicine at Mt. Sinai. Dr. Congress serves on the United Nations (UN) Team for the International Federation of Social Workers (IFSW), and is a past president of the New York City chapter of the National Association of Social Workers (NASW). Before entering academia, she was a practitioner, supervisor, and administrator in a community mental health clinic.

Health and Social Work:
Practice, Policy, and Research

Janna C. Heyman, PhD, LMSW
Elaine P. Congress, DSW, LCSW
Editors

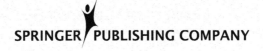

SPRINGER PUBLISHING COMPANY

Springer Publishing Company, LLC
11 West 42nd Street
New York, NY 10036
www.springerpub.com

Acquisitions Editor: Kate Dimock
Compositor: S4Carlisle Publishing Services

ISBN: 9780826141637
ebook ISBN: 9780826141644

Instructors' Materials: Qualified instructors may request supplements by emailing textbook@springerpub.com:
Instructors' Manual ISBN: 9780826141651
Instructors' PowerPoints ISBN: 9780826141668

Library of Congress Cataloging-in-Publication Data
Names: Heyman, Janna C., editor. | Congress, Elaine P., editor.
Title: Health and social work : practice, policy, and research / Janna C. Heyman and Elaine P. Congress, editors.
Description: New York : Springer Publishing Company, [2018] | Includes bibliographical references and index.
Identifiers: LCCN 2017056497 | ISBN 9780826141637 | ISBN 9780826141644 (ebook) | ISBN 9780826141651 (instructors' manual) | ISBN 9780826141668 (instructors' PowerPoints)
Subjects: | MESH: Social Work | Health Policy | Health Services Accessibility | Research | United States
Classification: LCC HV687 | NLM W 322 | DDC 362.1/0425--dc23 LC record available at https://lccn.loc.gov/2017056497

Contact us to receive discount rates on bulk purchases.
We can also customize our books to meet your needs.
For more information please contact: sales@springerpub.com

*To our students and all social workers, who inspire us every day
with their commitment and interest in health and health care. Their
recognition of health issues and health disparities and the need to
integrate practice, policy, and research motivated us to write this book.*

*To our husbands, Neil J. Heyman and the late Robert T. Snyder,
and our families, who always encouraged and supported us in our
academic endeavors and pursuit of promoting good health and well-being
and providing equal access to health and health care for all.*

Contents

Contributors

Priscilla D. Allen, PhD, LMSW Sister Michael Professor of Aging and Geriatrics and Associate Director, Life Course and Aging Center, Louisiana State University, Baton Rouge, Louisiana

James Amarante, LMSW, MS Research Assistant, Fordham University Graduate School of Social Service, New York, New York

Ellen Belluomini, PhD, LCSW Assistant Professor, Brandman University, Irvine, California

Cathy Berkman, PhD, MSW Associate Professor and Director of Palliative Care Fellowship, Fordham University Graduate School of Social Service, New York, New York

Kelsey H. Blumenstock, LMSW Research Assistant, Fordham University Graduate School of Social Service, New York, New York

Carolyn Brouard Bachelor Student, Department of Psychology & Counseling, Centenary University, Hackettstown, New Jersey

Derek Brian Brown, PhD, LMSW Assistant Professor, Department of Social Work, School of Health Professions, Long Island University–Brooklyn Campus, Brooklyn, New York

Julie A. Cederbaum, PhD, MSW, MPH Associate Professor, University of Southern California, Suzanne Dworak-Peck School of Social Work, Los Angeles, California

Elaine P. Congress, DSW, LCSW Associate Dean and Professor, Fordham University Graduate School of Social Service, New York, New York

Vincent Corcoran, BS Research Assistant, Fordham University Graduate School of Social Service, New York, New York

Jaih Craddock, MSW, MA Doctoral Candidate, University of Southern California, Suzanne Dworak-Peck School of Social Work, Los Angeles, California

Jose E. Crego, LCSW, LADC Director, Springfield Vet Center, Department of Veterans Affairs, West Springfield, Massachusetts

Meredith Doherty, LCSW Doctoral Candidate, Department of Social Welfare, City University of New York Graduate Center, New York, New York

Michelle Falcon, LMSW, MPH   Client Care Coordinator, Henry Street Settlement, New York, New York

Myra Glajchen, DSW, MSW   Director of Medical Education, MJHS Institute for Innovation in Palliative Care, New York, New York

Ralph Gregory, LMSW   Senior Advisor, Fordham University Graduate School of Social Service, Children and Families Institute, New York, New York

Janna C. Heyman, PhD, LMSW   Professor and Endowed Chair, Henry C. Ravazzin Center on Aging and Intergenerational Studies, Fordham University Graduate School of Social Service, New York, New York

Robert H. Keefe, PhD, ACSW, LMSW   Associate Professor, School of Social Work, University at Buffalo, State University of New York, Buffalo, New York

Peggy L. Kelly, LMSW, MPA   Research Coordinator, Fordham University Graduate School of Social Service, New York, New York

Sandra D. Lane, PhD, MPH   Professor, Laura J. and L. Douglas Meredith Professor of Public Health and of Anthropology, Syracuse University, Syracuse, New York

Tina Maschi, PhD, LCSW, ACSW   Associate Professor, Fordham University Graduate School of Social Service, New York, New York

Jeanne Matich-Maroney, PhD, LCSW-R   Associate Professor, Department of Social Work, Iona College, New Rochelle, New York

Sara Matsuzaka, MSW   Doctoral Candidate, Fordham University Graduate School of Social Service, New York, New York

Keith Morgen, PhD, LPC, ACS   Associate Professor, Department of Psychology & Counseling, Centenary University, Hackettstown, New Jersey

Manoj Pardasani, PhD   Senior Associate Dean and Associate Professor, Fordham University Graduate School of Social Service, New York, New York

Gary M. Reback, LMSW   Research Assistant, Fordham University Graduate School of Social Service, West Harrison, New York

Abigail M. Ross, PhD, MSW, MPH   Assistant Professor, Fordham University Graduate School of Social Service, New York, New York

Erik M. P. Schott, EdD, LCSW   Clinical Associate Professor, University of Southern California, Suzanne Dworak-Peck School of Social Work, Los Angeles, California

Jonathan B. Singer, PhD, LCSW   Associate Professor, Loyola University Chicago School of Social Work, Chicago, Illinois; Founder and Host, Social Work Podcast

Jaclyn Smith, BA   MA Candidate, Department of Psychology & Counseling, Centenary University, Hackettstown, New Jersey

Victoria Stanhope, PhD, MSW, MA   Associate Professor of Social Work, Silver School of Social Work, New York University, New York, New York

Gary L. Stein, JD, MSW   Professor, Wurzweiler School of Social Work, Yeshiva University, New York, New York

Lynn Videka, PhD   Dean and Collegiate Professor of Social Work, School of Social Work, University of Michigan, Ann Arbor, Michigan

Madeline K. Wachman, MSW, MPH   Program Manager, Center for Innovation in Social Work and Health, Boston University, Boston, Massachusetts

Linda White-Ryan, PhD, LCSW, RN   Assistant Dean, Fordham University Graduate School of Social Service, New York, New York

Sharon L. Young, PhD, LCSW   Associate Professor, Department of Social Work, Western Connecticut State University, Danbury, Connecticut

Foreword

Social work has a long-standing commitment to health care and the recognition of the inextricable link to quality of life and well-being across the life span. Our professional values and ethical principles provide important context related to the challenges of the affordability and accessibility of quality health care for all. While there have been remarkable gains in medical science that include cures and advances in disease treatment, sadly too many Americans continue to experience poor health outcomes. From the early days of our profession, attention was given to the need to improve care for vulnerable and at-risk populations. During the progressive era, settlement houses were known for establishing clinics to address the prominent health challenges of the era. This emphasis on meeting the health care needs of poor and marginalized populations has continued and has been supported by practice, policy, and research aimed at improving outcomes, especially for those who have experienced lifelong and generational disparities associated with racism, homophobia, and other stigmatizing conditions that negatively impact access and affordability as well as the health care experience.

Today's social workers must continue to close the pernicious gaps in health care that prematurely claim the lives of individuals and the associated impact on their families and communities. My father, a World War II veteran, succumbed to the complications of diabetes at the age of 57 years over 35 years ago. He is an exemplar of disparities that travel across the life span and create cumulative disadvantages. Although the gap is closing, the Centers for Disease Control and Prevention reports that there is an overall 4 year lower life expectancy for Blacks versus Whites. This gap widens based on gender and geographical locations. David Katz, President of the American College of Lifestyle Medicine, states, "Social justice is among the more important determinants of health outcomes, and disparities are very revealing about social justice and equity in public health."

It is my hope that within my lifetime, I will see the gap removed and the improvement in health care for all groups. This generation of social workers has the opportunity, despite the potential disruptions to the Patient Protection and Affordable Care Act (ACA), to realize continued health gains that will address the needs of most vulnerable populations. This will be done by our engagement in culturally competent practice that reaches out to marginalized groups and determines best approaches to engaging them in prevention and compliance. For example, social workers will be instrumental in helping the one in seven persons who are unaware that they have HIV to get tested and treated. By understanding their resistance to testing, social workers can help to develop outreach programs that break through the barriers that prevent testing. Additionally, social workers can organize support groups that educate individuals and family members to better respond to HIV in the family. Practice initiatives like this can make a difference. Coupling practice innovations with evidenced-based assessments provides social workers with valued leadership positions on interdisciplinary teams.

Additionally, policy initiatives that give primacy to enhanced prevention and treatment can also contribute to closing the equity gap. The ACA is an example of such legislation. For example, adding coverage for prevention services and coverage of preexisting conditions offer needed support, especially for historically oppressed and marginalized groups. It is important for social workers in health care to advocate for legislation that seeks to address pernicious inequities. Finally, eradicating social injustice in health care requires research that documents disparate outcomes. Understanding where gaps have closed and where they continue to exist allows us as social workers to use our keen sense of culture and environment. For example, there are critical questions that relate to modifying behaviors to prolong quality of life. Understanding the social determinants of health and the sometimes hidden barriers to better care is critically important. The government-sanctioned disparities such as the Tuskegee syphilis experiment, involuntary sterilization, and more still remain in the hearts and minds of many African Americans and continue to breed distrust in the health care system. Findings such as those in the 2002 Institute of Medicine "Unequal Treatment" report documented disparities in the treatment of cardiac patients and the premature amputation of lower extremities for African Americans suffering from diabetes. My father possibly fell victim to this undesirable life-changing event. I am convinced that my father fell victim to medical care that was "race-based" rather than person-centered. While it is wonderful to see the changes that have come about from this groundbreaking study, there is the nagging question of "what if" someone had stepped in earlier and addressed the disparities that compromised generations. Today, as social workers, we are empowered to stand up in the variety of health care practice settings that we serve and insist on equity. We can make a difference for our veterans, members of racial and sexual minorities, as well as other valued and marginalized members of our diverse society. The payoff is improved quality of life for many.

If we are to achieve health care equity, we must unlock the formula to translate knowing better to doing better. This is the next frontier of social work practice. This book offers valuable content that will provide new social work insights into practice, policy, and research, and their integration aimed at the elimination of disparities and achievement of health equity. I am grateful on both professional and personal levels to the contributors—I firmly believe that their insights will open eyes, hearts, and minds and lead to the highest standards of health care that honor the social work values of social justice and the dignity and worth of all persons. Our constituents deserve no less.

Sandra Edmonds Crewe, PhD, ACSW
Dean and Professor
Howard University School of Social Work

Preface

The pursuit of health and well-being is important to all people in the United States and globally. Historically, the settlement house movement was committed to promoting better health for recently arrived immigrants. The social work profession has continued to focus on this goal by working with diverse populations in many different health and behavioral health settings—inpatient, outpatient, and community-based. This is accomplished by collaborating with other health care professionals in partnership with individuals, families, groups, and communities served.

As we go to press, the United States is spending 17.8% of its gross domestic product on health care (Centers for Medicare & Medicaid Services, 2016) and only 9% on social services (Bradley & Taylor, 2013). The enhancement of social services is needed to help improve health and positive health outcomes. In collaboration with other health care professionals, social workers need to address issues of access, quality of care, prevention, and social justice to further advance the health care field. As health care is expanding, the U.S. Department of Labor Bureau of Labor Statistics (2016) has predicted there will be increased employment opportunities for social workers in health-related fields. Education and training to ensure social workers are prepared to meet this need are critical.

We were inspired to write this book, *Health and Social Work: Practice, Policy, and Research,* by the interest expressed by our students regarding health and social work. We quickly became aware of how challenging it was to consider each theme separately, so each chapter also speaks to the interconnections between practice, policy, and research and the way in which they are integrated to inform the health care field. Case examples are provided throughout the book to further enhance an understanding of these issues. Questions at the end of each chapter are used to generate further reflection and critical thought on chapter content.

Part I of the book includes chapters that address general topics of social work ethics and social determinants of health. In Part II, specific areas such as health promotion and public health, integrated behavioral health care, palliative and end-of-life care, substance misuse and abuse, and correctional health and psychosocial care are discussed. Part III focuses on specific populations, including children and family health, older adults and their families, immigrants and refugee health, LGBT health, health for people with disabilities, veterans, and health for persons with HIV/AIDS. An intersectionality lens is used throughout to promote a greater understanding of clients' multiple statuses of gender, race, ethnicity, socioeconomic status, education level, sexual orientation, and gender identification. A discussion of the greater power and privilege of social workers and other professionals in the health care field affects the health and well-being and the lives of clients.

Although we are the primary creators of this book, we have shared this journey with the many contributors who have provided information about health care and social work. First, we would like to thank all our contributors from across the United States who, with their extensive academic and practice experience in the health field, made outstanding contributions to this book.

We would like to acknowledge the social workers who have worked tirelessly in the field to help individuals, families, and communities in addressing health care. Without their significant efforts, the profession would not be where it is today.

We also want to acknowledge our dean at Fordham University Graduate School of Social Service, Dr. Debra McPhee, who is very committed to advancing the role of social workers in health care and provided continual support and encouragement. Several colleagues, Martha Bial, Shirley Gatenio Gabel, Ralph Gregory, Peggy Kelly, and Linda White-Ryan, served as consulting editors to help us prepare the book for publication. Special thanks to Karen Dybing who worked extensively with the formatting and the final editing for this book. We also would like to thank Fordham University doctoral student Sara Matsuzaka, who is the co-author of the chapter on intersectionality (Chapter 4), and MSW student Lindsay Poulos, as well as Kelsey Blumenstock and Gary Reback who provided additional material and support for the book.

We would like to acknowledge our Springer editor, Debra Riegert, who provided important guidance to us from the initial birth of the idea through submission of our manuscript. We also want to extend special thanks to Mindy Chen, assistant editor at Springer, who was always available for any question that we had and was able to speedily advise us how to proceed. We would also like to recognize the extensive support of Rose Mary Piscitelli, Senior Editor, and Vinolia Benedict Fernando, and their production team who provided valuable support to us.

As our book heads toward publication, there are still many unsettled and remaining questions about health and health care. There are continuing challenges about changing federal and state health care policies and how this will affect health care, especially for those from low socioeconomic status and/or vulnerable populations. The good news is that there are breakthroughs in terms of new treatments that will cure or minimize the negative symptoms of many illnesses and chronic conditions. In spite of all the advances, while life expectancy is increasing in the United States, there are still many health disparities that need to be addressed. While there has been progress in the field, there still are challenges confronting social workers and the individuals, families, groups, and communities they serve.

As always, social workers will continue to engage as a profession, as well as join with other health care professionals, in advocacy efforts to work toward our common goal of promoting good health and well-being for all.

Elaine Congress
Janna Heyman

REFERENCES

Bradley, E. H., & Taylor, L. A. (2013). *The American health care paradox: Why spending more is getting us less*. New York, NY: Public Affairs.

Centers for Medicare & Medicaid Services. (2016). The nation's health dollars, calendar year 2015. Retrieved from https://www.cms.gov/Research-Statistics-Data-and -Systems/Statistics-Trends-and-Reports/NationalHealthExpendData/Downloads/ PieChartSourcesExpenditures2015.pdf

U.S. Department of Labor Bureau of Labor Statistics. (2016). Social workers. *Occupational outlook handbook*. https://www.bls.gov/ooh/community-and-social-service/ social-workers.htm

PART I

The Changing Landscape and Social Workers' Roles

1

Introduction to Health and Social Work

Janna C. Heyman and Linda White-Ryan

Throughout history, social work has played a significant role in the changing health care delivery system. From the settlement house movement to today, social work professionals are an important part of the fabric of health care, serving diverse individuals across the life span, practicing in a range of health care settings, advocating to improve access, and addressing the growing needs of the most vulnerable populations. This chapter highlights the history of health and social work, including the roles of social workers when working with diverse populations. It underscores the unique contributions social workers make and the challenges they face in practice, policy, and research.

Over the past decade, the health care system in the United States has undergone substantial changes, often driven by the need to improve quality of care, contain escalating costs, increase access, and improve health care outcomes (Institute of Medicine [IOM], 2015). From 2009 to 2014, health care spending had slowed in the United States, but has recently begun to rise again (Organisation for Economic Co-operation and Development [OECD], 2016). Cross-national comparisons of health care spending indicate that the United States still exceeds other countries, spending 17.8% of its gross domestic product (GDP) on health care (Centers for Medicare and Medicaid Services [CMS], 2016). The 2010 Patient Protection and Affordable Care Act (ACA) has been described as "the most important health care legislation enacted in the United States since the creation of Medicaid and Medicare in 1965" (Obama, 2016, p. 525). Since the enactment of the ACA, access to health care has improved, with the percentage of uninsured individuals declining from 16.0% in 2010 to 8.9% in the first 6 months of 2016 (Zammitti, Cohen, & Martinez, 2016). Davis, Stremikis, Squires, and Schoen (2014) compared the United States with 11 industrialized countries. In this report, the United States ranked "last or near last in dimensions of access, efficiency and equity" (p. 1) and ranked fifth in quality of care.

Even though health care spending is higher when compared to other countries, globally, the United States lags behind in critical health care indicators. In 2014, life expectancy was estimated at 78.8 years at birth for the United States, ranking 43rd in comparison to other countries (IOM, 2014). Disparities in life expectancies by race and ethnic groups (Arias, 2016), educational attainment (Laditka & Laditka, 2015), income (Chetty et al., 2016), and living in a rural community (Singh & Siahpush, 2014) still are prominent concerns.

Similarly, while there has been a decrease in the infant mortality rate globally, the United States' infant mortality rate is 5.82 per 1,000 (Kochanek, Murphy, Xu, & Tejada-Vera, 2016), which is still higher than comparable countries (OECD, 2016). In 2014, the age-adjusted death rate was 724.6 per 100,000 (Kochanek et al., 2016); however, racial and ethnic disparities are still significant (National Center for Health Statistics, 2016). The age-adjusted death rate was 1.2 times greater for the non-Hispanic Black population than for the non-Hispanic White population (Kochanek et al., 2016). In addition to racial and ethnic disparities, health disparities are also found in education, sex, place of residence, and sexual orientation (Adler et al., 2016).

Another measure of health is disease burden which adjusts for years of life lost due to premature death and years of productive life lost to poor health or disability. Disease burden dropped 16% between 1990 and 2015; however, disease burden rates in the United States are still 25% higher than comparable countries on average (Kamal & Cox, 2017).

While health care spending in the United States is high, spending on social services to meet the growing needs of the vulnerable populations is low. Bradley and Taylor (2013) found that as a country, the United States spent "less than 10 percent of its GDP on social services" (p. 14). This includes retirement and disability benefits, supportive housing, and employment programs. Yet, if one takes a holistic approach to care, the provision of social services can help to prevent and support individuals with health care needs. With this in mind, health problems and solutions need a "system-oriented" approach (Emanuel et al., 2012; McGinnis et al., 2016). Social workers can play a critical role in advocating and collaborating with individuals, families, communities, and other professionals to shape the future of health and health care. Before addressing social workers' role in today's health care, it is extremely valuable to understand the historical perspective of health and social work.

BACKGROUND/HISTORICAL PERSPECTIVE

The intersection of social work and health can be traced back to the Elizabethan Poor Laws of 1601 and Colonial America. In fact, the almshouses were first built to house individuals who were poor, disabled, or who did not have a family to care for them. One of the first almshouses was established in Boston in the mid-1600s. In 1713, William Penn established an almshouse near Philadelphia to serve the Quaker population. In New York, the Poor House of the City of New York, later known as Bellevue Hospital, was built in 1737 (Burrows & Wallace, 1998). In subsequent years, urbanization and industrialization significantly changed the face of America. By the 1830s, most American cities had adopted institution-based poor relief (Bourque, 2010). In 1847, health care was further shaped by the establishment of the American Medical Association (AMA), which focused on developing and establishing uniform standards for ethics, education, training, and practice.

The church-based and secular charity organizations continued to recognize ways to address poverty and immigration issues. The scientific approach to charity led to investigation and registration for individuals in need of charity. In fact, in 1877, the first American Charity Organization Society (COS) was established in Buffalo, New York. COSs grew throughout the country.

In further response to industrialization and immigration, the settlement house movement focused on social reform and the environmental causes of poverty. According to Trattner (1999), "the goal was to bridge the gap, between the classes and races, to eliminate the sources of distress, and to improve urban living and working conditions" (p. 163). In 1889, Jane Addams and Ellen Gates Starr established Hull House in Chicago. It became the center for civic and social engagement, research, and advocating for the health and well-being of residents affected by the conditions of the industrial districts in the city (Lundblad, 1995). In 1893, Lillian Wald founded Henry Street Settlement, the first settlement house in New York City. Social work involvement in public health is also traced back to the settlement house movement, with its focus on sanitation and disease control (Popple & Leighninger, 2011; Ruth & Sisco, 2008).

During the same time, Richard Cabot, who studied earlier with Jane Addams, set up an all-volunteer social service unit in Massachusetts General Hospital in Boston in 1905. Cabot recognized the importance of social and mental problems when addressing the medical needs of the patient. In one of his books, *Social Service and the Art of Healing*, he wrote a chapter titled, "Team-Work of Doctor, Educator, and Social Worker and the Resulting Changes in the Three Professions" (Cabot, 1909), which recognized the importance of different professions. Cabot considered the "nonsomatic factors," such as living conditions and nutrition, as central to care. Richard Cabot worked with Garnet Pelton and Ida Cannon to organize a formal social work department working with outpatients at Massachusetts General Hospital. Johns Hopkins Medical Center in Baltimore (Abrams, n.d.) was one of the first inpatient units. The emergence of hospital social work in both settings advanced the health care field (Wenocur & Reisch, 1989).

With the growth of hospital social work, public health, and the expansion of the settlement house movement throughout the country, reformers, including many social workers, shaped the Progressive Party platform in 1912 (Miringoff & Opdycke, 1986; Trattner, 1999). This advanced the emergence of social insurance, child welfare, and labor policies. At this time, The Flexner Report, *Medical Education in the United States and Canada* (1910), was released (Duffy, 2010) and in 1915 Flexner questioned social work as a profession. The debate regarding this report was challenged and continued for years. Social workers continued to define the profession and played an integral role in the provision, delivery of services, and interventions to address individuals' physical and mental health care needs.

During the 1920s, there was a significant shift, resulting from the stock market crash in 1929, and the Great Depression. Hunger, unemployment, and losses became the face of America. Marches, mass rallies, and demands for relief measures were in the forefront of the news. In 1932, President Franklin Delano Roosevelt was elected and he began to address the state of the nation. The New Deal created a large relief package, often known as the alphabet programs, such as Federal Emergency Relief Act (FERA) and Works Progress Administration (WPA). This also included creation of the 1935 Social Security Act that provided for old-age and survivor insurance, old-age assistance, aid to dependent children, and aid to the blind, and shaped the health care delivery system. Although some of its provisions were initially thought of as temporary programs, the Social Security Act has its place in history and today.

In 1948, health as a human right was included in Article 25 of the Universal Declaration of Human Rights (UDHR) as one's "right to a standard of living adequate for the health and well-being of himself and his family, including . . . medical care and necessary social services" (United Nations, 1948, "Article 25"). It was reiterated in Article 12 of the International Covenant on Economic, Social and Cultural Rights (ICESCR) that states everyone has "the right . . . to the enjoyment of the highest attainable standard of physical and mental health" (Office of the United Nations High Commissioner for Human Rights [OHCHR], 1966, "Article 12"), as well as in the American Declaration of the Rights and Duties of Man; the International Convention on the Elimination of All Forms of Racial Discrimination; the Convention on the Elimination of All Forms of Discrimination against Women; the Convention on the Rights of the Child; the International Convention on the Protection of the Rights of All Migrant Workers and Members of Their Families; and the Convention on the Rights of Persons with Disabilities. The right to health is also recognized by national constitutions around the world (OHCHR & World Health Organization [WHO], n.d.).

The WHO, the UN's organization charged with promoting health, defined health in its 1946 preamble of its Constitution as "a state of complete physical, mental and social well-being and not merely the absence of disease or infirmity" and is one of the "... fundamental rights of every human being without distinction of race, religion, political belief, economic or social condition" (International Health Conference, 2002, p. 1). Further discussion of the right-based approach is addressed later in this chapter.

During the 1960s, health and social welfare initiatives grew again. President Kennedy's focus on poverty and social justice was significant. It was the work of Martin Luther King, Jr. as a civil rights leader and organizer that reshaped America. His "I Have a Dream" speech helped to change the nation and more fully recognize its struggles and injustices. President Kennedy supported King's work and civil rights, but it wasn't until after his assassination that many civil rights and anti-poverty programs were started. It was President Johnson who launched the War on Poverty, and Medicare and Medicaid were added to the Social Security Act in 1965. These significant legislative actions paved the way for addressing the health care needs of the future. Social work and its involvement in public health also continued to grow in the 1960s.

The 1980s shaped public health nationally. Acquired immune deficiency syndrome (AIDS) was first documented in 1981. Through the work of leaders and activists, including Jonathan Mann, the first director of the Global AIDS Program at the WHO, they helped to educate others about the disease. Mann stressed the rights of individuals and inequities in health care and focused on prevention to limit the spread of the disease (Fee & Parry, 2008).

The growth of new issues in health care and models of health care delivery ebbed and flowed (Black, 1984; Globerman & Bogo, 2002; Keigher, 1997). Priorities on addressing health care for population groups were further shaped. For example, in substance abuse, new programs were developed that enhanced the growth of both inpatient and outpatient programs to help persons with alcohol and substance abuse problems.

In 1990, a landmark act, the Americans with Disabilities Act (ADA), was signed into law by President George H. W. Bush. This act prohibits discrimination and guarantees equal opportunities for people with disabilities (U.S. Department of Justice, n.d.). By extending civil rights protections to persons with disabilities, the ADA provided individuals the same rights and opportunities as everyone.

Under President Clinton, there was a significant move to reshape health care and address the needs of the uninsured. As First Lady, Hillary Rodham Clinton led the Task Force on National Health Care Reform, comprised of government representatives, policy advisors, and health care experts, to develop a comprehensive plan to provide universal health care in the United States. After significant debate, the proposal was defeated.

In February 2001, President George W. Bush announced the New Freedom Initiative to promote increased access to educational and employment opportunities for people with disabilities. It was considered one of the first comprehensive studies of the nation's public and private mental health service delivery systems. The report emphasized how consumers, along with service providers, "will actively participate in designing and developing the systems of care in which they are involved" (U.S. Department of Health and Human Services, 2003, p. 12). Patient-centered care was supported throughout the New Freedom report and the 2001 IOM release of *Crossing the Quality Chasm: A New Health System for the Twenty-First Century*. Social workers advocated and encouraged the profession to lead initiatives in this area.

The IOM report (2001) and support nationwide led to the development of the "Triple Aim," a framework designed by the Institute for Health care Improvement, which focuses on (a) improving the patient's experience of care; (b) addressing population health; and (c) reducing per capita costs (Berwick, Nolan, & Whittington, 2008; Lewis, 2014). To address these priorities, integrated behavioral health in primary care developed throughout the country. Social workers are vital members of the interdisciplinary/interprofessional health care teams and collaborate with patients and other health care professionals to address these issues.

President Obama's 2010 ACA increased access to health care in some of the following ways: (a) providing subsidies to help lower-income individuals reduce out-of-pocket costs; (b) expanding coverage for young adults up to age 26 under their parents' plan; (c) expanding Medicaid by raising the eligibility guideline to 138% of the poverty level for states opting to expand Medicaid; (d) requiring all insurers to offer 10 categories of essential health benefits, such as maternity care and mental health services; and (e) requiring insurers to cover individuals regardless of preexisting conditions. The ACA had an employer mandate that required larger companies to provide affordable insurance. The ACA also required all Americans to buy health insurance or pay a tax penalty. (It is important to note that in December 2017, President Trump signed into law the Tax Cut and Jobs Act, Public Law 115-97, that removes the mandate for individual insurance coverage.) Further, it restricted insurers from charging older adults more than three times what younger individuals are charged, as well as prohibiting insurers from setting a limit on coverage payment levels. Other components of the ACA reflect rights-based approaches to health care in that it sought to improve access to health care, and emphasize preventive measures such as exercise and education, as well as recognize the interdependence of physical and behavioral health and aim to facilitate the interconnections between them.

After enactment of the ACA, there was extensive debate about repealing and replacing the Act. In March 2017, the House released the American Health Care Act, and it was approved in May 2017. In June 2017, after a series of closed-door sessions, the Senate released its version of a health care reform proposal, the Better Care Reconciliation Act. In July 2017, a "skinny repeal" was proposed in the Senate to scale back parts of the ACA. After extensive debate, on July 28, 2017, the Senate proposal was voted down. In the coming years, new proposals or refinement will further impact the future of health care in the United States.

The Centers for Medicare and Medicaid (2017) documented 8.8 million individuals enrolled at HealthCare.gov as of December 15, 2017. Even with high individual enrollment, there continues to be concern about the impact of the removal of the individual insurance mandate under the new Tax Cut and Jobs Act, Public Law 115-97. It is possible that by discontinuing the ACA health insurance mandate, it may change the population pools for the insurance exchanges and may significantly impact it.

THE RIGHT TO HEALTH CARE

According to Gatenio Gabel (personal communication, December 27, 2017),

> the rights-based approach to health that evolved in decades following WW II is much more than access to health care services and includes the services, education, and developing an environment that helps us live a fulfilling life. The ICESCR refers to these factors as the underlying determinants of health (OHCHR & WHO, n.d.). . . . The point is that from a rights-based approach, health intersects and is interdependent with other human rights. A rights-based approach to health also emphasizes that

services that help individuals obtain well-being cannot be limited or made exclusive to certain populations (OHCHR & WHO, n.d.). The right to health must be universal, non-discriminatory, and inclusive. . . . A rights-based approach also values the process and advocates that the population should participate in health-related decision-making at all levels of government. Facilities, goods and services should also respect medical ethics, be gender-sensitive and culturally appropriate. In other words, they should be medically and culturally acceptable and accessible to all. The rights-based approach in many ways is similar to the social work approach because at the foundation of both approaches is respect for the dignity and worth of all individuals.

There is extensive discussion in today's society about the right to health care (RTHC). The United Nations Sustainable Development Goals (SDGs) that apply to developed as well as developing countries list one of its goals as "good health and well being." The goal of ensuring healthy lives and promoting well-being of people at all ages has very specific targets including reducing maternal and infant mortality and increasing life expectancy (WHO, 2017). As discussed previously, when compared to other developed countries the United States's record on these health outcomes could be improved. The International Federation of Social Workers (IFSW) on Health states that

. . . health is an issue of fundamental human rights and social justice and binds social work to apply these principles in policy, education, research and practice. All people have an equal right to enjoy the basic conditions which underpin human health. These conditions include a minimum standard of living to support health and a sustainable and health promoting environment. All people have an equal right to access resources and services that promote health and address illness, injury and impairment, including social services. IFSW will demand and continue to work for the realisation of these universal rights through the development, articulation and pursuit of socially just health and social policies. (IFSW, 2012, p. 1)

This statement was approved at the IFSW General Meeting in Salvador de Bahia, Brazil, August 14, 2008 and it emphasized the importance of health as a human right internationally.

According to DaSilva (2016), international human rights law recognizes the right to health and it underscores both moral and legal principles. He states, "Moral theories seek to identify reasons people have a moral RTHC (and explain why it should be fulfilled through the law). Legal theories explain why legal authority must be used to recognize a RTHC principles" (DaSilva, 2016, p. 379). According to the WHO (2012), the goal of universal health care is a "practical expression of the concern for health equity and the right to health" (p. 3). The rights-based approach to health should be in the forefront. Gatenio Gabel (2016) states that a rights-based approach "requires consideration of the universally recognized principles of human rights: the equality of each individual as a human being, the inherent dignity of each person and the rights to self-determination, peace and security" (p. x). There have been efforts in some states to advocate for publicly funded health care as a basic human right (McGill & MacNaughton, 2016).

As a profession, social work has a history of advocating and ensuring human rights and social justice. The primary mission of the National Association of Social Workers (NASW) Code of Ethics is "to enhance human well-being and help meet the basic human needs of all people, with particular attention to the needs and empowerment of people who are vulnerable, oppressed, and living in poverty" (NASW, 2017, p. 1). The Code emphasizes the importance of promoting social justice and social change. Yet, in society, there are still practices that violate human rights. Social workers need to collaborate with other professionals, individuals, and communities to confront these and address problems such as inequities in health care and issues of access and affordability for all persons.

THE CHANGING FOCUS ON HEALTH CARE

Spending on health care in the United States has often focused on treatment with less emphasis on prevention. Noncommunicable, preventable chronic conditions can be attributed to more than 75% of the $3.2 trillion spent each year on medical care (CMS, 2016), with only 3% spent on prevention and public health (CMS, 2016). New initiatives have targeted reducing costs, development of new care models, and prevention (IOM, 2015). To address these challenges, McGinnis et al. (2016) explored how to rethink health care investments. They stressed the importance of renewed focus since often:

> . . . our incentives, are too narrow and too late: despite an increasingly strong and specific understanding of the preventable elements in the development of our health challenges—social, behavioral, environmental—our investments are primarily directed to their biomedical manifestations, well after the problems have taken root. (p. 2)

Investing in the health and well-being of individuals, families, organizations, and communities is critical. Social workers are well positioned to assist in this process. The ecological and life models within the profession have continued to support the person-in-environment perspective (Germain & Gitterman, 1980). Social work's ecological approach with its focus on the person-in-environment emphasizes the importance of understanding an individual, family, or community within the environmental contexts in which those people live and function. This perspective has historical roots in the profession of social work and includes an emphasis on personal and environmental change (Kondrat, 2013). The rights-based approach further empowers social workers to advocate across systems for holistic approaches to health (Gatenio Gabel, 2016).

As health care expenditures are a significant part of the U.S. economy, the challenge is to determine how to restructure delivery and payment in order to improve quality of, and access to, care. Social workers should take a place at the table to develop and enhance innovative approaches and models of health care service delivery.

Figure 1.1 illustrates some of the important considerations for health and health care for members of society. Throughout this book many of these areas are discussed, particularly as they impact health and health care. Although not exhaustive, these eight areas are:

- Access
- Continuum of services
- Cost
- Empowerment
- Equality
- Outcomes
- Prevention
- Quality of life

While one can view these areas as discrete, they can also interact with each other. For instance, providing *access* to health is essential, but so is ensuring access to a *continuum of*

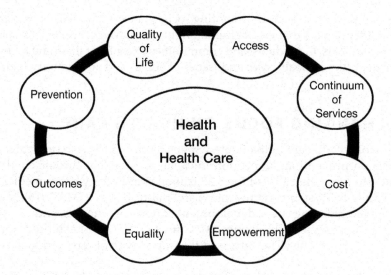

Figure 1.1 Ensuring health and health care.

services, and these two areas can overlap with one another. Another consideration is the breadth and depth of issues related to these eight areas. For example, the *cost* of health can also be captured in very broad terms, but can also have multiple layers, including the cost of lost lives that may have been prevented, cost of health care as part of the GDP, as well as cost of caregiving, which can significantly impact both the lives of many caregivers and the individuals they care for.

To further illustrate *access and equity,* one can look at the ACA. While the ACA (Patient Protection and Affordable Care Act, 2010) reduced the number of individuals without health care, there are still large gaps in coverage. For example, undocumented immigrants continue to lack coverage and many individuals lack coverage for chronic diseases. On the other hand, even when individuals do have insurance, they may also have difficulty in accessing health care. For example, some individuals on Medicaid have difficulty finding physicians who accept their coverage. Also, for many rural communities, there is a shortage of health care professionals, which creates further difficulties with access. Satellite clinics and other models of health care delivery in primary care settings can be critical to access to health care. While some people think that access is the same as having health insurance, access is a much broader issue. Yet, it is important to recognize that access is strongly correlated with better health care outcomes (Parento & Gostin, 2013).

Outcomes such as life expectancy, infant mortality, and other health indicators have significant racial and ethnic disparities. The right to health care demands that everyone should be able to enjoy health and well-being to the greatest extent possible. *Equality* must be ensured for all individuals. Ensuring *quality of life*, which is of the utmost importance, deserves to be promoted for all without exception. Achieving positive health outcomes for all individuals, families, and communities, in an inclusive and nondiscriminatory manner, needs to be in the forefront. *Empowering* individuals to make their own decision presumes collaborative roles for social workers in working with individuals, families, and communities and is a basic principle of the rights-based approach. Professionals foster empowerment "by providing a climate, a relationship, resources, and procedural means through which people can enhance their own lives" (Simon, 1990, p. 32). Respecting the rights of individuals and empowering them to make decisions about their care setting is another example of how these areas intersect.

Prevention is a frequently overlooked aspect of health care with greater attention placed on treatment. Social workers can play an important role in educating about the risk and protective factors to empower the client-bases they serve to advocate for equality in health care services that reduce risk factors and improve health. Significant advances in public health have focused on prevention, including work in disease infection and control, environmental sustainability, and suicide prevention (Turnock, 2007). Social workers stress the importance of primary prevention, which emphasizes preventing disease and injury before it occurs. This is well aligned with the profession's person-in-environment perspective. As recognized in the past (Gilbert, 1982) and present (DeVylder, 2016; Silverman, 2008), social workers need to collaborate with individuals, families, and communities to be the catalysts for change to increase the focus on prevention. The 145-year-old American Public Health Association (APHA) has long promoted prevention as an important policy in addressing health issues (APHA, 2017) and representatives from the large Public Health Social Work section of APHA serve on the Governing Council.

The NASW (2016) underscores prevention into its practice standards for social workers. In addition, the Council on Social Work Education (CSWE) has included prevention in its 2015 Education Program Accreditation Standards (EPAS). As stated in the EPAS 2.0, in order to promote human and social well-being, generalist practitioners need to "use a range of prevention and intervention methods in their practice with diverse individuals, families, groups, organizations, and communities based on scientific inquiry and best practices" (p. 11). Attention on prevention is also consistent with the goals of the American Academy of Social Work and Social Welfare's Grand Challenges Initiative.

Social work encompasses a strengths-based, person-centered perspective, which utilizes holistic, biological, psychological, social, and spiritual perspectives. As highlighted in CSWE EPAS (2015), "engagement is an ongoing component of the dynamic and interactive process of social work practice with, and on behalf of, diverse individuals, families, groups, organizations, and communities" (p. 8). The importance of engagement is paramount. Assessment that includes collecting comprehensive information is also an important step in the process. Collaboration and respect for cultural values and beliefs is an important part of the process. Social workers are often on the frontline in addressing health and health care for individuals, families, communities, and the larger system of care.

These areas, discussed here as well as described in Figure 1.1, are expanded upon throughout each of the chapters in this book.

CONCLUSION

Social workers have long held important roles in health and health care. The changing landscape of health care calls for advocacy and advances in the field. The right to health care is a pivotal human right and continues to be in the forefront. Social workers can help to change the health care delivery system that embraces collaboration with the individuals, families, communities, and other disciplines to ensure good health for all members of society. Social workers recognize the dignity and worth of all people as well as the influence of the environment on human life. As a profession involved in direct practice, advocacy work, policy development, and research, it is critical to improve the health care system on all levels, including a strong focus on prevention. The recognition of health care disparities that continue to exist in society is a major concern of social workers responding to the needs of vulnerable populations. The values of the profession today still reflect the early values of social workers that emphasize the right to equality and access to health and health care.

As agents of change, social workers have the important function of becoming involved in economic and policy development—collaborating and advocating for initiatives that demand education, prevention, and treatment, leading to the promotion of health and health care for all. This book underscores the critical importance of health for all members of society and the significant role of social work in the field.

REFERENCES

Abrams, J. M. (n.d.). Psychiatry social work at the Johns Hopkins Hospital. Retrieved from http://www.hopkinsmedicine.org/psychiatry/about/anniversary/social _work_history.html

Adler, N., Cutler, D., Fielding, J., Galea, S., Glymour, M., Koh, H., & Satcher, D. (2016). Addressing social determinants of health and health disparities (Discussion Paper). In *Vital Directions for Health and Health Care Series*. Washington, DC: National Academy of Medicine. Retrieved from https://nam.edu/wp-content/uploads/2016/09/ Addressing-Social-Determinants-of-Health-and-Health-Disparities.pdf

American Public Health Association. (2017). Policies and advocacy. Retrieved from https://www.apha.org/policies-and-advocacy

Arias, E. (2016). Changes in life expectancy by race and Hispanic origin in the United States, 2013–2014. *NCHS Data Brief 244*. Hyattsville, MD: National Center for Health Statistics.

Berkwick, D. M., Nolan, T. W., & Whittington, J. (2008). The Triple Aim: Care, health, and cost. *Health Affairs, 27*(3), 759–769. doi:10.1377/hlthaff.27.3.759

Black, R. B. (1984). Looking ahead: Social work as a core health profession. *Health & Social Work, 9*(2), 85–95.

Bourque, M. (2010). Almhouses. In *Encyclopedia for urban studies* (pp. 18–19). Thousand Oaks, CA: Sage.

Bradley, E. H., & Taylor, L. A. (2013). *The American health care paradox: Why spending more is getting us less*. New York, NY: Public Affairs.

Burrows, E., & Wallace, M. (1998). *Gotham: A history of New York City to 1898*. New York, NY: Oxford University Press.

Cabot, R. C. (1909). *Social service and the art of healing*, New York, NY: Moffat, Yard, and Company.

Centers for Medicare and Medicaid Services. (2016). The nation's health dollar ($3.2 trillion), calendar year 2015: Where it came from. Retrieved from https://www.cms .gov/Research-Statistics-Data-and-Systems/Statistics-Trends-and-Reports/ NationalHealthExpendData/Downloads/PieChartSourcesExpenditures2015.pdf

Centers for Medicare and Medicaid Services. (2017). Weekly enrollment snapshot: Week seven. Retrieved from https://www.cms.gov/Newsroom/MediaReleaseDatabase/ Fact-sheets/2017-Fact-Sheet-items/2017-12-21.html

Chetty, R., Stepner, M., Abraham, S., Lin, S., Scuderi, B., Turner, N., . . . Cutler, D. (2016). The association between income and life expectancy in the United States, 2001–2004. *Journal of the American Medical Association, 315*(16), 1750–1766. doi:10.1001/jama.2016.4226

Congressional Budget Office. (2017). H.R. 1628, American Health Care Act: Cost estimates. Retrieved from https://www.cbo.gov/publication/52752

Council on Social Work Education. (2015). *Educational policy and accreditation standards.* Alexandria, VA: Author. Retrieved from https://www.cswe.org/getattachment/ Accreditation/Accreditation-Process/2015-EPAS/2015EPAS_Web_FINAL.pdf.aspx

DaSilva, M. (2016). A goal-oriented understanding of the right to health care and its implications for future health rights litigation. *Dalhousie Law Journal, 39*(2), 377–395.

Davis, K., Stremikis, K., Squires, D., & Schoen, C. (2014). *Mirror, mirror on the wall: How the performance of the U.S. health care system compares internationally.* New York, NY: The Commonwealth Fund. Retrieved from http://www.commonwealthfund.org/~/ media/files/publications/fund-report/2014/jun/1755_davis_mirror_mirror_2014 _exec_summ.pdf

DeVylder, J. (2016). Preventing schizophrenia and severe mental illness: A grand challenge for social work. *Research on Social Work Practice, 26*(4), 449–459.

Duffy, T. P. (2010). The Flexner Report—100 years later. *Yale Journal of Biology and Medicine, 84*(3), 269–276.

Emanuel, E., Tanden, N., Altman, S., Armstrong, S., Berwick, D., deBrantes, F., . . . Spiro, T. (2012). A systemic approach to containing health care spending. *New England Journal of Medicine, 367*(10), 949–954. doi:10.1056/NEJMsb1205901

Fee, E., & Parry, M. (2008). Jonathan Mann, HIV/AIDS, and human rights. *Journal of Public Health Policy, 29*(1), 54–71. doi:10.1057/palgrave.jphp.3200160

Gatenio Gabel, S. (2016). *A rights-based approach to social policy analysis.* Basel, Switzerland: Springer International.

Germain, C., & Gitterman, A. (1980). *The life model of social work practice.* New York, NY: Columbia University Press.

Gilbert, N. (1982). Policy issues in primary prevention. *Social Work, 27,* 293–297.

Globerman, J., & Bogo, M. (2002). The impact of hospital restricting on social work education. *Health and Social Work, 27*(1), 7–16.

Institute of Medicine. (2001). *Crossing the quality chasm: A new health system for the twenty-first century.* Washington, DC: National Academies Press.

Institute of Medicine. (2014). *U.S. health in international perspective: Shorter lives, poorer health.* Washington, DC: National Academies Press.

Institute of Medicine. (2015). *Vital signs: Core metrics for health and health care progress.* Washington, DC: National Academies Press.

International Federation of Social Workers. (2012). Health. Retrieved from http://ifsw .org/policies/health

International Health Conference. (2002). Constitution of the World Health Organization. 1946. *Bulletin of the World Health Organization, 80*(12), 983–984.

Kamal, R., & Cox, C. (2017). *U.S. health system is performing better, though still lagging behind other countries.* Menlo Park, CA: Kaiser Family Foundation. Retrieved from http://www.healthsystemtracker.org/brief/u-s-health-system-performing-better -though-still-lagging-behind-countries/?post_types=brief#item-start

Keigher, S. M. (1997). What role for social work in the new health care practice paradigm? *Health & Social Work, 22,* 149–155.

Kochanek, K. D., Murphy, S. L., Xu, J., & Tejada-Vera, B. (2016). Deaths: Final data for 2014. *National Vital Statistics Reports, 65*(4). Retrieved from https://www.cdc.gov/ nchs/data/nvsr/nvsr65/nvsr65_04.pdf

Kondrat, M. E. (2011). *Person-in-environment*. Oxford, UK: Oxford University Press.

Laditka, J., & Laditka, S. (2015). Associations of educational attainment with disability and life expectancy by race and gender in the United States: A longitudinal analysis of the Panel Study of Income Dynamics. *Journal of Aging and Health, 28*(8), 1403–1425.

Lewis, N. (2014). A primer on defining the Triple Aim. Retrieved from http://www .ihi.org/communities/blogs/_layouts/15/ihi/community/blog/itemview .aspx?List=81ca4a47-4ccd-4e9e-89d9-14d88ec59e8d&ID=63

Lundblad, J. (1995). Jane Addams and social reform: A role model for the 1990s. *Social Work, 40*(5), 661–669.

McGill, M., & MacNaughton, G. (2016). The struggle to achieve the human rights to health care in the United States. *Southern California Law Journal, 25*, 625–685.

McGinnis, J. M., Berwick, D. M., Daschle, T. A., Diaz, A., Fineberg, H. V., Frist, W. H., . . . Lavizzo-Mourey, R. (2016). Systems strategies for better health throughout the life course (Discussion Paper). In *Vital Directions for Health and Health Care Series*. Washington, DC: National Academy of Medicine. Retrieved from https://nam.edu/ wp-content/uploads/2016/09/Systems-Strategies-for-Better-Health-Throughout -the-Life-Course.pdf

Miringoff, M. L., & Opdycke, S. (1986). *American social welfare policy: Reassessment and reform*. Englewood Cliffs, NJ: Prentice-Hall.

National Association of Social Workers. (2016). *NASW standards for social work practice in health care settings*. Washington, DC: Author.

National Association of Social Workers. (2017). Code of ethics. Retrieved from https:// www.socialworkers.org/About/Ethics/Code-of-Ethics

National Center for Health Statistics. (2016). *Health, United States, 2015: With special feature on racial and ethnic health disparities*. Hyattsville, MD: Author.

Obama, B. (2016). United States health care reform: Progress to date and next steps. *Journal of the American Medical Association, 316*(5), 525–532. doi:10.1001/jama.2016.9797

Office of the United Nations High Commissioner for Human Rights. (1966). International covenant on economic, social and cultural rights. Retrieved from http://www.ohchr .org/EN/ProfessionalInterest/Pages/CESCR.aspx

Office of the United Nations High Commissioner for Human Rights & World Health Organization. (n.d.). The right to health. Fact sheet no. 31. Retrieved from http:// www.ohchr.org/Documents/Publications/Factsheet31.pdf

Organisation for Economic Co-operation and Development. (2016). OECD economic sur-veys: United States 2016. Retrieved from http://www.oecd-ilibrary.org/economics/ oecd-economic-surveys-united-states-2016/executive-summary_eco_surveys-usa-2016-2-en

Parento, E. W., & Gostin, L. O. (2013). Better health, but less justice: Widening health disparities after National Federation of Independent Business v. Sebelius. *Notre Dame J.L. Ethics & Public Policy, 27*, 481–512.

Patient Protection and Affordable Care Act. (2010). 42 U. S. C. § 18001.

Popple, P. R., & Leighninger, L. (2011). *Social work, social welfare and American society* (8th ed.). New York, NY: Pearson.

Ruth, B. J., & Sisco, S. (2008). Public health. In T. Mizrahi & L. E. Davis (Eds.), *Encyclopedia of social work* (20th ed., pp. 476–483). Oxford, UK: Oxford University Press.

Silverman, E. (2008). From ideological to competency based: The rebranding and maintaining of medical social work's identity [Commentary]. *Social Work, 53*, 89–91.

Simon, B. L. (1990). Rethinking empowerment. *Journal of Progressive Human Services, 1*, 27–39.

Singh, G., & Siahpush, M. (2014). Widening rural-urban disparities in life expectancy, U.S., 1969–2009. *American Journal of Preventive Medicine, 46*(2), e19–e29. doi:10.1016/j.amepre.2013.10.017

Trattner, W. (1999). *From poor law to welfare state* (6th ed.). New York, NY: Free Press.

Turnock, B. J. (2007). *Essentials of public health.* Sudbury, MA: Jones & Bartlett.

United Nations. (1948). Universal Declaration of Human Rights. Retrieved from http://www.ohchr.org/EN/UDHR/Documents/UDHR_Translations/eng.pdf

U.S. Department of Health and Human Services. (2003). *New Freedom Commission on Mental Health. Achieving the promise: Transforming mental health care in America* (Final Report; DHHS Pub. No. SMA-03-3831). Rockville, MD: Author.

U.S. Department of Justice. (n.d.). Information and technical assistance on the Americans with Disabilities Act. Retrieved from https://www.ada.gov/ada_intro.htm

Wenocur, S., & Reisch, M. (1989). *From charity to enterprise: The development of American social work in a market economy.* Urbana: University of Illinois Press.

World Health Organization. (2012). *Positioning health in the post-2015 development agenda* (WHO Discussion Paper). Geneva, Switzerland: Author.

World Health Organization. (2017). SDG #3 targets. Retrieved from http://www.who.int/sdg/targets/en

Zammitti, E. P., Cohen, R. A., & Martinez, M. E. (2016). *Health insurance coverage: Early release of estimates from the National Health Interview Survey, January-June 2016.* Report prepared for the National Center for Health Statistics, Hyattsville, MD. Retrieved from https://www.cdc.gov/nchs/data/nhis/earlyrelease/insur201611.pdf

2

Ethics and Values in the Health Field

Elaine P. Congress

Social work values and ethics continually guide policy, practice, and research in the health care field. Using the lens of social work values, this chapter begins with examining social work policies and government policies on health care. Identifying ethical challenges and dilemmas and applying a model of ethical decision making for practitioners is also addressed. The chapter closes with the need for continued research on ethics to enhance social workers' understanding of this important area.

POLICIES/CODES OF HEALTH CARE PROFESSIONALS

What values and ethics influence policy in the health care field? The Hippocratic oath that guides medical practice stresses the importance of doing no harm and non-maleficence continues to be the mantra of those in the medical and health-related professions. Social workers often use this principle in guiding their practice in the health field. This also relates to respect for the worth and dignity of each person, as social workers believe that this approach is the best way to minimize doing harm. Social work as well as other professions in the health field (nursing, physical therapy, rehabilitation counseling) have different codes of ethics to guide professional practice (Kangasniemi, Pakkanen, & Korhonen, 2015). Other codes also address the importance of respect for the dignity and worth of each patient (Kangasniemi et al., 2015).

But how is this policy translated into practice during the modern age with so many complicated choices? How can one navigate a health environment with many possibilities each with different consequences?

SOCIAL WORK CODE OF ETHICS

Since social work is a value-based profession, it is essential for social workers to look at what standards the profession has developed to guide policy, practice, and research in the health field. The National Association of Social Workers (NASW) Code of Ethics provides the primary framework for ethical practice for social workers (NASW, 2017). While the NASW Code does not specifically mention the word "health," its values and principles can be applied to health care practice (Table 2.1).

Table 2.1 NASW Values and Ethical Principles

Value	Ethical Principle
Service	Social workers' primary goal is to help people in need and to address social problems.
Social justice	Social workers challenge social injustice.
Dignity and worth of the person	Social workers respect the inherent dignity and worth of the person.
Importance of human relationships	Social workers recognize the central importance of human relationships.
Integrity	Social workers behave in a trustworthy manner.
Competence	Social workers practice within their areas of competence and develop and enhance their professional expertise.

Source: Adapted from the National Association of Social Workers. (2017). Code of ethics. Retrieved from https://www.socialworkers.org/About/Ethics/Code-of-Ethics

All of these values and ethical principles are incorporated into social work practice in the health field. Social workers continually promote a social justice mission, are committed to service for all people who need health care regardless of their ability to pay, and often become involved in internal and external advocacy initiatives to expand health care benefits to all. All patients/clients in a health care setting, regardless of national origin, ethnicity, age, disability, or social/economic class, are treated with dignity and respect. Finally, all social workers in the health care field continually try to develop their competency by taking advantage of in-service or external continuing education opportunities to increase their knowledge and skills.

SOCIAL WORK ETHICAL STANDARDS IN HEALTH CARE

Perlman (1975) said that a value has small worth unless it can be actualized in practice. What type of guidance does the NASW Code of Ethics with its general values and principles provide for social work practitioners in the health care field? While the Code addresses major issues, it does not provide direct guidance about the particular challenges that practitioners in the health field face. The NASW, however, has developed standards for social work practice in health settings that do outline ethical principles for social workers in the health field (NASW, 2016).

The first standard in this 13-standard document explicitly describes how social work values and ethics affect practice in the health field:

Standard 1. Ethics and Values

Social workers practicing in health care settings shall adhere to and promote the ethics and values of the social work profession, using the NASW Code of Ethics as a guide to ethical decision making. (NASW, 2016, p. 16)

The following interpretation is provided:

> *The primary mission of the social work profession is to enhance human well-being and help meet the basic human needs, with special attention to the needs of people and communities who are vulnerable, oppressed, or living in poverty. Social workers have an ethical obligation to address the health care needs of these groups and advocate for change to ensure access to quality care. The profession's mission is rooted in core values that have been embraced by social workers throughout the profession's history and highlight social work's distinct purpose and perspective. These values—service, social justice, dignity and worth of the person, importance of human relationships, compassion, integrity and competence—constitute the foundation of social work and underlie the practice of social work in health care settings. The NASW* Code of Ethics *establishes the ethical responsibilities of all social workers with respect to their own practice, clients, colleagues, employees and employing organizations, the social work profession, and society. Acceptance of these responsibilities—which include upholding a client's right to privacy and confidentiality and promoting client self-determination—fosters competent social work practice in health care settings. In a health care system characterized by technological advancement and rapid change in care delivery and financing of health care services, ethical dilemmas among and between clients, families, health care professionals, and organizations are potentially numerous and complex. The NASW* Code of Ethics *and prevailing clinical bioethics provide a foundation for social workers to manage such dilemmas. Health care social workers have the responsibility to know and comply with local, state, federal, and tribal legislation, regulations, and policies, addressing topics such as guardianship; parental rights; advance directives; and reporting requirements for abuse, neglect, exploitation, suicide, and threat of harm to others. When an ethical dilemma or conflict occurs, the health care social worker is expected to employ available mechanisms, including social work supervision, peer review, institutional ethics committees, and external consultation, to resolve the dilemma. (NASW, 2016, pp. 16–17)*

Ethical standards in health care similar to the Code of Ethics, however, set forth general principles but do not provide much specific guidance about navigating ethical dilemmas and decision making in health care practice.

DISTRIBUTIVE JUSTICE PRINCIPLES

What principles can be used to guide ethical practice for social workers in health care? The principles of distributive justice (Congress, 1999; Reamer, 2001) can be helpful in understanding the dilemmas that arise in health care. Four principles—equality, need, compensation, and contribution—are often used to develop health care policies and programs.

Social workers believe that all have an equal right to health care, but know that socioeconomic differences frequently create inequities in access and treatment. When there are limited options, how can a resource be divided equally? For example, a social worker in a hospital had only one available opening in a skilled nursing facility, but four clients who were waiting for immediate discharge to an outpatient facility.

Need is also an important criterion that is often used to determine how to distribute a scarce resource. Ethical dilemmas arise on the macro, mezzo, and micro levels about who has the greatest need. For example, what macro government decisions are made about funding? Are decisions made in terms of age as, for example, an assessment is made that adolescents may have greater need for a new program than seniors? On a mezzo level, especially in a time of cutbacks, agencies frequently make decisions about which programs to keep and which to eliminate. Unfortunately, current management decisions are often made in terms of financial viability with minimal consideration of need (Reisch, 2014). On a micro level, health care practitioners continually struggle with how to serve first, especially when there are many clients all needing immediate help. For example, in a very busy large metropolitan hospital, a social worker recently debated about whom to see first, a family with a 5-year-old child who was just diagnosed with leukemia, or a 55-year-old single person with no support system who, following hospitalization for a heart attack, now needs to be discharged immediately.

In health care practice, does a triage system develop? The concept of triage began during World War II when decisions were continually made about whom to save among seriously injured solders. Sometimes not the most seriously injured patient received the greatest medical attention, but rather the one who would survive. Do social workers in the health field also prioritize need in this way by giving more immediate attention to the patient who can be helped, not the one who is terminally ill (Congress, 1999)?

A third principle is that of compensation based on the belief that certain populations who have often received severe deprivation in the past should now receive special compensation. Affirmative Action programs provide an example of this principle in action. Applying this principle to the health field, should certain populations who have been previously disadvantaged receive special attention for their health care, especially if it can be established that their current need is great?

A fourth principle of distribution and possibly the most controversial is that of contribution. Should someone receive access to health care and treatment based on what they have contributed to society? The 2010 Patient Protection and Affordable Care Act (ACA) requires organizations with more than 50 employees to provide health care to their employees. Those who have the skills and are documented have the option to work in a larger organization and thus have greater access to health care. The underlying but unspoken belief is that their contribution is more. Another example of how contribution is used to distribute limited health care resources is that those who have contributed the most to society (or sometimes to fund-raising efforts) can afford luxurious accommodations in hospitals and 24-hour health care attendants as outpatients.

Where there is limited availability, distribution of transplanted organs is also an area of concern. While social workers believe that distribution of limited resources should have equal access, this seems to be related to status and socioeconomic factors. For example, about 20 years ago, many in health care were appalled to learn that a famous baseball star, Mickey Mantle, received a liver transplant despite having compromised health (Congress, 1999). Also, decisions about giving heart transplants are made in terms of availability to take medicines on a regular basis and thus unfortunately many homeless people are excluded (personal communication).

COMPETING ETHICAL PRINCIPLES

In an attempt to navigate among so many competing principles, Loewenberg and Dolgoff (2000) developed the following hierarchy:

1. Autonomy and freedom (self-determination)
2. Equality and inequality
3. Least harm
4. Privacy and confidentiality

5. Protection of life
6. Quality of life
7. Truthfulness and full disclosure

A later study by Dolgoff, Loewenberg, and Harrington (2009) found that there was little consistency about how social workers rank these often competing principles.

Context is viewed as very important in deciding which principle should prevail. For example, promoting the right to self-determination and preserving life are two major principles that may be in conflict. Understanding the context, however, can help the social worker understand how protection of life may be more important when working with a healthy 18-year old with suicidal intent, while promoting self-determination and quality of life might be paramount in social work practice with a 80-year-old man suffering from terminal lung cancer.

PRACTICE

What are current practice challenges in the health field? Administrators in health care identified the following issues, ranging from macro financial to clinical micro dilemmas (Larson, 2013):

1. Balancing care quality and efficiency
2. Improving access to care
3. Building a sustaining health care workforce of the future
4. Addressing end-of-life issues
5. Allocating limited medications and donor organs

Health care providers have the desire to provide quality services, but often struggle with the need to reduce costs. At times, the best treatment option is not always the least expensive as sometimes a health care provider wants to readmit but knows that there will be a penalty as the patient has one of the six diseases designated for outpatient care. At other times, a social worker may believe that an undocumented person is in need of health care, but the individual may lack funds to pay.

Current practice in health care supports a patient's right to self-determination. This may be compromised, however, because of the complexity of medical care and the limited time doctors and other health professionals have to spend with patients. Another challenge is the increasing number of those seeking health care who may not speak and understand English well. Using children as interpreters is not a good option because they often are kept from school to accompany parents to medical appointments or they may be asked to participate in health care discussions that are not appropriate. Since there are problems when a child or relative is used to translate, there have been efforts to support and develop skilled translation services in the health field (Drugan & Tipton, 2017).

Health Care Challenges—Beginning of Life

On the borders of life and age there are dilemmas. There are macro issues based on policy and legal decisions, but also practice issues that confront clinicians in the health care field.

When does life begin? The right for women to plan their families—even when it involves termination of pregnancy—was established in the United States by the 1973 *Roe v. Wade* Supreme Court landmark decision. Over the years, there have been modifications based on length of gestation, mother's health, age, and financial status, and the laws governing abortion differ from state to state. Some who argue that life begins at conception have introduced funding reductions to agencies like Planned Parenthood that provide educational and service programs around family planning for women and their families. While NASW has supported a woman's right to choose (Bailey, 2004), individual social workers may have differing views about this issue that may make it challenging for them to work in a multiservice health facility.

What is the age at which neonatal infants can survive? One hundred years ago, children who were born prematurely would not have survived at all, and 50 years ago they may have survived but often with severe visual and other handicaps. Now infants even under one pound or with severe physical problems can be saved. The costs of neonatal and sometimes lifelong intensive care for the premature pose challenging ethical questions (Murakas & Parsi, 2008).

Health Care Challenges—End of Life

The population in the United States, as well as around the world, is increasing (Population Reference Bureau, 2008). Older people as well as younger people, even those with life-threatening illnesses, live much longer than previously. People are asked to make health decisions for themselves before their health is so compromised that they lose the capacity to make their own decisions. All states recognize some form of living will, advance directives, or proxy (American Bar Association, 2017).

How does this policy decision affect those in direct practice? Self-determination is seen as an important ethical principle in the health care field. Patients are now asked to consider using Advanced Health Care Directives for themselves about what medical measures should be used and also to name health care proxies to make health decisions for them if they are unable to do so. This illustrates an important way by which patients are given the right to exercise self-determination and participate in making their own health care decisions.

Informed Consent

Another ethical concern and challenge for the health care social worker is enhancing informed consent for all clients. There are numerous examples in medical history of disadvantaged and vulnerable populations not being afforded informed consent. The often-cited Tuskegee Syphilis Experiment from 1932 to 1972 is a classic example of a minority group that was not given the option to exercise informed consent because information about effective treatment was withheld.

The NASW Code of Ethics addresses informed consent by advising social workers to "use clear and understandable language to inform clients of the purpose of the service, risks related to the services, limits to services because of the requirements of third-party payer, relevant costs, reasonable alternatives, clients' right to refuse or withdraw consent, and the time frame covered by the consent" (NASW, 2017, p. 8).

Informed consent requires three main elements: presumption of competence, voluntary action, and disclosure before consent. Presumption of competence implies that a client can gather diverse information, exercise judgment, and make a decision that may differ from that of the practitioner (Palmer & Kaufman, 2003). Minors and individuals ruled incompetent by the courts are presumed unable to provide informed consent. This is not an inflexible policy, though, because minors, people with mental illnesses, individuals with disabilities, and individuals affected by dementia are increasingly given the option of exercising informed consent to the extent of their ability. Ensuring that all people are deemed competent to make their own decisions is vitally important. There may be an erroneous perception that people who do not understand English and/or have limited education may not be competent to make their own decisions. The use of professional interpreters and explanations of medical conditions and procedures in simple vocabulary may help those with limited education or English to make competent health care decisions.

In order for patients to be ruled incompetent to make decisions, there must be a court decision that is not based on diagnosis or language difference.

Another important aspect of informed consent involves voluntary action without duress or coercion. Voluntary action may be hampered when there are institutional pressures to prevent clients from making independent decisions. Some patients/clients may be overly influenced by the authority of the health care provider and thus are not able to exercise independent judgment. This may be especially true for populations of individuals who have been stigmatized, oppressed, and prevented previously from making their own decisions. Also, all too often, clients are prescribed medications with serious side effects without being informed of the full extent of the medications' possible side effects. Care must be taken that clients are able to refuse taking medications without undue threats that doing so will be detrimental to their health.

A final condition for informed consent is that consent must be preceded by the disclosure of adequate information. All possible risks and side effects must be reviewed and understood before clients can be expected to provide informed consent, even though such disclosure may lead clients to refuse treatment. In working with clients, social workers must ensure that they have complete understanding of possible consequences and risks of different types of treatment. For example, the American Psychiatric Association reported that nearly 50% of individuals with severe and persistent mental illnesses may develop permanent neurological symptoms, such as tardive dyskinesia, as a result of the medications they take (Swenson, 1997). While it was hoped that the new type of antipsychotic medication would not lead to such a large incident of tardive dyskinesia, this has not been the case (Vox, 2010). Yet many psychiatric patients and their families from poor minority populations may be pressured to take very strong psychotropic medications without having had the possible risks made clear to them.

Ethical Challenge—Cultural Difference in Health Beliefs

Another challenge for the health care practitioner occurs when clients have differing health beliefs. The NASW Code of Ethics stresses the importance of cultural competency. Social workers should "be able to demonstrate competence in the provisions of services that are sensitive to clients' cultures and to differences among people and cultural groups" (NASW, 2017, pp. 9–10). Culturally competent practice involves more than speaking the client's language or having knowledge about a client's specific culture. It involves understanding and accepting how culture has shaped the client's health beliefs. With all clients, but perhaps especially with clients from different cultures, social workers should work toward maximizing clients' self-determination. With clients from diverse backgrounds, the social worker needs to be continually aware of the power dynamics that enter into any social work relationship, especially when working with individuals from backgrounds that have been traditionally oppressed.

Cultural Humility

A new perspective in culturally competent work is adopting a stance of cultural humility in working with clients from different cultural backgrounds (Ashford, 2008). Cultural humility has been defined as an approach that begins with greater self-reflection on the part of the practitioner in terms of the power differences. Learning from clients about their cultures is paramount rather than the traditional cultural competency approach whereby practitioners had preconceived ideas about the cultures of their clients and sought to increase their skills in this area. Beginning first in the medical field where doctors first learned in multicultural trainings about the importance of listening to clients from different fields and not imposing practitioner beliefs on clients (Tervalon & Murray-Garcia, 1998), this approach is very relevant for social workers in the health care field when clients from different cultures are encouraged to share their own beliefs about health, well-being, disease, and health care.

Intersectionality

Incorporating a cultural humility approach with an understanding of power dynamics that impact the practitioner/client relationship, social work education and practice has now focused on intersectionality (Council on Social Work Education [CSWE], 2015). The social work practitioner in the health care field has to be cognizant of the multiple identities that should be recognized in working with clients with diverse identities of gender identification, race, ethnicity, age, social/economic class, religion, educational level, sexual orientation identities many of which may be devalued and stigmatized in society (see Chapter 4, Intersectionality, Social Work, and Health).

Westernized Health Care Approach—Prevention, Diagnosis, and Treatment

Those who work in health care quickly learn that people from different cultures may approach health prevention, diagnosis, and treatment in different ways. Most social workers in the United States are very aware of the importance of prevention, how diet, exercise, not smoking, and regular health screenings can contribute to improved health. Yet many, especially those who come from countries in the developing world, may not have this concept of prevention. For some, health care might have been minimal and only sought when there are health emergencies.

Most social workers in the United States believe in a Westernized system of medical care that includes regular physical examinations, x-rays, MRIs, CAT scans, blood tests, and surgery when necessary. For physical complaints, people seek consultation with physicians; for mental/behavioral health problems, they consult psychiatrists, psychologists, and social workers. Many immigrants, especially those from developing countries, may see the physical and mental as very connected. Mental health symptoms may be defined in physical terms, as for example "dolor de cabeza" (pain in the head) referring not to a physical headache, but rather to anxiety related to a stressful living situation.

Challenges With Clients From Different Backgrounds

While social workers work to maximize choice for their clients, they may face special challenges when clients' heath beliefs differ radically from those of the employing agency. Although social workers strive to maximize their clients' rights to self-determination, the NASW Code of Ethics also states that social workers have an ethical responsibility to their employer (NASW, 2017). Social workers may face a dilemma in advocating for their patient's right to choose alternative health care when there is a marked difference in the health policies and practices of their employing institutions.

What if the immigrant's behavior seems contrary to accepted medical practice? What should the social worker do if the relative of a hospitalized patient continues to bring in food that is antithetical to a prescribed diet? What if the hospital policy proscribes a clear discussion about end-of-life decisions and a client refuses this discussion stating that it will bring bad luck? Research suggests that many minorities are particularly wary of making end-of-life decisions (Gutheil & Heyman, 2005).

While social workers are respectful of clients' rights to pursue their own choices, what if the choices are potentially quite harmful? What about a patient with a serious health problem that insists that the only cure for her illness is taking a special tonic that she received in a local botanica?

For example, consider the case of a 50-year-old female patient recently diagnosed with leukemia who told her social worker that she had decided not to pursue medical treatment. Instead, she believed that taking a special preparation her grandmother made would cure her. Using professional judgment, the social worker could argue that self-determination should be compromised because there is risk of "serious, foreseeable and imminent harm to a client or other identifiable person" (NASW, 2017, p. 7). How direct should the social worker be in encouraging the client to follow prescribed medical treatment? Although most adults might have the right to make individual decisions about their health care, court proceedings can be initiated to declare clients incompetent to make their own health decisions. A court proceeding to declare a person incompetent is used most frequently for older people and people with mental and developmental disabilities where their judgment is severely compromised and much less frequently with adults who do not choose a specific type of medical intervention.

Goldberg (2000) sees a dilemma for social workers who strive to respect the beliefs of all cultures but also support the basic human right to health and well-being. Although social workers are respectful of differing health beliefs, a conflict can arise if the practice is potentially life-threatening. This is especially challenging if the patient is a child. For example, what about a parent who refuses to let her child be immunized because she fears he will develop autism? What is the appropriate ethical stance for a social worker if a parent chooses to consult a faith healer rather than a surgeon for a child with a brain tumor? Should the parents be referred to Child Protective Services because they did not pursue recommended medical treatment for their child?

Challenges—Interdisciplinary Work and Interdisciplinary Committees

Although social workers in the health field have always worked with professionals in other disciplines, interdisciplinary work can be very challenging (Sherman, 2013; Wynia, Kishore, & Belar, 2014). This may be a new area for many beginning social workers since most social work schools, as well as other professional schools like medicine and nursing, spend most of the time focusing on their unique professional identities, rather than learning about how to successfully work with those from other disciplines.

A formal way in which social workers work with other health care professionals is through interdisciplinary ethics committees. Reamer (2006) outlines some issues that arise in these committees, but notes that social workers who participate in such groups usually become well respected team members (Cole, 2012; Reamer, 2006). Since health care has moved from the hospitals to the community, there may be additional challenges in assembling a team of health care professionals.

Ethics Audit

Since there are so many ethical challenges that may arise in health care and growing out of a concern for risk management, Reamer has proposed an Ethics Audit to help social workers assess ethical practice within their health care organization. The Social Work Ethics Audit promotes ethical practice in health settings and minimizes ethics-related risks (Kirkpatrick, Reamer, & Sykulski, 2016).

Ethical Dilemmas and Decision Making

Faced with ethical dilemmas in health care, how do social workers make difficult decisions? Over the years, social workers have proposed many models for ethical decision making (Congress, 1999, 2000; Lowenberg & Dolgoff, 2000; Reamer, 1990). Reamer (1990) provides six guidelines and Loewenberg and Dolgoff (2000) suggest an "Ethical Principle Screen" that places seven ethical principles in a hierarchy.

The ETHIC model developed by this author (Congress, 1999, 2000) took into consideration that social workers in the health field are often overworked with little time to address ethical dilemmas in practice (Figure 2.1). How much do social workers engage in a process of ethical decision making? It has been suggested that social workers rarely, if ever, engage in a process of ethical decision making (McAuliffe, 2005).

Recognizing that social workers have limited time to engage in a decision-making process, a short, easy guide to ethical decision making was created (Congress, 2000). The ETHIC model consists of these five steps:

EXAMINE

What personal, social, agency, client, social, professional, and cultural values affect this ethical dilemma?

THINK

What ethical standards from the NASW Code of Ethics and the NASW Standards for Practice in the Health Care field apply to this issue? What government laws and policies, as well as agency practices and regulations, are relevant?

HYPOTHESIZE

What would be the consequences of pursuing different courses of action? Scenarios that focus on the risks as well as the advantages of alternative decisions can be developed to help in the decision-making process.

IDENTIFY

Who will be the most harmed and helped if different decisions are made? As social workers, it is often best to consider these choices in terms of social work's commitment to the most vulnerable.

CONSULT

The first person to consult for social workers is often their direct supervisor, but in the health field there are many others with whom one can consult. Sometimes these consultations take place in a structured way through regularly scheduled case consultations or interprofessional ethics committees.

POLICY

International Social Work Ethics and Health

Social workers in the health field in the United States are often impacted by health issues of those around the world, such as the increasing number of immigrants and refugees that access health care and the concern that deadly new viruses such as Ebola and swine flu are only a plane ride away. Thus, social workers need to have a global perspective in addressing health concerns. The International Federation of Social Workers (IFSW) in cooperation with the International Association of Social Workers has adopted a statement of ethical standards for social workers (IFSW, 2012).

While this document is similar to the NASW Code of Ethics and the Practice Standards in Health Care, it does not specifically address ethical decision making for practitioners. However, it does stress a rights approach for addressing policy and practice issues in the health field. The right to good health and what is needed to achieve it is considered a basic human right (Olsen & Chatterjee, 2014).

When adopting a global perspective on ethics and health, the United Nations (UN) Sustainable Development Goals (SDG) provide guidance in this area. A specific goal (Goal 3) in this document focuses on good health and well-being for all (UN, n.d.). A main part of this goal has been maternal health, child health, and decreasing HIV, malaria, tuberculosis, infectious and chronic diseases around the world. Other SDGs focus on related health goals such as no poverty (Goal 1), zero hunger (Goal 2), and clean water and sanitation (Goal 6).

Health care policy in the United States limits access to health care based on the ability to pay. There is concern that it does not seem to incorporate a rights-based approach and the newest proposed federal health care policy may move even further from a rights-based approach to health. However, there are some positive indications that social work values have been adopted into U.S. health care policies.

Confidentiality is an important ethical standard for social workers and the NASW Code of Ethics has 18 standards related to this theme, more than any other area (Rock & Congress, 1999). The federal Health Insurance Portability and Accountability Act of 1996 (HIPAA) and the ACA stress the importance of maintaining confidentiality for patients/clients receiving health care. The use of technology for medical records adds new confidentiality challenges (American College of Health care Executives, 2016) and these concerns have been addressed in the social work literature (NASW, 2017; Reamer, 2013).

E Examine values
  - Personal
  - Agency
  - Family
  - Social
  - Cultural
  - Client
  - Professional

T Think about
  - Code of Ethics
  - Laws and regulations
  - Agency policies

H Hypothesize about consequences of different decisions

I Identify
  - Who is most vulnerable
  - Who will be helped or harmed

C Consult with
  - Supervisors
  - Colleagues

Figure 2.1 ETHIC model of decision making.

Another major area in which social work ethical standards seem to have been incorporated into American health care policy is in terms of informed consent. Over the last 50 years, the need to secure informed consent of patients has become an accepted part of medical practice. All patients have the right to have medical procedures and possible consequences spelled out to them. This corresponds positively with social work's ethical standard on honesty and integrity in relating to clients (NASW, 2017).

Healthy People 2020 Policy

Involving patients in identifying what are their health problems played a major role in United States Department of Health and Human Services's Healthy People 2020 (USDHHS, 2010). This document is an interesting illustration about how the social work ethical principle of respect and inclusion of all was incorporated into conducting this large U.S. government survey, as it involved implementing an extensive stakeholder feedback process that was unparalleled in government (USDHHS, 2010). This federal government agency received more than 8,000 comments from professional public health experts, health organizations, as well as the general public regarding the selection of Healthy People 2020 objectives.

On the basis of these comments, a number of new topic areas were added, such as:

1. Adolescent Health
2. Blood Disorders and Blood Safety
3. Dementias, Including Alzheimer's Disease
4. Early and Middle Childhood
5. Genomics
6. Global Health
7. Health-Related Quality of Life and Well-Being
8. Health Care–Associated Infections
9. Lesbian, Gay, Bisexual, and Transgender Health
10. Older Adults
11. Preparedness
12. Sleep Health
13. Social Determinants of Health

An ongoing focus of Healthy People 2020 has been the elimination of health disparities and inequities. Health disparities refers to the differences in illnesses, chronic health conditions, and mortality that occur across racial, ethnic, and economically oppressed groups, of which people of color often are the most at risk (Pollard & Scommegna, 2013). Because of social workers' ongoing commitment to promoting social justice, this topic is of particular concern to those in the health field (Keefe & Jurkowski, 2013).

Since unequal access to health care based on race and ethnicity has been a contributing factor to health disparities (Smedley, Stith, & Nelson, 2003), working to overcome disparate health care access and to improve health outcomes for all people is an important area for social workers in the health field (Keefe & Jurkowski, 2013).

Healthy People 2020 (USDHHS, 2010) recognizes that the goal of reducing health inequities and disparities cannot be limited only to health in the United States, but must include other countries as well. As a result, global health has become a new topic area and is listed as one of the Healthy People 2020 core topics.

Addressing Health Disparities

Addressing health disparities is an important ethical concern for social workers who are keenly aware of how life expectancy is related to race, ethnicity, and social/economic class. Although the gap is reducing, African Americans consistently show poorer life expectancies than Caucasians; for example, a non-Hispanic White woman or man in the United States may live to 79 years of age while African Americans have a life expectancy of only 75.6 years (Tavernise, 2016). Income, social/economic class, and access to health care are also contributing factors to differences in health and those of higher social/economic class have life expectancies of about 5 years higher than poor Americans (Waldron, 2007).

How much do current U.S. health policies address health care disparities? The ACA did extend health care coverage to more than 20 million people who were previously denied (Sifferin, 2014). Yet many people face continuing challenges in accessing health care and this negatively affects health outcomes. In contrast to most other developed countries with a single payee system, the United States has financial and employment issues that detrimentally affect people's access to health care. As mentioned, under the current ACA, those who work in organizations with under 50 employees or above Medicaid standards for their state may not have any health insurance coverage, and marginalized populations such as undocumented immigrants still lack any health care coverage. There is also evidence that all immigrants, even those who are citizens, may still lack coverage as 21% of foreign-born Latinos who are now U.S. citizens still lack health care, while only 14% of all native born citizens do (Krogstad & Lopez, 2014).

Policy—Access to Health Care

As this book goes to press, there is concern that the number of people covered for health care will be decreased. According to the Congressional Budget Office (CBO), the passage of this bill might result in 13 million people losing health care insurance. Those who would not be covered are predominately the poor who cannot afford the higher health care premiums or now that Medicaid standards have increased in many states may not have their health needs covered through Medicaid.

Policy decisions continually affect practice as this Case Example 2.1 illustrates.

Case Example 2.1

Robert, a 50-year-old married father of two children, lost his job when the factory where he worked closed. At that time he also lost his health insurance, so he has not been able to go to the doctor for over a year. He has a persistent cough, but treats it with over-the-counter medications. When he went with his children to a community health fair, Joanne, a social worker in the health field, encouraged Robert to go to the outpatient clinic for evaluation of his cough. Unfortunately, however, he lacked health care insurance and was not eligible for Medicaid. The clinic's policy was not to accept clients who did not have Medicaid or were not self-paying. This created an ethical dilemma for Joanne as she wanted to adhere to agency policy, but felt that her main responsibility was to provide service to a client who needed it.

Policy—Health Care Move to the Community

Another recent policy decision that has affected practice is the move from the hospital to the community. Many surgical procedures are now provided on an ambulatory basis and hospital stays have been greatly reduced. This move has been compared to deinstitutionalization in the mental health field in the 1950s and 1960s that spearheaded the move from psychiatric hospitals to community treatment. With new Medicaid guidelines, hospitals are penalized by additional fees if patients they have treated are rehospitalized within 1 month of discharge (Rau, 2016).

Expanded treatment options in the community are viewed as a positive way to treat patients as it provides greater opportunity for involvement with families in the care and support of medically fragile patients. There are many advantages to this move from hospital to community care. While in the hospital doctors and nurses ruled, in the community clients had much more say in their health care decisions. Another positive is increased demand for social workers to provide guidance, education, and community support for clients with poor health and their families. While health care provided primarily in the community increases opportunities for social workers, as well as is more supportive of clients' rights to make their own decisions, there are new dilemmas.

Are people, especially frail older adults who may live alone in the community, able to secure needed medical and support services? How is confidentiality maintained in the community clinic? There may be additional challenges in maintaining confidential records in a community setting. Also there may be ongoing difficulties in communication between the hospital and those involved in community care.

RESEARCH

There are many ethical questions that need further research. While there are many ongoing research studies of new medications and treatments for different medical diseases, there is much less focus of research of ethical issues and dilemmas in health care settings and how they are addressed. Much of the literature has focused on identifying problems (Allen, 2011; McCormick et al., 2014; McIntosh & Hoek, 2006).

Social workers may struggle with ethical dilemmas in the health care workplace, but the conflictual issues and the methods they use to address them are rarely the focus of research studies. Crigger, Fox, Rosell, and Rojjanasrirat (2017), however, did look at health care professionals' experiences with ethics consultations and used their findings to develop a theory to guide professionals in making ethical decisions.

Another exception is Lillemoen and Peterson's (2012) study on identifying ethical dilemmas that arise in the workplace. Lack of knowledge and skills was seen as contributing to workers' difficulty in identifying and addressing ethical challenges in the workplace. Case studies have been proposed as an important way to help the social work health professional learn more about and navigate difficult dilemmas (McCormick et al., 2014).

CONCLUSION

There is good and bad news in the study of ethics and health. A general most discouraging fact is that among developing countries, the United States does not have a good record in terms of infant mortality, heart and lung disease, sexually transmitted infections, adolescent pregnancies, injuries, homicides, and rates of disability. Longevity rates are also not encouraging as a recent study of 17 high-income countries found that the average U.S. citizen can be expected to live almost 4 years less than those who lived in other high-income countries (Woolf & Aron, 2013). The good news, however, from a social work ethical perspective is that although many in the United States have limited access to health care and there are major health disparities, especially for minority populations, health care policies often reflect social work principles of self-determination, inclusion, and confidentiality. In addition, the move of health care from the hospital to the community provides greater opportunities for social workers to put into practice looking at clients in terms of their environment as well as enabling clients to make individual decisions about their care. Another positive development in the health care field is the growing number of social workers who want to enter the health field and have opportunities to make a difference in the future of health care.

CHAPTER DISCUSSION QUESTIONS

1. How does the social worker make ethical decisions in health care when faced with an ethical dilemma?
2. What is the social worker's ethical obligation in working in agencies or systems that limit access to health care?
3. With limited time and resources, how does a social worker prioritize who receives attention first?
4. How do current social workers actualize social work principles of confidentiality in the modern age of technology and community care?
5. What is the most effective way that social workers can participate in interdisciplinary teams?

CASE EXAMPLE AND DISCUSSION QUESTIONS

Case Example 2.2

Jessica, a licensed social worker, has worked for a major hospital for the last 5 years, two of which have been in a community-based outpatient facility. Her newest client is Carmen, a 40-year-old Latina woman who was recently diagnosed with type 2 diabetes. Carmen and her five children, ranging in age from 2 to 18, moved into a shelter for the homeless last year when Carmen's husband became abusive. Several ethical dilemmas surrounding Jessica's work with Carmen arose.

The first involved agency policy and the client's need for ongoing treatment, while the other dilemma involved client self-determination. Jessica first began with an examination of what were relevant values. She looked at her own beliefs in that she could not understand how a person could have had five children and continue to live with a man who was abusive and not supporting his family. Jessica also recognized that she felt that a person should take more responsibility for her own health care and became concerned when Carmen reported eating a large piece of cake at a family party.

Jessica was also aware of agency policy and how this impacted her work with Carmen. The hospital had very strict guidelines for only providing medical care if clients were covered by Medicaid or self-paying. Carmen had a part-time job in a neighborhood pizzeria, so her income was slightly above Medicaid standards, and she could not afford medications to treat her diabetes. In the shelter, a conflict developed when Carmen continued to see her estranged spouse and the shelter had very strict rules about visits from male guests. In terms of values, Carmen really questioned taking pills for her diabetes. Her aunt had given her a special medication from the botanica and she thought it would work just as well if not better.

(continued)

Case Example 2.2 *(continued)*

Questions for Discussion

1. Values

    How do Carmen's and Jessica's values differ? What health care agency and shelter values affect this case?

2. Policies

    What laws and agency regulations are relevant in this case?

3. Scenarios

    What would be the consequence of Jessica telling Carmen that she must abide by agency rules about male visitors or insisting that Carmen follow the health procedures of her employing agency? What are other alternative courses of action?

4. Vulnerability

    Who is the most vulnerable in this case example and how much should this affect Jessica's ethical decision making?

5. Consultation

    Who should Jessica speak with about this case?

REFERENCES

Allen, K. (2011). Health care social workers and ethics committees. *The New Social Worker, 18*(4), 4–7. Retrieved from http://www.socialworker.com/feature-articles/ethics-articles/Health_Care_Social_Workers_and_Ethics_Committees/

American Bar Association. (2017). Living wills, health care proxies, & advance health care directives. Retrieved from https://www.americanbar.org/groups/real_property_trust_estate/resources/estate_planning/living_wills_health_care_proxies_advance_health_care_directives.html

American College of Healthcare Executives. (2016). Health information confidentiality. Retrieved from https://www.ache.org/policy/hiconf.cfm

Ashford, J. (2008). *Human behavior in the social environment: A multidimensional perspective* (3rd ed.). Belmont, CA: Cengage.

Bailey, G. (2004). Respecting the right to choose from the president. *NASW News*. Retrieved from https://www.socialworkers.org/pubs/news/2004/04/bailey.asp

Cole, P. (2012). You want me to do what? Ethical practice within interdisciplinary collaborations. *Journal of Social Work Values and Ethics, 9*(1), 26–38.

Congress, E. (1999). *Social work values and ethics: Identifying and resolving professional dilemmas.* Belmont, CA: Wadsworth.

Congress, E. (2000). What social workers should know about ethics: Understanding and resolving practice dilemmas. *Advances in Social Work, 1*(1), 1–25.

Council on Social Work Education. (2015). *Educational policy and accreditation standards for baccalaureate and master's social work programs.* Alexandria, VA: Author. Retrieved from https://www.cswe.org/getattachment/Accreditation/Accreditation-Process/2015-EPAS/2015EPAS_Web_FINAL.pdf.aspx

Crigger, N., Fox, M., Rosell, T., & Rojjanasrirat, W. (2017). Moving it along: A study of health care professionals' experience with ethics consultations. *Nursing Ethics, 24*(3), 279–291. doi:10.1177/0969733015597571

Dolgoff, R., Loewenberg, F. M., & Harrington, D. (2009). *Ethical decisions for social work practice* (8th ed.). Belmont, CA: Brooks/Cole.

Drugan, J., & Tipton, R. (2017). Translation, ethics and social responsibility. *The Translator, 23*(2), 119–125.

Goldberg, M. (2000). Conflicting principles in multicultural social work. *Families in Society, 81*, 12–21.

Gutheil, I. A., & Heyman, J. C. (2005). Communication between older persons and their health care agent: Results of an intervention. *Health & Social Work, 30*(2), 107–116.

International Federation of Social Workers. (2012). Statement of ethical principles. Retrieved from http://ifsw.org/policies/statement-of-ethical-principles

Kangasniemi, M., Pakkanen, P., & Korhonen, A. (2015). Professional ethics in nursing: An integrative review. *Journal of Advanced Nursing, 71*(8), 1744–1757. doi:10.1111/jan.12619

Keefe, R., & Jurkowski, E. (Eds.). (2013). *Handbook for public health social work.* New York, NY: Springer Publishing.

Kirkpatrick, W., Reamer, F., & Sykulski, M. (2016). Social work ethics audits in health care settings: A case study. *Health and Social Work, 31*(3), 225–228.

Krogstad, J., & Lopez, M. (2014). Hispanic immigrants more likely to lack health insurance than U.S.-born. Retrieved from http://www.pewresearch.org/fact-tank/2014/09/26/higher-share-of-hispanic-immigrants-than-u-s-born-lack-health-insurance

Larson, J. (2013). Five top ethical issues in health care. *AMN Health Care.* Retrieved from https://www.amnhealthcare.com/latest-healthcare-news/five-top-ethical-issues-healthcare

Lillemoen, L., & Petersen, R. (2012). Ethical challenges and how to develop ethics support in primary health care. *Journal of Humanities and Social Sciences, 5*(6), 14–18.

Loewenberg, F. M., & Dolgoff, R. (2000). *Ethical decisions for social work practice* (6th ed.). Itasca, IL: F.E. Peacock.

McAuliffe, D. (2005). I'm still standing: Impacts & consequences of ethical dilemmas for social workers in direct practice. Retrieved from https://www.researchgate.net/publication/29464251_I%27m_Still_Standing_Impacts_and_Consequences_of_Ethical_Dilemmas_for_Social_Workers_in_Direct_Practice

McCormick, A., Stowell-Weiss, P., Carson, J., Tebo, G., Hanson, I., & Quesada, B. (2014). Continuing education in ethical decision making using case studies from medical social work. *Social Work in Health Care, 3*(4), 344–363.

McIntosh, B., & Hoek, R. V. (2006). Negotiating the path of ethical decision-making in health care social work. *Critical Social Work, 7*(2). Retrieved from http://www1.uwindsor.ca/criticalsocialwork/negotiating-the-path-of-ethical-decision-making-in-health-care-social-work

Murakas, J., & Parsi, K. (2008). The cost of saving the tiniest lives: NICUs versus prevention. *AMA Journal of Ethics, 10*(10), 655–658.

National Association of Social Workers. (2016). NASW standards for social work practice in health care settings. Retrieved from https://www.socialworkers.org/LinkClick.aspx?fileticket=fFnsRHX-4HE%3D&portalid=0

National Association of Social Workers. (2017). Code of ethics. Retrieved from https://www.socialworkers.org/About/Ethics/Code-of-Ethics/Code-of-Ethics-English

Olsen, J., & Chatterjee, A. (2014). Interprofessional global health education. In K. Libel, S. M. Berthold, R. Thomas, & L. Healy (Eds.), *Advancing human rights in social work education* (pp. 353–368). Alexandria, VA: CSWE Press.

Palmer, N., & Kaufman, M. (2003). The ethics of informed consent: Implications for multicultural practice. *Journal of Ethnic and Cultural Diversity in Social Work, 12*(1), 1–26.

Perlman, H. (1975). Self-determination: Reality or illusion? In F. McDermott (Ed.), *Self-determination in social work* (pp. 65–89). London, UK: Routledge and Kegan Paul.

Pollard, K., & Scommegna, P. (2013). The health and life expectancy of older Blacks and Hispanics in the U.S. Retrieved from http://www.prb.org/Publications/Reports/2013/life-expectancy-blacks-Hispanics

Population Reference Bureau. (2008). Human population: Population growth (Chart: World population growth, 1950–2050). Retrieved from http://www.prb.org/Publications/Lesson-Plans/HumanPopulation/PopulationGrowth.aspx

Rau, J. (2016). Medicare's readmission penalties hit new high. Retrieved from http://khn.org/news/more-than-half-of-hospitals-to-be-penalized-for-excess-readmissions

Reamer, F. (1990). *Social work values and ethics.* New York, NY: Columbia University Press.

Reamer, F. (2001). *Social work ethics audit: A risk management tool.* Washington, DC: NASW Press.

Reamer, F. (2006). *Social work values and ethics* (2nd ed.). New York, NY: Columbia University Press.

Reamer, F. (2013). Social work in a digital age: Ethical and risk management challenges. *Social Work, 58*(2), 163–172.

Reisch, M. (2014). Ethical practice in an unethical environment. In S. Banks (Ed.), *Ethics* (pp. 51–56). Bristol, UK: Policy Press.

Rock, B., & Congress, E. (1999). The new confidentiality for the 21st century in a managed care environment. *Social Work, 44*(3), 253–262.

Sherman, R. (2013). Why interdisciplinary teamwork in health care is challenging. *Emerging RN Leader.* Retrieved from http://www.emergingrnleader.com/?s=Why+interdisciplinary+teamwork+in+health+care+is+challenging

Sifferin, A. (2014). 20 million Americans get insurance under Obamacare, report says. *Time.* Retrieved from http://time.com/2950961/obamacare-health-care-obama

Smedley, B. D., Stith, A. Y., & Nelson, A. R. (2003). *Unequal treatment: Confronting racial and ethnic disparities in health care.* Washington, DC: National Academies Press.

Swenson, L. (1997). *Psychology and law for helping professions.* Pacific Grove, CA: Brooks/Cole.

Tavernise, S. (2016, May 8). Black Americans see gains in life expectancy. *The New York Times.* Retrieved from https://www.nytimes.com/2016/05/09/health/blacks-see-gains-in-life-expectancy.html?_r=0

Tervalon, M., & Murray-Garcia, J. (1998). Cultural humility versus cultural competence: A critical distinction in defining physician training outcomes in multicultural education. *Journal of Health Care for the Poor and Underserved, 9*(2), 117–125.

United Nations. (n.d.). Goal 3: Ensure healthy lives and promote well-being for all at all ages. Retrieved from http://www.un.org/sustainabledevelopment/health

U.S. Department of Health and Human Services. (2010). Healthy People 2020. Retrieved from http://www.healthypeople.gov/2020/default.aspx

Vox, F. (2010). Tardive dyskinesia rates remain high with atypical antipsychotics. *Reuters Health Information.* Retrieved from http://www.mindfreedom.org/kb/psychiatric-drugs/antipsychotics/neuroleptic-brain-damage/tardive-dyskinesia/tardive-dyskinesia-atypicals

Waldron, H. (2007). Trends in mortality differentials and life expectancy for male social security-covered workers by socioeconomic status. *Social Security Bulletin, 67*(3). Retrieved from https://www.ssa.gov/policy/docs/ssb/v67n3/v67n3p1.html

Woolf, S. H., & Aron, L. (Eds.). (2013). *U.S. health in international perspective: Shorter lives, poorer health.* Washington, DC: National Academies Press. Retrieved from https://www.nap.edu/read/13497/chapter/1

Wynia, M., Kishore, S., & Belar, C. (2014). A unified code of ethics for health professionals: Insights from an IOM workshop. *Journal of the American Medical Association, 311*(8),799–800.

3

Social Determinants of Health

Janna C. Heyman, Peggy L. Kelly, Gary M. Reback, and Kelsey H. Blumenstock

The World Health Organization (WHO) defines social determinants of health as "the circumstances in which people are born, grow up, live, work, and age, and the systems put in place to deal with illness. These circumstances are in turn shaped by a wider set of forces: economics, social policies, and politics" (WHO, 2017, p. 1). The U.S. Department of Health and Human Services (USDHHS) points out that factors such as access to healthy foods, safe neighborhoods, and education are predictors of better health. Accordingly, as part of the USDHHS's Office of Disease Prevention and Health Promotion (ODPHP), the 10-year agenda for improving the nation's health, currently known as Healthy People 2020, focuses on "social and physical environments that promote good health for all" (ODPHP, 2017a). In addition, Healthy People 2020 also developed five key areas of social determinants of health, including: economic stability (poverty, employment, food insecurity, and housing instability); education (high school graduation, enrollment in higher education, language and literacy, and early childhood education and development); social and community context (social cohesion, civic participation, discrimination, and incarceration); health and health care (access to health care, access to primary care, and health literacy); and neighborhood and built environment (access to foods that support healthy eating patterns, quality of housing, and crime and violence, and environmental conditions; see Table 3.1).

The term "social determinants of health" entered the common vernacular with the formation of the Commission on Social Determinants of Health by WHO in 2005, which was charged to address the social factors leading to ill health and health inequities. The subsequent report of the Commission provided critical background information for the 2011 World Conference on Social Determinants of Health, which resulted in the Rio Political Declaration on Social Determinants of Health. The declaration was endorsed by member states and noted that health inequalities are unacceptable and arise from societal conditions that can, and should, be corrected (WHO, 2017).

In the United States, efforts to address inequity in health across population groups began in the 1990s, first with the establishment of the Office of Women's Health in 1991. The passage of the Women's Health Equity Act of 1996 addressed the exclusion of women from medical research, as well as the lack of knowledge of women's health care needs. Then, in 1998, the USDHHS established the Initiative to Eliminate Racial and Ethnic Disparities in Health. This initiative targeted six major areas for improved health outcomes for diverse populations: infant mortality, cancer, cardiovascular disease, diabetes,

Table 3.1 Social Determinants of Health

Economic Stability	Education	Social and Community Context	Health and Health Care	Neighborhood and Built Environment
• Poverty • Employment • Food insecurity • Housing instability	• High school graduation • Enrollment in higher education • Language and literacy • Early childhood education and development	• Social cohesion • Civic participation • Discrimination • Incarceration	• Access to health care • Access to primary care • Health literacy	• Access to foods that support healthy eating patterns • Quality of housing • Crime and violence • Environmental conditions

Source: Summary created from the Office of Disease Prevention and Health Promotion. (2017b). Social determinants of health. Retrieved from https://www.healthypeople.gov/2020/topics-objectives/topic/social-determinants-of-health

HIV/AIDS, and infectious disease. Mental health, especially suicide, was also included as a primary concern as part of this initiative. Another important milestone was the passage of the Minority Health and Health Disparities Research and Education Act of 2000, which required all of the institutes and centers of the National Institutes of Health to include strategic plans that take into consideration health disparities (Moniz, 2010).

One of the reasons why it is important to consider the social determinants of health is that it points to major discrepancies in the health status of the population. Chetty et al. (2016) examined data on race and ethnicity-adjusted life expectancy at age 40 by income, sex, and geographic area to determine factors associated with a difference in life expectancy. They found that those with higher incomes had greater longevity, with a significant difference in life expectancy between the richest 1% and the poorest 1% of people. In addition to race and ethnicity, health disparities are also evident according to differences in education, sex, place of residence, and sexual orientation (Adler, Glymour, & Fielding, 2016). Furthermore, Moniz and Gorin (2010) refer to research showing that "medical care has played a limited role in reducing mortality in Western nations, whereas factors such as increased income, improved nutrition, and public health efforts play a greater role in the extension of human life" (p. 284). These factors take into consideration health as a biopsychosocial phenomenon, in which thoughts, feelings, and moods can affect the onset of disease, the course of disease, and the management of disease.

The Centers for Disease Control and Prevention's (CDC) Health Disparities and In-equality Report highlights four findings that demonstrate the enormity of health disparities (CDC, 2013a, 2013b). First, non-Hispanic Blacks are 50% more likely to die of heart disease or stroke than non-Hispanic Whites. Second, Hispanics and non-Hispanic Blacks have a higher prevalence of adult diabetes than Asians and non-Hispanic Whites. In addition, adults without a college degree and those with lower household incomes have a higher prevalence of diabetes. Third, non-Hispanic Blacks have double the infant mortality rate of non-Hispanic Whites, and rates are higher for those living in the South and Midwest.

Fourth, men are four times more likely to commit suicide than women, regardless of age or race, and the rates are highest among American Indian/Alaskan Natives and non-Hispanic Whites. The CDC's findings also align with those from a meta-analysis of nearly 50 studies that found that social factors such as low education, racial segregation, low social support, poverty, and income inequality accounted for over a third of total deaths annually in the United States (Galea, Tracy, Hoggatt, DiMaggio, & Karpati, 2011).

PRACTICE

The National Association of Social Workers (NASW) points out that social determinants of health have a long history within the profession of social work (Rine, 2016). The NASW Code of Ethics Preamble (2017) asserts, "Fundamental to social work is attention to the environmental forces that create, contribute to, and address problems in living" (p. 1). This is reflected in social work's person-in-environment perspective, the biopsychosocial assessment model, and the framing of social determinants of health as a social justice issue. A connection between social work and the social determinants of health was made in the Social Work Grand Challenges introduced by the American Academy of Social Work and Social Welfare in January 2015. One of social work's challenges for the future is to remain a key player in the health care field, especially as practice approaches and best practices continue to emerge.

The Council on Social Work Education (CSWE, 2017) calls on the profession to address social determinants of health and eradicate health disparities to improve overall health and health care in communities across the country. CSWE uses a competency-based, outcomes orientation with nine competencies or criteria. It is moving toward a more collective, holistic, and interdependent approach to ensure that the foundation of all professional practice is infused with the values of serving all populations and eradicating disparities and inequities.

All social workers are ethically responsible to consider the impact of the social determinants of health. Key social work roles range from preventive and wellness services (individuals, families, and groups) to large-scale interventions (Rine, 2016). Social workers utilize the skills of engagement with individuals to develop a trusting relationship with the individual/ family/group/community. Assessment includes collecting information to understand the client base's history, experiences, and perspectives. Collaboration between the social worker and the client base to set goals and objectives is an important aspect of the helping process. A strength-based, nonjudgmental approach is critical to social work practice and respect for the client is equally important. Social workers need to have skill sets related to competency in diversity and differences. Cultural responsivity is crucial and the social worker's awareness of personal positionality is vital to the social worker's relationship with individual/families/ group/community. Evaluation of the goals and objectives is an important part of the process and provides information about whether achieving the goals is successful.

Case Example 3.1

The social worker at a community mental health clinic welcomed Chhay into his office. Chhay complained that she had stomachaches and trouble sleeping, but the medical doctor found nothing wrong and therefore had referred her to the clinic. Chhay is 17 years old, a Khmer single mother who has two children, 22 months and 6 months old. They all live with Chhay's grandmother, uncle, her younger sister, and an older male cousin. The social worker explored with Chhay how long had she been having pain and what transpired in her life at the time the pain and trouble sleeping developed.

(continued)

Chhay responded she was having financial problems and was feeling overwhelmed about supporting her children. The social worker and Chhay collaborated to set some goals and objectives. At the end of the session, the social worker made arrangements to see Chhay again the following week.

Case Example 3.1 illustrates issues related to diversity and difference and the importance of meeting the clients where they are. Employing the social work skills of engagement and person-in-environment perspective, the social worker worked with the client to identify the source of her problems and to link her to appropriate financial, food, and other resources. The social worker can also teach the client skills to help alleviate stress and can continue to engage the client in future work.

While Case 3.1 illustrates a micro level example, another example of social determinants of health can be shown in working in a community. Social workers may facilitate community assessment among disparate groups and help define shared problems and common goals. This requires active listening, and excellent communication and networking skills. Community social workers can aid in the creation of grassroots activities and programs, and assist in lifting up community voices. Provision of linkages to outside power bases, resources, and the media are other potential roles. Using education to combat ideological oppression and empowering the community to be the primary agent of change are the core of community work.

Agency social workers often experience a broad range of roles. Social service agency clinicians often attain supervisory positions that call for a new perspective to handle managerial and administrative work. Social workers must develop skills related to planning, budgeting, grant writing, program evaluation, human resources management, and coordination of activities to achieve agency goals. Administrators and agency leaders must also address issues of sustainability, organizational climate, staff retention, public relations, and attraction of clients. One way to handle this effectively is to collaborate with community stakeholders and to build professional partnerships. In any partnership there is a need to address resources and decision-making power.

Good practice thus entails a thorough knowledge of one's workplace setting, the intricate web of power relationships, and infrastructure. It also requires skills in building both intra- and interagency relationships. Of note is the increasingly critical role of the expanding use of technology, not only in data collection and analysis, but in actual service delivery and the implementation of interprofessional teams.

POLICY

Evidence has been amassed over the past few decades that demonstrates that social, political, economic, and cultural environments all have an impact on health outcomes (Carey & Crammond, 2015). This is further bolstered by research, which has shown that medical health care on its own cannot remedy the detrimental effects of poor social environments (Embrett & Randall, 2014). The National Academy of Medicine has reinforced this point in stating that caring for health cannot be confined to the health care system, as it must also encompass other systems such as education, employment, justice, and transportation (McGinnis et al., 2016). As a result of this evidence, calls have come for changes in policy, at both the national and international levels, to address the social determinants of health.

Some of the challenges in the U.S. health care system have already been discussed (see Chapter 1, Introduction). Healthy People 2020 defines health disparities as "a particular type of health difference that is closely linked with social or economic disadvantage" (USDHHS, 2008, p. 46). Disparities have been found to be prevalent by race, ethnicity, and socioeconomic groups, with the greatest differences apparent between African Americans and Whites (McGinnis et al., 2016). Education has also been shown to be one of the greatest predictors of mortality (Hummer & Hernadez, 2013).

So what is being done to address these problems with the U.S. health care system, and how can consideration of the social determinants of health play a role? The CDC, for its part, has introduced a wide range of programs that recognize the importance of the social determinants of health to the well-being of the population. These programs cut across sectors such as housing, education, and transportation, and work in partnership with communities. Among these are the built environment and health initiative that links public health with community design decisions in an effort to design and build healthy communities. Another initiative is the Racial and Ethnic Approaches to Community Health, known as REACH, which aims to reduce racial and ethnic health disparities by establishing community-based programs that are culturally tailored to serve African Americans, American Indians, Hispanics, Asian Americans, Alaskan Natives, and Pacific Islanders (CDC, 2016). Although these programs hold promise, more needs to be done to fully embrace the social determinants of health perspective in national policy.

As part of the National Academy of Medicine's Vital Directions for Health and Health Care Initiative, Adler, Cutler, et al. (2016) focus on the social determinants of health and health disparities by drawing attention to the United States's underinvestment in social services, and describe how this plays a role in the country's lagging health indicators. Adler, Cutler, et al. (2016) assert: "The best available evidence suggests that a health policy framework addressing social and behavioral determinants of health would achieve better population health, less inequality, and lower costs than our current policies" (p. 1). Accordingly, they suggest a "rebalancing" of the nation's health priorities to focus on preventing social conditions and behavioral choices that can lead to damaging health outcomes. More specifically, they offer a three-pronged policy approach geared toward diminishing health disparities and improving health: (a) address the contribution that economic and social policies, such as education and transportation, make to health; (b) promote policies that encourage healthy behaviors and reduce risky behaviors; and (c) improve access to, and the quality and efficiency of, clinical health care services, particularly to disadvantaged populations.

Since the social determinants of health are so closely aligned with social and economic policies, it is worthwhile to explore some of these policies in greater depth. For instance, there is the federal minimum wage, the threshold of which currently stands at $7.25 per hour—where it has been since it was last increased in 2009 (U.S. Department of Labor, n.d.-b). Someone would have to work 40 hours a week, for 50 weeks a year, to earn just $14,500 per year, which is below the poverty level for a family of two. Since poverty is a predictor of poor health and premature mortality, raising the minimum wage to a more sustainable level could translate into better health outcomes. One study by Komro, Livingston, Markowitz, and Wagenaar (2016) found that increasing the federal minimum wage by $1 was associated with a decline in low birth weight births and postneonatal deaths. And in a study that lent support to the effort in New York City to raise the minimum wage to $15 per hour, Tsao et al. (2016) projected that there would have been up to 5,500 fewer premature deaths from 2008 to 2012 had the minimum wage been $15 per hour, with most of the deaths that would have been prevented coming from lower-income communities among people of color. In New York State, increases in the minimum wage are currently being phased in.

Other important policies relate to family caregiving, whether it involves parents caring for young children or children caring for elderly parents. The Family and Medical Leave Act (FMLA) of 1993 enables workers to take up to 12 weeks of unpaid leave for conditions such as caring for a newborn child, caring for a seriously ill spouse, child, or parent, or for one's own serious health condition (U.S. Department of Labor, n.d.-a). Businesses with 50 or more employees must comply with the law; as a result, many people working for small employers are not covered by the law. Aside from expanding the FMLA to cover more workers, the law could also have a greater impact on health, particularly maternal and infant health, if it provided for paid maternity leave, as is common in many other developed countries.

Similarly, more can be done to assist family members who provide care to older adults. The National Family Caregiver Support Program, which is under Title III-E of the Older Americans Act, is a federal program that provides services to families who care for frail older relatives, as well as grandparents and other relatives age 55 and over who are raising children. Among the program's provisions are: providing information to caregivers about services; giving assistance to caregivers to access these services; providing counseling, support and training to caregivers to assist in their caregiving roles; and respite care for caregivers (Generations United, n.d.). Another program for caregivers is the Child and Dependent Care Tax Credit, also known as the Elderly Dependent Care Credit, which enables an individual or family to receive tax credits to cover costs of expenses such as home care or adult day care (Paying for Senior Care, 2017). Although these programs are somewhat modest in their reach, they can provide some much needed assistance to burdened caregivers, who, according to the CDC's National Health Interview Survey (2014), tend to experience declines in physical health, moderate to severe stress, and significant financial strain as a result of their caregiving responsibilities.

Care provided by qualified professionals, especially to young children, can also have a positive effect on health and well-being. D'Onise, Lynch, Sawyer, and McDermott (2010) conducted a systemic review of preschool interventions, including the popular Head Start program, to assess their impact on health outcomes from 1980 to 2008. They found some indications of reductions in obesity, better social competence, improved mental health, and greater crime prevention among children in center-based care. Knudsen, Heckman, Cameron, and Shonkoff (2006) also found that low-income children who attended a pre-K derived social and cognitive benefits over the long term, with savings generated on remedial education, incarceration, and teen pregnancies.

For people with disabilities, the landmark Americans with Disabilities Act (ADA) of 1990 prohibits discrimination, provides equal opportunities, and guarantees that people with disabilities can participate fully in the mainstream of American life (U.S. Department of Justice, n.d.). By extending civil rights protections to people with disabilities, the ADA offers these individuals the same rights and opportunities as everyone else so that they can become full and active participants in society. Chapter 1, Introduction, provides more details on the terms and provisions of the ADA. Despite efforts of the law to prohibit discrimination against people with disabilities, more work needs to be done. In fact, just 17.5% of people with disabilities were employed in 2015, many of them part-time, compared to 65.0% of those without a disability (U.S. Bureau of Labor Statistics, 2016b). To gain a better understanding of the impact that the ADA has had as a social policy, the National Institute on Disability and Rehabilitation Research (NIDRR) is funding a 5-year systemic review of existing ADA research. Disability advocates have complained that much of the cited research on the ADA has been anecdotal and descriptive, thereby making it difficult to either fully assess the law's impact, or to be particularly useful to policy makers. The systemic review, therefore, is intended to accomplish the following:

build a foundation of knowledge on the ADA; inform policy making, research, and information dissemination about the law; and contribute to capacity building of ADA regional centers (Harris et al., 2014).

Health policies with respect to people who have encountered the criminal justice system also need to be carefully reviewed. See Chapter 10, Criminal Justice, for a comprehensive overview of the issue. With the highest incarceration rate in the world, the United States needs to pay greater attention to the adverse effects of incarceration on health, especially for youth involved in the juvenile justice system. Incarceration results in higher rates of infectious disease transmission, including viral hepatitis, HIV/AIDS, and tuberculosis (Drucker, 2013), yet the care offered to inmates often fails to meet their needs, especially for women. Moreover, incarcerated youth, despite having greater health care needs, are confronted with inadequate health care services, especially for mental health and substance abuse treatment (Braverman & Murray, 2011), as well as prenatal care for girls. Strengthening mental health services, pursuing alternative sentencing strategies, and family preservation programs could help to improve the health conditions of many people who have encounters with the criminal justice system (Adler, Cutler, et al., 2016).

In addition to these economic and social policies, the social determinants of health are also influenced by environmental policies and conditions. Climate change can have an impact on air pollution and air quality, extremes in temperature and weather, natural disasters, and rising sea levels and flooding, all of which can influence people's health and well-being (Dekker, 2014). For example, pollution and decreased air quality can contribute to respiratory and cardiovascular disease, and compound conditions such as asthma. Furthermore, weather extremes can destroy crops, which could limit the availability, or drive up the cost of, nutritious food, especially for low-income families. The United States's policy with respect to climate change has gone through a period of flux, as there is not universal agreement as to what is the best approach to take to combat global warming. For instance, the United States originally joined 194 other nations in signing the Paris Climate Accord, which addresses greenhouse gas emission mitigation, adaptation, and financing, but subsequently withdrew from the agreement in favor of pursuing a more nationally based approach. The impact of such a major policy shift on the social determinants of health will likely become evident over time.

RESEARCH

Research on social determinants of health crosses a range of different issues. For example, the Robert Wood Johnson Foundation (2011) identified some of the more significant social determinants of health that affect low-income neighborhoods. These include lack of access to affordable housing, limited access to the playgrounds and recreation needed for healthy childhood development, and unsafe streets that limit opportunities for walking, bicycling, jogging, and other healthy activities. In addition, the Robert Wood Johnson Foundation (2011) included cigarette and alcohol advertising overtly targeted to minors, lead paint, polluted air, and other unhealthy in-home contaminants. Many inner city and poor rural neighborhoods also lack access to healthy and nutritious food. These neighborhood hazards are associated with: lower life expectancy (Chetty et al., 2016; Egen, Beatty, Blackley, Brown, & Wykoff, 2017); higher levels of obesity (Myers, Slack, Martin, Broyles, & Heymsfield, 2016); and higher prevalence of chronic illnesses (Ward, Jemal, Cokkinides, & Singh, 2004; Ziliak & Gundersen, 2014).

According to the American Public Health Association (2017), education is linked to health for all ages. In a report on income and disparities related to educational attainment, the U.S. Census Bureau (2017) reported that 58% of all Americans, but 68% of African

Americans and 77% of Latinos, have only a high school diploma. The U.S. Bureau of Labor Statistics (2016a) reported that the less than high school educated have a 7.4% unemployment rate and a median income of $504 per week, while those with a bachelor's degree have a 2.4% unemployment rate and a median income of $1,380 per week. The Bureau of Labor Statistics data show the strong relationship between education and income and make clear the power that education has to raise millions out of poverty.

Additionally, the CDC (2013c) reported that 8.1% of those with less than a high school education are problem drinkers compared to 4.2% of college graduates. The CDC also stated that 29% of those with less than a high school education smoke cigarettes compared to 10.2% of college graduates. The CDC connects these poor lifestyle choices to cancer, heart disease, diabetes, and other life shortening chronic illnesses.

With respect to access, the introduction of the ACA in 2010 meant that 14 million uninsured Americans were able to obtain health insurance (Ryan, Abrams, Doty, Shah, & Schneider, 2016). Ryan et al. (2016) also reported that the percentage of uninsured African Americans dropped from 31% to 14% between 2010 and 2016 and the percentage of uninsured Latinos dropped from 48% to 32% during that same period. Unfortunately, Braveman and Gottlieb (2014) reported that "The United States spends more money per capita on health care than any other nation on Earth, but ranks at or near the bottom among affluent nations on key measures of health such as life expectancy and infant mortality" (p. 20). Chetty et al. (2016) added that despite the significantly greater access to health care under the ACA, the life expectancy of the bottom half of income earners has almost remained stagnant, while the top half continues to show steady increases.

Research into health access as a social determinant of health has focused on the need to move away from the current treatment-centered approach toward a more progressive patient-centered approach (Berkman, Sheridan, Donahue, Halpern, & Crotty, 2011; Braveman & Gottlieb, 2014; Charmel & Frampton, 2008; Smith, Saunder, Stuckhardt, & McGinnis, 2014). Smith et al. (2014) explained that a patient-centered approach is the key to reducing the cost and increasing the quality of health care, especially in low-income communities. The authors explained that patient-centered care is a collaborative process that occurs when "patients, families, and caregivers are full active participants in the health care delivery process" (p. 1). Social workers have a vital role to play in helping transform health care into a patient-centered model (Bravemen & Gootlieb, 2014).

Tangible benefits of a patient-centered approach have been demonstrated (Charmel & Frampton, 2008; Smith et al., 2014). A 5-year study, which compared two hospitals, one with a patient-centered approach and one with a traditional approach, found that in five consecutive annual surveys, the patient-centered hospital demonstrated shorter average stays, fewer adverse health events, and higher patient satisfaction. The patient-centered hospital included sensitivity training for staff, patient, and family education groups, one-on-one sessions, trained case managers, and the like (Charmel & Frampton, 2008). Smith et al. (2014) added that patient-centered hospitals also reported better staff morale, lower cost of care per patient, and fewer malpractice cases.

Improved health literacy is an additional important component of a patient-centered approach, which Smith et al. (2014) explained as "an individual's ability to obtain, understand, and apply health information to make appropriate health decisions" (p. 3). In a systematic review of 96 studies on health literacy, Berkman et al. (2011) reported that poor health literacy is associated with negative outcomes including: increased hospitalization and emergency room usage; less compliance with medical instructions; less use of preventive measures, such as mammograms, colonoscopies, and flu shots; and poorer overall health status with higher mortality rates. The study underscored the importance of including an emphasis on health literacy education in any patient-centered approach.

The issue of housing is addressed in a large-scale survey of low-income families. Cutts et al. (2011) defined housing instability as being homeless, living in overcrowded conditions, and needing to move frequently. The survey results showed that "housing insecurity is associated with poor health, lower weight, and developmental risk among young children" (p. 1). Fenelon et al. (2017) conducted a longitudinal study to compare the mental and physical health of public housing residents with those on a waiting list for public housing. The study found that the stress of housing instability measurably affected both the physical and mental health of those on the waiting list compared to those in stable housing. These studies demonstrate the need for housing stability in promoting more positive health outcomes for those in living poverty.

The U.S. Department of Agriculture (USDA, 2016) reports that 21% of those living below the U.S. poverty level report low food security, while 16% report very low food security. Using data from the 1999–2010 National Health and Nutrition Examination Survey (NHANES), Ziliak and Gunderson (2014) found that food insecurity may lead to: higher risk of birth defects; increased risk of asthma; higher hospitalization rates; more occurrences of oral health problems; and higher probability of behavioral and mental health problems, among others. Additionally, the Economic Policy Institute (2015) reported that 62% of those in poverty are either unemployed or part-time employed. Benach et al. (2014) conducted a meta-analysis of perceived job insecurity and found that those with precarious employment had higher incidences of depressive and anxiety disorders, worse self-reported health, and higher use of health services than those with steady employment. The Robert Wood Johnson Foundation (2013) explained that stable, higher paying jobs offer private health insurance, which not only provides a high level of health care choice, but also emphasizes health education and preventive medicine as tools to stay healthy.

Research also indicates several community contexts that are determinants of health; these may include social cohesion, civic participation, discrimination, and incarceration (USDHHS, 2008). Irrespective of socioeconomic status, communities that treat each other with respect, repay acts of kindness, and work together for the common good of all develop social trust, which many researchers identify as an important determinant of health (Gilbert, Quinn, Goodman, Butler, & Wallace, 2013; Helliwell & Putnam, 2004; Herian, Tay, Hamm, & Diener, 2014; Kim & Kawachi, 2006). A meta-analysis of 39 studies relating social context to health found that reciprocity and trust were the two community factors most strongly associated with better perceived health (Gilbert et al., 2013). Furthermore, Helliwell and Putnam (2004) concluded that in many low-income communities, "living in a high trust community seems to improve health . . . in addition to the even more powerful effect of a trustworthy community on subjective well-being" (p. 1443).

Civic participation is also an important component of healthy communities. Civic participation may take the form of volunteer work, political engagement, attending houses of worship, and other community activities (Kim & Kawachi, 2006). Research shows that communities with higher levels of civic engagement demonstrate higher levels of happiness and better health outcomes even when controlling for demographics and socioeconomic status (Heliwell & Putnam, 2004). Heliwell and Putnam (2004) found a connection between high levels of civic participation and high levels of trust, concluding that the health benefits of social cohesion and civic participation are additive. In a large study of urban residents, Kim and Kawachi (2006) found better self-rated health among those who participated in formal group activities, particularly in urban areas with higher population density.

CONCLUSION

By deepening the understanding of social determinants of health and the major health care disparities that result, social workers can improve the health circumstances of vulnerable populations. As pointed out in the Introduction to this book, more spending on health care does not necessarily lead to better outcomes. To achieve positive health outcomes, it is critical for social workers to advocate for policies that can address and promote health for all members of society.

CHAPTER DISCUSSION QUESTIONS

1. Explain the social determinants of health and how they inform practice, policy, and research.

2. How are vulnerable populations impacted by social determinants of health?

3. What can social workers do to address social determinants of health in micro, mezzo, and macro practice?

CASE EXAMPLE AND DISCUSSION QUESTIONS

Case Example 3.2

An elementary school (K-6) is housed on the grounds of a housing project in a deteriorating downtown urban center. The building's capacity was surpassed years ago and three trailers have been parked next to it to handle the overflow of classes. The student: teacher ratio is 33:1; 82% of the students qualify for free or reduced price lunch; and 14% of the students are homeless.

A teacher asked Karen, one of two school social workers, to meet a 9-year-old male student, John. For several weeks, John had been inattentive in class, sometimes fell asleep at his desk, frequently neglected to do his homework, and was at risk of failing. His teacher had been unable to get in touch with John's mother, despite sending home three notes asking the mother to see her.

Karen met with John in her office. During the meeting she explored with John how he was feeling about school. John shrugged and looked down. Karen then asked which class he liked best, and John quickly looked up and said, "Lunch." Karen then suggested she and John ask his mother to join them, but John said she probably wouldn't because she doesn't speak English and now works two jobs. John then said he had to leave; he had to pick up his younger sisters and take them home.

Questions for Discussion

1. As the school social worker, what is the first thing you would do in conducting an assessment with John?

(continued)

Case Example 3.2   *(continued)*

2.   What are some ways you can engage John and his mother?

3.   What other resources, both in the school and its surrounding community, would be helpful to John and his mother?

REFERENCES

Adler, N., Cutler, D., Fielding, J., Galea, S., Glymour, M., Koh, H., & Satcher, D. (2016). Addressing social determinants of health and health disparities (Discussion Paper). In *Vital Directions for Health and Health Care Series*. Washington, DC: National Academy of Medicine. Retrieved from https://nam.edu/wp-content/uploads/2016/09/Addressing-Social-Determinants-of-Health-and-Health-Disparities.pdf

Adler, N., Glymour, M., & Fielding, J. (2016). Addressing social determinants of health and health inequalities. *Journal of the American Medical Association, 316*(16), 1641–1642. doi:10.1001/jama.2016.14058

American Public Health Association. (2017). Education attainment linked to health throughout lifespan: Exploring social determinants of health. Retrieved from http://thenationshealth.aphapublications.org/content/46/6/1.3.full

Benach, J., Vives, A., Amable, M., Vanroelen, C., Tarafa, G., & Muntaner, C. (2014). Precarious employment: Understanding an emerging social determinant of health. *Annual Review of Public Health, 35*, 229–253. doi:10.1146/annurev-publhealth-032013-182500

Berkman, N. D., Sheridan, S. L., Donahue, K. E., Halpern, D. J., & Crotty, K. (2011). Low health literacy and health outcomes: An updated systematic review. *Annals of Internal Medicine, 155*(2), 97–107. doi:10.7326/0003-4819-155-2-201107190-00005

Braveman, P., & Gottlieb, L. (2014). The social determinants of health: It's time to consider the causes of the causes. *Public Health Reports, 129*(1 Suppl. 2), 19–31. doi:10.1177/00333549141291S206

Braverman, P., & Murray, P. (2011). Health care for youth in the juvenile justice system. *Pediatrics, 128*(6), 1219–1235. doi:10.1542/peds.2011-1757

Carey, G., & Crammond, B. (2015). Action on the social determinants of health: Views from inside the policy process. *Social Science and Medicine, 128*, 134–141. doi:10.1016/j.socscimed.2015.01.024

Centers for Disease Control and Prevention. (2013a). CDC health disparities and inequalities report—United States 2013. *Morbidity and Mortality Weekly Report, Supplement, 62*(3), 1–187.

Centers for Disease Control and Prevention. (2013b). Conclusion and future directions: CDC health disparities and inequalities report—United States, 2013. *CDC Health Disparities and Inequalities Report—United States, 2013, 62*(3), 184–186.

Centers for Disease Control and Prevention. (2013c). Health behaviors of adults: United States, 2008–2010. U.S. Department of Health and Human Services, Series 10, Number 257.

Centers for Disease Control and Prevention. (2014). National Health Interview Survey. Retrieved from https://www.cdc.gov/nchs/nhis/

Centers for Disease Control and Prevention. (2016). Retrieved from https://www.cdc .gov/socialdeterminants/cdcprograms/index.htm

Charmel, P. A., & Frampton, S. B. (2008). Building the business case for patient-centered care. *Health care Financial Management, 62*(3), 80–85.

Chetty, R., Stepner, M., Abraham, S., Lin, S., Scuderi, B., Turner, N., . . . Cutler, D. (2016). The association between income and life expectancy in the United States, 2001–2014. *Journal of the American Medical Association, 315*(16), 1750–1766. doi:10.1001/jama.2016.4226

Council on Social Work Education. (2017). Ensuring access to care and protecting under-served and vulnerable populations: Principles for health-care public policy. Retrieved from https://cswe.org/getattachment/Advocacy-Policy/Health-care-Principles -Feb-2017.pdf.aspx

Cutts, D. B., Meyers, A. F., Black, M. M., Casey, P. H., Chilton, M., Cook, J. T., & Rose-Jacobs, R. (2011). US housing insecurity and the health of very young children. *American Journal of Public Health, 101*(8), 1508–1514. doi:10.2105/AJPH.2011.300139

Dekker, S. (2014). Climate change and social determinants of health: Innovating climate policy. International Center for Climate Governance, Reflection No. 19. Retrieved from http:// www.iccgov.org/wp-content/uploads/2015/05/19_ICCG_Reflection_February_2014.pdf

D'Onise, K., Lynch, J., Sawyer, M., & McDermott, R. (2010). Can preschool improve child health outcomes? A systemic review. *Social Science and Medicine, 70*(9), 1423–1440. doi:10.1016/j.socscimed.2009

Drucker, E. (2013). *A plague of prisons: The epidemiology of mass incarceration in America.* New York, NY: The New Press.

Economic Policy Institute. (2015). Poor people work: A majority of poor people who can work do. Retrieved from http://www.epi.org/publication/poor-people-work -a-majority-of-poor-people-who-can-work-do/

Egen, O., Beatty, K., Blackley, D. J., Brown, K., & Wykoff, R. (2017). Health and social conditions of the poorest versus wealthiest counties in the United States. *American Journal of Public Health, 107*(1), 130–135.

Embrett, M., & Randall, G. (2014). Social determinants of health and health equity policy research: Exploring the use, misuse, and nonuse of policy analysis theory. *Social Science and Medicine, 108,* 147–155.

Fenelon, A., Mayne, P., Simon, A. E., Rossen, L. M., Helms, V., Lloyd, P., . . . Steffen, B. L. (2017). Housing assistance programs and adult health in the United States. *American Journal of Public Health, 107*(4), 571–578.

Galea, S., Tracy, M., Hoggatt, K., DiMaggio, C., & Karpati, A. (2011). Estimated deaths attributable to social factors in the United States. *American Journal of Public Health, 101*(8), 1456–1465.

Generations United. (n.d.). National Family Caregiver Support Program. Retrieved from http://www.gu.org/OURWORK/PublicPolicy/GrandfamiliesPolicy/NationalFam-ilyCaregiverSupportProgram.aspx

Gilbert, K. L., Quinn, S. C., Goodman, R. M., Butler, J., & Wallace, J. (2013). A meta-analysis of social capital and health: A case for needed research. *Journal of Health Psychology, 18*(11), 1385–1399. doi:10.1177/1359105311435983

Harris, S., Gould, R., Ojok, P., Fujiera, G., Jones, R., & Olmstead, A. (2014). Scoping review of the Americans with Disabilities Act: What research exists, and where do we go from here? *Disabilities Studies Quarterly, 34*(3). doi:10.18061/dsq.v34i3.3883

Helliwell, J. F., & Putnam, R. D. (2004). The social context of well-being. *Philosophical Transactions-Royal Society of London Series B: Biological Sciences, 359*(1449), 1435–1446. doi:10.1098/rstb.2004.1522

Herian, M. N., Tay, L., Hamm, J. A., & Diener, E. (2014). Social capital, ideology, and health in the United States. *Social Science & Medicine, 105*, 30–37. doi:10.1016/j.socscimed.2014.01.003

Hummer, R. A., & Hernandez, E. M. (2013). The effect of educational attainment on adult mortality in the United States. *Population Bulletin, 68*(1), 1.

Kim, D., & Kawachi, I. (2006). A multilevel analysis of key forms of community- and individual-level social capital as predictors of self-rated health in the United States. *Journal of Urban Health, 83*(5), 813–826. doi:10.1007/s11524-006-9082-1

Knudsen, E., Heckman, J., Cameron, J., & Shonkoff, J. (2006). Economic, neurobiological, and behavioral perspectives on building America's future workforce. *Proceedings of the National Academy of Sciences of the United States of America, 103*(27), 10155–10162.

Komro, K., Livingston M., Markowitz, S., & Wagenaar, A. (2016). The effect of an increased minimum wage on infant mortality and birth weight. *American Journal of Public Health, 106*(8), 1514–1516. doi:10.2105/AJPH.2016.303268

McGinnis, J., Berwick, D., Daschle, T., Diaz, A., Fineberg, H., Frist, W., ... Lavizzo-Mourey, R. (2016). *System strategies for better health throughout the life course: A vital direction for health and health care* (Discussion Paper). In *Vital Directions for Health and Health Care Series*. Washington, DC: National Academy of Medicine.

Moniz, C. (2010). *Social work and the social determinants of health perspective: A good fit*. Silver Spring, MD: National Association of Social Workers.

Moniz, C., & Gorin, S. (2010). *Health and mental health care policy: A biopsychosocial perspective* (3rd ed.). Boston, MA: Allyn & Bacon.

Myers, C. A., Slack, T., Martin, C. K., Broyles, S. T., & Heymsfield, S. B. (2016). Change in obesity prevalence across the United States is influenced by recreational and health care contexts, food environments, and Hispanic populations. *PLoS One, 11*(2), 1–13. doi:10.1371/journal.pone.0148394

National Association of Social Workers. (2017). Code of Ethics. Retrieved from https://www.socialworkers.org/About/Ethics/Code-of-Ethics

Office of Disease Prevention and Health Promotion. (2017a). About healthy people. Retrieved from https://www.healthypeople.gov/2020/About-Healthy-People

Office of Disease Prevention and Health Promotion. (2017b). Social determinants of health. Retrieved from https://www.healthypeople.gov/2020/topics-objectives/topic/social-determinants-of-health

Paying for Senior Care. (2017). Federal tax credit for elderly dependent care. Retrieved from https://www.payingforseniorcare.com/longtermcare/resources/dependent_care_tax_credit.html

Rine, C. (2016). Social determinants of health: Grand challenges in social work's future: Guest editorial. *National Association of Social Workers, 41*, 143–145.

Robert Wood Johnson Foundation. (2011). Neighborhood and health. Retrieved from http://www.rwjf.org/content/dam/farm/reports/issue_briefs/2011/rwjf70450

Robert Wood Johnson Foundation. (2013). Health policy snapshot: Public health and prevention. Retrieved from http://www.rwjf.org/content/dam/farm/reports/issue_briefs/2013/rwjf403360

Ryan, J., Abrams, M. K., Doty, M. M., Shah, T., & Schneider, E. C. (2016). How high-need patients experience health care in the United States. Findings from the 2016 Commonwealth Fund Survey of High-Need Patients. *Issue Brief, Commonwealth Fund, 43,* 1–20.

Smith, M., Saunders, R., Stuckhardt, L., & McGinnis, J. M. (2014). *Best care at lower cost.* Washington, DC: National Academies Press.

Tsao, T., Konty, K., Van Wye, G., Barbor, O., Hadler, J., Linos, N., & Bassett, M. (2016). Estimating potential reductions in premature mortality in New York City from raising the minimum wage to $15. *American Journal of Public Health, 106*(6), 1036–1041. doi:10.2105/AJPH.2016.303188

U.S. Bureau of Labor Statistics. (2016a). Employment projections. Retrieved from https://www.bls.gov/emp/ep_chart_001.htm

U.S. Bureau of Labor Statistics. (2016b). Persons with a disability: Labor force characteristics—2016. USDL-16-1248, News Release, U.S. Department of Labor. Retrieved from http://www.bls.gov/news.release/pdf/disabl.pdf

U.S. Census Bureau. (2017). Educational attainment in the United States: 2015. Retrieved from https://www.census.gov/content/dam/Census/library/publications/2016/demo/p20-578.pdf

U.S. Department of Agriculture. (2016). Statistical supplement to household food security in the United States in 2015. Retrieved from https://www.ers.usda.gov/webdocs/publications/79436/ap-072.pdf?v=42622

U.S. Department of Health and Human Services. (2008). Recommendations for the framework and format of Healthy People 2020: Phase I Report. The Secretaries Advisory Committee on National Health Promotion and Disease Prevention Objectives for 2020. Phase I: Recommendations for the framework and format of Healthy People 2020. Retrieved from http://www.healthypeople.gov/sites/default/files/PhaseI_0.pdf

U.S. Department of Justice. (n.d.). Information and technical assistance on the Americans with Disabilities Act. Retrieved from https://www.ada.gov/ada_intro.htm

U.S. Department of Labor. (n.d.-a). Family and Medical Leave Act. Retrieved from https://www.dol.gov/whd/fmla/

U.S. Department of Labor. (n.d.-b). Minimum wage. Retrieved from https://www.dol.gov/whd/minimumwage.htm

Ward, E., Jemal, A., Cokkinides, V., & Singh, G. K. (2004). Cancer disparities by race/ethnicity and socioeconomic status. *CA: A Cancer Journal for Clinicians, 54*(2), 78–93. Retrieved from http://onlinelibrary.wiley.com/doi/10.3322/canjclin.54.2.78/epdf

World Health Organization. (2017). Social determinants of health. Retrieved from http://www.who.int/social_determinants/thecommission/finalreport/key_concepts/en/

Ziliak, J. P., & Gundersen, C. (2014). The health consequences of senior hunger in the United States: Evidence from the 1999–2010 NHANES. Retrieved from http://www.aaa1b.org/wp-content/uploads/2016/08/Health-Consequences-of-Food-Insecurity-final.pdf

4

Intersectionality, Social Work, and Health

Abigail M. Ross, Elaine P. Congress, and Sara Matsuzaka

In recent years, health researchers and practitioners have turned to intersectional approaches to practice, policy analysis, and the conduct of research to better understand the etiology of persistent and pervasive population-level inequities in health care access and health outcomes (Caiola, Docherty, Relf, & Barroso, 2014; Sen, Iyer, & Mukarjee, 2009). As a construct, intersectionality provides a useful framework for understanding how unequal distributions of power across social groups perpetuate poorer health outcomes and disenfranchisement from modern health care benefits in certain groups. Intersectional approaches are also consistent with values of dignity and worth of the person and social justice that undergird the Social Work Professional Code of Ethics (National Association of Social Workers, 2017). These are mechanisms through which social workers can (a) engage diversity and difference in practice and (b) advance human rights, social, economic, and environmental justice, and correspond to Competencies 2 and 3 in the 2015 Council on Social Work Education's (CSWE) Educational Policy and Accreditation Standards (EPAS). This chapter begins with a brief historical overview of intersectionality and a discussion of core elements of the construct as applied to the social determinants of health and health care. The authors then describe current innovations to social work practice, policy, and research that utilize intersectional approaches, and conclude with a discussion of current challenges and future directions for the social work profession.

BACKGROUND

Origins and Conceptualizations of Intersectionality

Coined by Kimberlé Williams Crenshaw (1991), intersectionality was developed within Black feminist discourses that confronted positivistic essentialist approaches within feminism in favor of a more experience-based epistemology (Simien, 2007). Black feminism challenged the invisibility of Black women's voices and interests within the feminist movement. The work of Crenshaw (1991) and other contemporaries was preceded by a long history of Black feminist efforts by activists and scholars such as Sojourner Truth, Anna Julia Cooper, Maria Stewart, Angela Davis, and Deborah King to address the multiplicity of challenges faced by women of color (Hill Collins, 1997, 2000).

The exact definition of intersectionality remains vague and a source of contention among scholars (Smooth, 2013). Hancock (2007) conceptualized intersectionality as a paradigm that functions both as an explanatory conceptual framework and as a methodological approach. As a framework, intersectionality provides a lens through which to examine and understand the complexity of a marginalized person's lived experience based on the influences of intersecting and interactive domains of self-identification combined with (or contrasted by) social categorization within societal systems of oppression and dominance (Davis, 2008; Galupo, Mitchell, & Davis, 2015; McCall, 2005; Shields, 2008). In particular, McCall (2005) suggested that "intersectionality is the most important theoretical contribution that women's studies, in conjunction with related fields, has made thus far" (p. 1771).

As an analytic method, intersectionality has the potential to improve understandings of the varied and dynamic configurations of identity and related oppression. Specifically, Black feminist contributions via intersectional analysis have shifted discourse around race and gender by challenging the notion that they are distinct constructs without overlapping systems of power and oppression (Crenshaw, 1991). This work has led to additional methodological advances (e.g., the Queer of Color Critique) that examine the complex associations among race/ethnicity, gender, and sexual identities within queer and transgender people of color (Ferguson, 2003). In social work, intersectionality has been described as the network of identities that formulate and determine experiences of both oppression and privilege within a given society (Halpern, 2017).

Core Assumptions

Intersectionality holds that the lived experiences of individuals are shaped by multiple dimensions of interlocking identity whereby social categories of race, ethnicity, gender, class, sexuality, citizenship, religiosity, and nation articulate one another within systems of oppression, dominance, and control (Hall, 1971). Intersectionality thus rejects essentialist universalizing views on lived experience. While variably defined (Hancock, 2007), there is general consensus on a number of core assumptions that characterize the construct:

- Lived experiences cannot be reduced to a single social identity category (Hill Collins, 2000; Crenshaw, 1991; Wing, 1997).
- Social identity categories (e.g., race, ethnicity, gender/gender expression, age, class, ability, sexuality) are nonadditive, interdependent, and mutually constituted (Hill Collins, 2000; Crenshaw, 1991; Wing, 1997).
- By definition, social identity categories are socially constructed and are associated with unequal social relationships among groups of people (Weber, 2006).
- Social identity categories are inseparable from social processes and societal structures, which in turn are shaped by power and are the mechanisms through which resources (e.g., health care) are distributed (Hankivsky et al., 2014).

The Case for Intersectionality in Health

A large body of research has elucidated the influence of social determinants of health on short- and long-term health outcomes (Smedley, Stith, & Nelson, 2003; World Health Organization [WHO], 2008; see Chapter 3). Social determinants of health include social identity categories such as race, ethnicity, gender/gender expression, socioeconomic status (SES), and sexual orientation, as well as conditions driven by circumstance, such as access to and quality of health care. In the United States, socially marginalized groups, such as racial/ethnic minorities, sexual minorities, and people with lower SES continue to experience suboptimal access to and quality of health care, as well as poorer health outcomes (Clarke et al., 2013; National Center for Health Statistics, 2012; Smedley et al., 2003; Vargas-Bustamante, Chen, Rodriguez, Rizzo, & Ortega, 2010). Over the past two decades, the urgent need to promote health and health equity has been highlighted throughout a number of national and international initiatives (Healthy People 2020, U.S. Department of Health and Human Services [USDHHS], 2011; WHO, 2008).

Despite these calls to action, research shows that disparities in leading health indicators have either remained unchanged over time or, in some cases, worsened (Sondik, Huang, Klein, & Satcher, 2010), perhaps due to an absence of intersectional approaches in health care service delivery and policy design. For example, research indicates that substance abuse treatment programs are insufficiently addressing the needs of sexual and gender minorities with substance use disorders (Lyons et al., 2015; Senreich, 2011). Sexual and gender minorities may face heteronormative barriers to effective care within substance abuse treatment based on gender-segregated structural components, the inability to continue hormone replacement therapy, exposures to stigma and discrimination, and cultural incompetence among staff (Eliason & Hughes, 2004). Exposure to such barriers can lead to potentially harmful outcomes for sexual and gender minority clients, such as treatment avoidance, leaving treatment prematurely, and/or relapse (Nuttbrock, 2012; Senreich, 2009).

PRACTICE

Social work practitioners in the health field are bound both by the NASW Code of Ethics (2017) as well as recently developed standards of social work practice in health care settings (Wheeler & McClain, 2016). These standards for Social Work Practice in Health Care Settings require both an

> . . . understanding [of] how one's own cultural values, beliefs, biases, experiences, and perceptions affect interactions with clients and colleagues, as well as recognition of how societal oppression and privilege related to cultural and linguistic diversity (such as racism, sexism, homophobia, ageism, or xenophobia) affect clients' biopsychosocial–spiritual well-being, access to and use of supports and services, and health outcomes. (Wheeler & McClain, 2016, p. 22)

Cultural Humility

While cultural responsiveness to clients has long been an important theme in social work practice and education, the focus on intersectionality is a relatively new development. As noted in the CSWE's Educational & Policy Accreditation Standards (CSWE, 2015), social work educators are advised to incorporate an intersectionality approach characterized by cultural humility:

> Educational Policy 3.0—Diversity. The program's expectation for diversity is reflected in its learning environment, which provides the context through which students learn about differences, to value and respect diversity, and develop a commitment to cultural humility. The dimensions of diversity are understood as the intersectionality of multiple factors including but not limited to age, class, color, culture, disability and ability, ethnicity, gender, gender identity and expression, immigration status, marital status, political ideology, race, religion/spirituality, sex, sexual orientation, and tribal sovereign status. (CSWE, 2015, p. 14)

A cultural humility perspective serves as an important segue into an intersectional approach that stresses the multiple identities of clients. Developed initially for medical education (Tervalon & Murray-Garcia, 1998), cultural humility is defined as "having an interpersonal stance that is other-oriented rather than self-focused, characterized by respect and lack of superiority toward an individual's cultural background and experience" (Hook et al., 2013, p. 353). In other words, the practice of cultural humility requires ongoing attention to and awareness of one's own biases, as well as recognition of the limitations of what one knows—or thinks one knows—about a client's culture (Tervalon & Murray-Garcia, 1998). Characterized by principles of lifelong learning and self-reflection, recognition of and changes in power imbalances in service of fostering collaborative and respectful relationships, and institutional accountability (Tervalon & Murray-Garcia, 1998), cultural humility has been positively associated with strength in therapeutic alliance and improved treatment outcomes (Hook, Davis, Owen, Worthington, & Utsey, 2013). It also has the potential to reduce instances of microaggressions that occur within the therapeutic relationship and more broadly in settings where care is delivered. It is especially useful in health care settings in particular, as cultural beliefs about health and illness and experiences with the health care system may influence the patient's and the family's willingness to seek or engage with care.

Liberation Health Social Work

Despite its natural fit with social work values and the profession's ethical standards, intersectionality is frequently avoided in social work education and training (Robinson, Cross-Denny, Lee, Rozas, & Yamada, 2016). Building on rich traditions of liberation psychology (Martin-Baro, 1994), popular education (Freire, 1974, 1998), and radical social work (Reynolds, 1973), liberation health social work (LHSW) is both a theory of human behavior and a method of practice (Belkin Martinez, 2014). As a theory of human behavior, one of the core assumptions of LHSW is that the problems of individuals, families, and communities cannot be understood in isolation from the societal conditions from which they developed. As a method of practice, LHSW not only strives to help clients understand the personal, cultural, and institutional factors that contribute to their problems, it also empowers them to act to change these social conditions (Belkin Martinez, 2014). In addition to maintaining the assumption that workable solutions for individuals, families, and communities are both individual and social, LHSW also recognizes the importance of ideology and thereby prioritizes the task of deconstructing dominant worldview messages. When unrecognized and internalized, dominant worldview messages (e.g., equating thinness with beauty) frequently result in object-like experiences (Freire, 1974). These object-like experiences may contribute to a passive sense of self that adversely affects a client's self-efficacy and inhibits personal agency. LHSW seeks to raise consciousness about dominant worldview messages that may be unconsciously internalized, so that experiences become more subject-like and individuals, families, and communities can thereby "liberate themselves from both internal and external oppressions" (Belkin Martinez, 2014, p. 22).

Gender, gender identity, and gender expression are of particular relevance for social workers in health care settings, as medical care for individuals who are intersex or have nonconforming gender identities invariably includes a psychosocial component. It is estimated that 6% of the U.S. population, or one in 189 Americans, do not identify with their birth gender (Crissman, Berger, Graham, & Dalton, 2017); there is some evidence that this number is growing in part due to increased acceptance of gender diversity in society (Landers & Kapadia, 2017). Findings from a recent study showed that the majority of those who identify as transgender (trans) were more likely to identify as people of color, fall below the poverty line, and lack a college education (Crissman, Berger, Graham, & Dalton, 2017). Challenges that trans people may encounter in the health care system were first identified over 15 years ago, but reiterated recently in terms of problematic access to care, possibly due to encountering discrimination by health care professionals (Lombardi, 2001, 2017). Ongoing training has been recommended as a way to manage these biases (Witten & Eyler, 2012).

The following case example illustrates the challenges that require an intersectional approach in working with a transgender client in a health care setting.

Case Example 4.1

Carlotta is a 25-year-old Latinx transgender woman (male to female [MTF]) who presents to the outpatient clinic for treatment of depression accompanied by feelings of hopelessness, worthlessness/low self-esteem, and passive suicidality ("maybe I would be better off dead"). Carlotta's gender pronouns are "she/her/hers." She initially came to a large city in the Southern United States about 10 years ago to visit a relative; she overstayed her visa and she became undocumented. Growing up in a large family in a rural community in Mexico, she was defined at birth as male and raised as male in her family's Catholic home. She was later ostracized from her family due to her gender identity and expression. She fears discrimination and violence were she to return to Mexico.

Since arriving in the United States, she has found it difficult to secure consistent work because of her immigration status, lack of education, and limited English proficiency. She was terminated from an "off the books" job because the boss received a negative comment from a customer about "the employee in a skirt who had deep voice." Carlotta would like to engage in hormone therapy and ultimately undergo gender reassignment surgery, but has not been able to acquire consistent health care that is responsive to her needs. She recently visited the emergency room (ER) in an attempt to acquire a referral for hormone therapy, but was told that she was not able to start a hormone regimen because of her untreated depressive symptoms. The ER team mispronounced (used "he" instead of "she") her three times and then discharged her with a referral to a local community center for treatment, where she was assigned to a White 50-year-old middle-class social worker. The social worker lives with her husband and two teenage children in a suburban community. The social worker considers herself bilingual as she had spent her junior year abroad in Madrid and had minored in Spanish in college.

When employing the liberation health method of practice, a LHSW would first attempt to see the problem as it is experienced in its totality by the client, subsequently analyze the personal, cultural, and institutional factors that contribute to the problem, and then act to change the problem. Personal factors are those that are consistent with a standard biopsychosocial assessment, including individual and developmental history, health and illness, trauma and loss, family conflict, and social support. Cultural factors include dominant worldview messages around race, gender, class, individualism, competition, sexual preference, ableism, consumerism, and stigma. For example, in Carlotta's case, her unconscious adoption of the xenophobic dominant worldview that equated "undocumented immigrants as illegal aliens" and lived experiences of transphobia contributed to feelings of dehumanization and worthlessness. Finally, institutional factors include health care, education, housing, and the criminal justice system that may be contributing to the problem. In Carlotta's case, the daunting nature of the health care system

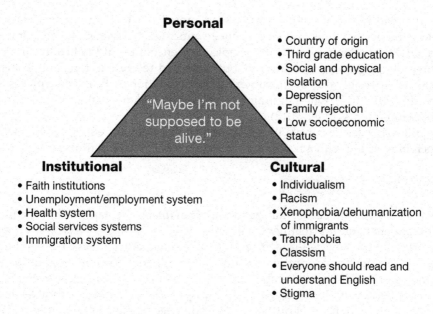

Figure 4.1 Carlotta's liberation health triangle.

combined with the relative lack of knowledge about trans health needs of the provider team contributed to her feelings of hopelessness. Carlotta's liberation health triangle, which identifies additional factors contributing to the problem, is depicted in Figure 4.1.

POLICY

On average, the United States spends more dollars per person on health care than any other country in the world, yet health outcomes are not commensurate with these expenditures. Access to and quality of health care are two of the most salient predictors of health outcomes. A recent study examining the relationship of health care access and quality to the outcome of amenable causes of mortality, defined as health conditions that would not result in death if effective medical care were obtained, showed that the United States ranked 35th of 195 countries on the health care access and quality index (HAQ), well below any other developed country (Barker et al., 2017). Within the United States, research shows that average life expectancy varies by more than 20 years across counties, with a high of 87 years in Summit County, Colorado, compared to 67 in Oglala Lakota County, South Dakota, home to a large Native American population (Dwyer-Lindgren et al., 2017). Results show that combined, health care factors (such as access and quality), SES, race/ethnicity, and malleable behavioral and metabolic risk factors explained 74% of county-level variation factors (Dwyer-Lindgren et al., 2017). Taken together, results of these studies show that people are dying from preventable causes with well-known treatments. Policy analysts attribute these numbers to a marked lack of investment in prevention as well as variable access to and quality of care, both of which are frequently contingent upon insurance coverage.

The passage of the Patient Protection and Affordable Care Act (ACA) represented a shift toward prevention and universal coverage through provisions requiring uncapped coverage of essential health benefits and the expansion of Medicaid eligibility in 31 states. Notably, the 10 categories of essential health benefits include preventive wellness services, chronic disease management, mental health, pediatric services, and maternity and newborn care. While some of these essential health benefits can be utilized by all (e.g., preventive wellness services), others expand coverage for nondominant or marginalized social identity categories (e.g., women, children, people with mental and physical disabilities/health problems) disproportionately, thereby attending to power differentials and incorporating an intersectional approach. The provision prohibiting caps to annual per-person expenditures is designed to provide individuals with more health benefits without additional financial burden.

Recent research indicates that gaining insurance coverage through the Medicaid expansions has decreased the probability of not receiving care by 20% to 25% (Glied, Ma, & Borja, 2017). In a survey of individuals who had acquired health insurance through marketplace exchanges or Medicaid expansion, over 50% of respondents reported they would not have been able to access or afford care prior acquiring coverage through the ACA expansion (Collins, Gunja, Doty, & Beutel, 2016). Early findings from another study also suggest that the ACA expansion has the potential to reduce, but not eliminate, health disparities among racial and ethnic groups (Hayes, Riley, Radley, & McCarthy, 2015).

Intersectionality-Based Policy Assessment Framework

While reductions in disparities in access to care and health outcomes across social identity groups indicate progress toward achieving equity, they cannot necessarily be attributed to intersectional approaches, as outcomes are frequently assessed across a single dimension (e.g., race, gender). Moreover, reductions in disparities are not necessarily an indicator of improved health outcomes within or across populations, structural change, or optimal health policy. Building on health impact (Cole & Fielding, 2007) and health equity impact assessment (Haber, 2010) tools, the Intersectionality-Based Policy Analysis (IBPA) framework is an innovative multidimensional approach to health policy analysis that seeks to elucidate specifically who benefits—and who is excluded—from health policy priorities and goals, as well as the intended and unintended consequences of subsequent resource allocation (Hankivsky, 2012; Hankivsky et al., 2014).

IBPA comprises eight general principles that guide 12 overarching questions; together these components shape the subsequent analysis. The 12 questions consist of five descriptive questions that are designed to elicit contextual information related to the policy issue in question and seven transformative questions that are intended to generate alternative solutions with attention to measurable impacts and outcomes (Hankivsky et al., 2014). Please see Table 4.1.

Originally developed and implemented in Canada (Hankivsky, 2012), IBPA has expanded to Europe through the SOPHIE Project, a multinational collaboration designed to generate new knowledge about the effects of European policies on health inequalities through innovative methodologies for international, national, and local policy evaluation (Palencia, Malmusi, & Borrell, 2014). While initially designed for health policy analysis, IBPA may be a useful tool for analysis of institutional and organizational policies as well.

In addition to policies related to health access, coverage, and quality of care, it is important to note the indirect health effects associated with the existence and application of social policies in systems that are not designed to address health explicitly. These are described extensively in Chapters 3, 10, and 13 of this book. In particular, the adverse

Table 4.1 Guiding Principles and Questions of IBPA

IBPA Guiding Principles	
Intersecting categories	
Multi-level analysis	
Power	
Reflexivity	
Time and space	
Diverse knowledge	
Social justice	
Equity	
IBPA Questions	
Descriptive	What knowledge, values and experiences do you bring to this area of policy analysis?
	What is the policy "problem" under consideration?
	How have representations of the "problem" come about?
	How are groups differentially affected by this representation of the "problem"?
	What are the current policy responses to the "problem"?
Transformative	What inequities actually exist in relation to the "problem"?
	Where and how can interventions be made to improve the "problem"?
	What are feasible short-, medium-, and long-term solutions?
	How will proposed policy responses reduce inequities?
	How will implementation and uptake be ensured?
	How will you know if inequities have been reduced?
	How has the process of engaging in an IBPA transformed: 1. Your thinking about relations and structures of power and inequity? 2. The ways in which you and others engage in the work of policy development, implementation and evaluation? 3. Broader conceptualizations, relations and effects of power asymmetry in the everyday world?

IBPA, Intersectionality-Based Policy Analysis.

effects on health of the school-to-prison pipeline phenomenon and disproportionate rates of arrest, imprisonment, and death of Black people at the hands of law enforcement in people of color, especially those of sexual minority status, suggest an absence of intersectional approaches. Importantly, there are positive health effects of socially inclusive policies, such as the Supreme Court decision to uphold legalization of gay marriage. Research shows a lower prevalence of adolescent suicide attempts in states that had legalizing same-sex marriage policies compared to those that did not (Raifman, Moscoe, Austin, & McConnell, 2017). Understanding the different formal and informal policies that negatively affect the health of groups with stigmatized statuses, as well as power dynamics inherent in social systems, is essential component of applying intersectional approaches to policy analysis.

RESEARCH

In order to move from a deficit-oriented focus on specific disparities to achieving broad-based health equity, Purnell et al. (2016) identify a number of action steps for improving health care research and service delivery. These include (a) increasing patient and stakeholder engagement in developing, testing, and disseminating interventions; (b) developing interventions that include and incorporate informal social networks and encompass the entire continuum of health care (e.g., prevention, primary care, specialty care); and (c) improving professionals' communication skills, cultural competence, and capacity to understand cultural differences in patient and family decision making.

The majority of studies embracing intersectionality as either a conceptual framework or a methodology has been conducted primarily using qualitative methodology (Bilge & Denis, 2010; Phoenix & Pattynama, 2006) and has focused on understanding intersectional lived experiences (Bowleg, 2013), as opposed to examining population-level health outcomes or testing interventions developed using intersectional approaches. Bauer (2014) has suggested that the absence of intersectional approaches in population health research, which is primarily quantitative in nature, is attributable to both measurement difficulties and limitations in statistical analytic techniques. Specifically, the complexity of simultaneously intersecting identities, social positions, and processes of oppression and privilege does not lend itself to categorical measurement that is inherent in quantitative analyses. As eloquently described by a research participant, "once you've blended the cake, you can't take the parts back to the main ingredients" (Bowleg, 2013, p. 754). Measurement difficulties are often accompanied by methodological challenges, including constraints regarding the number of variables that can be included in statistical computations and other potential stumbling blocks (e.g., regression model interaction scaling, structuring of risk modification analyses, inherent assumptions of equidistance and unilevel design germane to many statistical analytic techniques; Bauer, 2014). Greater use of statistical techniques such as multilevel regression analyses and effect-measure modifications may assist in bridging the translational gap between intersectionality theory and population health research methodology.

Community-Based Participatory Research

Importantly, findings from a number of studies suggested that participation in research by communities that are disproportionately affected by health disparities does have the potential to (a) improve community-level health outcomes and (b) influence policy change that advances health equity (Brown et al., 2003; Garcia, Minkler, Cardenas, Grills, & Porter, 2014; Minkler, 2010; Minkler, Garcia, Williams, LoPresti, & Lilly, 2010). Community-based participatory research (CBPR) is a collaborative approach to research that equitably involves community members, stakeholders, and researchers in all aspects of the research process (Israel, Schulz, Parker, & Becker, 1998). In short, CBPR can be conceptualized as a shift away from research *on* the community toward research *with* the community. CBPR enhances the utility, relevance, and uptake of interventions designed to improve health and well-being of individuals and communities (see Israel et al., 1998 and O'Fallon, Tyson, & Dearry, 2000, for reviews). The authors synthesize the "key principles of community-based research, examine its place within the context of different scientific paradigms, discuss rationales for its use, and explore major challenges and facilitating factors and their implications for conducting effective community-based research aimed at improving the public's health" (Israel et al., 1998, p. 173). The main principle of community-based research involves "the active engagement and influence of community members in all aspects of the research process" (Israel et al., 1998, p. 177). Furthermore, the need to "build on strengths and resources within the community" (p. 178), as well as a focus on partnerships and "a co-learning and empowerment process" (p. 179), is also stressed. With respect to translating CBPR findings to policy change and health outcomes, Cacari-Stone, Wallerstein, Garcia, and Minkler (2014) note the link between civic engagement and political participation that is critical for ensuring that the gap between research evidence and policy change is bridged.

CONCLUSION

Social workers and other health care providers are faced with increasing demands to provide culturally responsive care to diverse populations across a variety of settings (American Nursing Association, 2015; American Psychological Association, 2015; CSWE, 2015; Institute of Medicine, 2003; NASW, 2012). This chapter described innovative approaches to practice, policy, and research that have the potential to incorporate both the complexity of mutually constituted social identity categories as well as their interdependency with larger social contexts, including the U.S. health care system. At their core, each of these intersectional approaches seeks to center or amplify lived experiences with the goal of generating new knowledge in conjunction with transformative change.

While health and social science researchers have called for necessary paradigm shifts that do not rely exclusively on individualized interventions, but rather include population-level approaches that address social determinants of health, these alone are not sufficient. As noted, one of the core tenets of intersectionality is the assumption that power, transmitted through social structures and manifested via the inequitable distribution of resources, goods, and commodities, often results in systematic and recurrent oppression of groups who are already disadvantaged and living at the margins of society. Until health, health care, and health care coverage are treated as universal and inalienable human rights—as opposed to privileges for which only select groups are eligible, or commodities available only to those who can afford them—population-level disparities in health care access, utilization, and quality will continue to persist. Moreover, preventable adverse health outcomes—including disease onset, course/progression, and premature death—will continue to be widespread both in the United States and globally, and disparities in health outcomes will undoubtedly grow. Social workers are well positioned to continue to engage in intersectional practice, policy development and analysis, research, and advocacy efforts that will collectively produce this much needed ideological shift and result in the structural and systemic changes required to ensure health for all.

CHAPTER DISCUSSION QUESTIONS

1. How do the core assumptions of intersectionality relate to social work ethics and values?

2. How might you incorporate intersectional approaches into your social work practice?

3. What are some of the key challenges in intersectionality health research and service delivery?

4. How might an intersectional framework help social workers develop interventions that are equipped to address the social determinants of health?

5. Do you think U.S. health care policy embraces an intersectional framework? Why or why not?

CASE EXAMPLE AND DISCUSSION QUESTIONS

Case Example 4.2

Caroline is a 26-year-old Black female receiving supportive therapy within her university's counseling center. As a full-time student 2 months into her first semester of her Master's in Business Administration (MBA) program, she came to the counseling center with complaints of anxiety. Caroline identified that her current mental health challenges stem from a persistent fear of being exposed as "not good enough" for the MBA program. She referred to herself as a "fraud" and stated that she believes that she was "only let into the school" due to "probably an affirmative action thing" based on her racial/ethnic identity. Caroline's anxiety has recently escalated to the point that she has been skipping classes which, in turn, has been exacerbating her anxiety because she knows how absenteeism may affect her grades. The counselor used techniques rooted in cognitive behavioral therapy to explore how her thoughts were triggering her anxiety issues. Caroline acknowledged that her thought of being "not good enough" is not true based on her achieving a cumulative 3.8 GPA in college. However, she admitted that "knowing that it isn't true" still was not stopping her automatic thought from occurring and triggering her anxiety. In additional sessions, Caroline processed her childhood and adolescence during which she and her four younger sisters were raised by a single mother in a low-income community. She noted that they always struggled to get by financially, which led her to start working at an early age to support her family. She said that none of her friends from her neighborhood attended college and that they were all more focused on settling down and having children. She admitted to feeling like an outsider in her community, noting, "Where I'm from, women just don't do 'this.'"

Questions for Discussion

1. How might a clinician work with this patient to help her overcome her anxiety?

2. What kind of support network would help this patient work through her presenting issues?

3. How does Caroline's gender, race/ethnicity, and class, and their interactions, affect her thought of being "not good enough" within her MBA program?

REFERENCES

American Nurses Association. (2015). *Code of ethics for nurses with interpretative statements.* Silver Spring, MD: Author.

American Psychological Association. (2015). *Guidelines for psychological practice with transgender and gender nonconforming people.* Retrieved from https://www.apa.org/practice/guidelines/transgender.pdf

Barker, R., Fullman, N., Sorensen, R., Bollyky, T., McKee, M., Nolte, E., . . . Murray, C. J. L. (2017). Health care access and quality index based on mortality from causes amenable to personal health care in 195 countries and territories, 1990–2015: A novel analysis from the Global Burden and Disease Study 2015. *The Lancet, 389*(10091), 231–266. doi:10.1016/S0140-6736(17)30818-8

Bauer, G. R. (2014). Incorporating intersectionality theory into population health research methodology: Challenges and the potential to advance health equity. *Social Science and Medicine, 110*(6), 10–17. doi:10.1016/j.socscimed.2014.03.022

Belkin Martinez, D. (2014) Liberation health: An introduction. In D. Belkin Martinez and A. Fleck-Henderson (Eds.), *Social justice in clinical practice: A liberation health framework for social work* (pp. 1–28). London, UK: Routledge.

Bilge, S., & Denis, A. (2010). Introduction: Women, intersectionality and diasporas. *Journal of Intercultural Studies, 31*, 1–8. doi:10.1080/07256860903487653

Bowleg, L. (2013). "Once you've blended the cake, you can't take the parts back to the main ingredients": Black gay and bisexual men's descriptions and experiences of intersectionality. *Sex Roles, 68*(11–12), 754–767. doi:10.1007/s11199-012-0152-4

Brown, P., Mayer, B., Zavestoski, S., Luebke, T., Mandelbaum, J., & McCormick, S. (2003). The health politics of asthma: Environmental justice and collective illness experience in the United States. *Social Science Medicine, 57*(3), 453–464.

Cacari-Stone, L., Wallerstein, N., Garcia, N., & Minkler, M. (2014). The promise of community-based participatory research for health equity: A conceptual model for bridging evidence with policy. *American Journal of Public Health, 104*(9), 1615–1623. doi:10.2105/AJPH.2014.301961

Caiola, C., Docherty, S., Relf, M., & Barroso, J. (2014). Using an intersectional approach to study the impact of social determinants of health for African-American mothers living with HIV. *Advances in Nursing Science, 37*(4), 287–298. doi:10.1097/ANS.0000000000000046

Clarke, A. R., Goddu, A. P., Nocon, R. S., Stock, N. W., Chyr, L. C., Akuoko, J. A., & Chin M. H. (2013). Thirty years of disparities intervention research: What are we doing to close racial and ethnic gaps in health care? *Medical Care, 51*(11), 1020–1026. doi:10.1097/MLR.0b013e3182a97ba3

Cole, B. L., & Fielding, J. E. (2007). Health impact assessment: A tool to help policymakers understand health beyond health care. *Annual Review of Public Health, 28*, 393–412.

Collins, S. R., Gunja, M. Z., Doty, M. M., & Beutel, S. (2016, May). *Americans' experiences with ACA marketplace and Medicaid coverage: Access to care and satisfaction.* New York, NY: The Commonwealth Fund.

Council on Social Work Education. (2015). *Educational policy and accreditation standards.* Alexandria, VA: Author.

Crenshaw, K. (1991). Mapping the margins: Intersectionality, identity politics, and violence against women of color. In M. A. Finemane & R. Mykitiuk (Eds.), *The public nature of private violence* (pp. 93–118). New York, NY: Routledge.

Crissman, H., Berger, M., Graham, L., & Dalton, V. (2017). Transgender demographics: A household probability sample of US adults 2014. *American Journal of Public Health, 107*(2), 213–215. doi:10.2105/AJPH.2016.303571

Davis, K. (2008). Intersectionality as buzzword: A sociology of science perspective on what makes a feminist theory successful. *Feminist Theory, 9*(1), 67–85.

Dwyer-Lindgren, L., Bertozzi-Villa, A., Stubbs, R. W., Morozoff, C., Mackenbach, J. P., van Lenthe, F. J., . . . Murray, C. J. (2017). Inequalities in life expectancy among US counties, 1980 to 2014: Temporal trends and key drivers. *JAMA Internal Medicine, 77*(7), 1003–1011. doi:10.1001/jamainternmed.2017.0918

Eliason, M. J., & Hughes, T. (2004). Treatment counselor's attitudes about lesbian, gay, bisexual, and transgendered clients: Urban vs. rural settings. *Substance Use and Misuse, 39*(4), 625–644.

Ferguson, R. A. (2003). *Aberrations in black: Toward a queer of color critique.* Minneapolis: University of Minnesota Press.

Freire, P. (1974). Education as the practice of freedom. In *Education for critical social consciousness* (pp. 1–78). London, UK: Continuum.

Freire, P. (1998). *Pedagogy of freedom: Ethics, democracy and civic courage.* Latham, MD: Rowman & Littlefield.

Galupo, M. P., Mitchell, R. C., & Davis, K. S. (2015). Sexual minority self-identification: Multiple identities and complexity. *Psychology of Sexual Orientation and Gender Diversity, 2*(4), 355–364.

Garcia, A. P., Minkler, M., Cardenas, Z., Grills, C., & Porter, C. (2014). Engaging homeless youth in community-based participatory research: A case study from Skid Row, Los Angeles. *Health Promotion and Practice, 15*(1), 18–27. doi:10.1177/1524839912472904

Glied, S., Ma, S., & Borja, A. (May 2017). Effect of the Affordable Care Act on Health Care Access. *The Commonwealth Fund.* Retrieved from http://www.commonwealthfund.org/publications/issue-briefs/2017/may/effect-aca-health-care-access

Haber, R. (2010). Health equity impact assessment. *The Wellesley Institute.* Retrieved from http://www.wellesleyinstitute.com/wp-content/uploads/2011/02/Health_Equity_Impact_Assessment_Haber.pdf

Hall, S. (1971). Race, articulation and societies structured in dominance. In P. Essed, & D. T. Goldberg (Eds.), *Sociological theories race colonialism* (pp. 305–345). London, UK: Wiley-Blackwell.

Halpern, K. (2017). Identifying gaps in teaching intersectionality in higher education: A literature review. *Journal of Undergraduate Social Work Research, Inaugural Issue, 1*, 1–7.

Hancock, A.-M. (2007). Intersectionality as a normative and empirical paradigm. *Politics and Gender, 3*(2), 248–254.

Hankivsky, O. (2012). Women's health, men's health, and gender and health: Implications of intersectionality. *Social Science and Medicine, 74*(11), 1712–1720. doi:10.1016/j.socscimed.2011.11.029

Hankivsky, O., Grace, D., Hunting, G., Giesbrecht, M., Fridkin, A., Rudrum, D., . . . Clark, N. (2014). An intersectionality-based policy analysis framework: Critical reflections on a methodology for advancing equity. *International Journal of Equity in Health, 13*, 119. doi:10.1186/s12939-014-0119-x

Hayes, S., Riley, P., Radley, D., & McCarthy, D. (2015). Closing the gap: Past performance of health insurance in reducing racial and ethnic disparities in access to care could be an indication of future results. *The Commonwealth Fund*. Retrieved from http://www.commonwealthfund.org/~/media/files/publications/issue-brief/2015/mar/1805_hayes_closing_the_gap_reducing_access_disparities_ib_v2.pdf

Hill Collins, P. (1997). Defining Black feminist thought. In L. Nicholson (Ed.), *The second wave: A reader in feminist theory* (pp. 241–260). New York, NY: Routledge. ISBN: 9780415917612

Hill Collins, P. (2000). *Black feminist thought: Knowledge, consciousness, and the politics of empowerment* (2nd ed.). New York, NY: Unwin Hyman.

Hook, J., Davis, D., Owen, J., Worthington, E., & Utsey, S. (2013). Cultural humility: Measuring openness to diverse clients. *Journal of Counseling Psychology, 60*(3), 353–366. doi:10.1037/a0032595

Institute of Medicine. (2003). *Health professions education: A bridge to quality*. Washington, DC: National Academies Press.

Israel, B., Schulz, A., Parker, E., & Becker, A. (1998). Review of community-based research: Assessing partnership approaches to improve public health. *Annual Review of Public Health, 19*, 173–202.

Landers, S., & Kapadia, F. (2017, February). The health of the transgender community: Out, proud, and coming into their own. *American Journal of Public Health, 107*(2), 205–206. doi:10.2105/AJPH.2016.303599

Lombardi, E. (2001, June). Enhancing transgender health care. *American Journal of Public Health, 91*(6), 869–872.

Lombardi, E. (2017). Enhancing transgender health care. *American Journal of Public Health, 107*(2), 230–231. doi:10.2105/AJPH.2016.1072230

Lyons, T., Shannon, K., Pierre, L., Small, W., Krusi, A., & Kerr, T. (2015). A qualitative study of transgender individuals' experiences in residential addiction treatment settings: Stigma and inclusivity. *Substance Abuse Treatment, Prevention, and Policy, 10*, 17. doi:10.1186/s13011-015-0015-4

Martin-Baro, I. (1994). *Writings for a Liberation Psychology: Essays 1985–1989*. In A. Aron, & S. Corne (Eds.), Cambridge, MA: Harvard University Press.

McCall, L. (2005). The complexity of intersectionality. *Signs, 30*(3), 1771–1800.

Minkler, M. (2010). Linking science and policy through community-based participatory research to study and address health disparities. *American Journal of Public Health, 100*(Suppl. 1), S81–S87. doi:10.2105/AJPH.2009.165720

Minkler, M., Garcia, A., Williams, J., LoPresti, T., & Lilly, J. (2010). Sí se puede: Using participatory research to promote environmental justice in a Latino community in San Diego, California. *Journal of Urban Health, 87*(5), 796–812. doi:10.1007/s11524-010-9490-0

National Association of Social Workers. (2012). Governance: National Committee on Lesbian, Gay, Bisexual, and Transgender Issues. Retrieved from http://www.socialworkers.org/governance/cmtes/nclgbi.asp

National Association of Social Workers. (2017). Code of ethics. Retrieved from https://www.socialworkers.org/About/Ethics/Code-of-Ethics

National Center for Health Statistics. (2012). *Health, United States, 2011: Special feature on socioeconomic status and health*. Hyattsville, MD: Author. Retrieved from http://www.cdc.gov/nchs/data/hus/hus11.pdf

Nuttbrock, L. A. (2012). Culturally competent substance abuse treatment with transgender persons. *Journal of Addictive Diseases, 31*(3), 236–241. doi:10.1080/10550887.2012.694600

O'Fallon, L., Tyson, F., & Dearry, A. (2000). *Successful models of community-based participatory research: Final report.* Research Triangle Park, NC: National Institute of Environmental Health Sciences.

Palencia, L., Malmusi, D., & Borrell, C. (2014). *Incorporating intersectionality in evaluation of policy impacts on health equity: A quick guide.* Barcelona, Spain: Project SOPHIE. Retrieved from http://www.sophie-project.eu/pdf/Guide_intersectionality_SOPHIE.pdf

Phoenix, A., & Pattynama, P. (2006). Intersectionality. *European Journal of Women's Studies, 13,* 187–192.

Purnell, T., Calhoun, E., Golden, S., Halladay, J., Krok-Schoen, J., Appelhans, B., & Cooper, L. (2016). Achieving health equity: Closing the Gaps in health disparities, interventions, and research. *Health Affairs, 35*(8), 1410–1415. doi: 10.1377/hlthaff.2016.0158

Raifman, J., Moscoe, E., Austin, B., & McConnell, M. (2017). Same-sex marriage legalization in suicide attempts among high school students. *JAMA Pediatrics, 171*(4), 350–356. doi:10.1001/jamapediatrics.2016.4529

Reynolds, B. (1973). *Between client and community.* New York, NY: Oriole Press.

Robinson, M., Cross-Denney, B., Lee, K., Rozas, L., & Yamada, A. (2016). Teaching note— Teaching intersectionality: Transforming cultural competence content in social work education. *Journal of Social Work Education, 52*(4), 509–517.

Sen, G., Iyer, A., & Mukherjee, C. (2009) A methodology to analyse the intersections of social inequalities in health. *Journal of Human Development Capabilities, 10*(3), 397–415.

Senreich, E. (2009). A comparison of perceptions, reported abstinence, and completion rates of gay, lesbian, bisexual, and heterosexual clients in substance abuse treatment. *Journal of Gay and Lesbian Mental Health, 13,* 145–169.

Senreich, E. (2011). The substance abuse treatment experiences of a small sample of transgender clients. *Journal of Social Work Practice in the Addictions, 11,* 295–299.

Shields, S. A. (2008). Gender: An intersectionality perspective. *Sex Roles, 59,* 301–311. doi:10.1007/s11199-008-9501-8

Simien, E. (2007). Doing intersectionality research: From conceptual issues to practical Examples. *Politics & Gender, 3*(2), 36–43.

Smedley, B. D., Stith, A. Y., & Nelson, A. R. (2003). *Unequal treatment: Confronting racial and ethnic disparities in health care.* Washington, DC: National Academies Press.

Smooth, W. (2013). Intersectionality from theoretical framework to policy intervention. In R. A. Wildon (Ed.), *Situating intersectionality* (p. 12). New York, NY: Palgrave.

Sondik, E. J., Huang, D. T., Klein, R. J., & Satcher, D. (2010). Progress toward the Healthy People 2010 goals and objectives. *Annual Review of Public Health, 31*(1), 271–281. doi:10.1146/annurev.publhealth.012809.103613

Tervalon, M., & Murray-Garcia, J. (1998). Cultural humility versus cultural competence: A critical distinction in defining physician training outcomes in multicultural education. *Journal of Health Care for the Poor and Underserved, 9*(2), 117–125.

U.S. Department of Health and Human Services. (2011). Healthy People 2020. Retrieved from https://www.healthypeople.gov/2020/topics-objectives

Vargas-Bustamante, A., Chen, J., Rodriguez, H. P., Rizzo, J. A., & Ortega, A. N. (2010). Use of preventive care services among Latino subgroups. *American Journal of Preventive Medicine, 38*(6), 610–619.

Weber, L. (2006). Reconstructing the landscape of health disparities research: Promoting dialogue and collaboration between feminist intersectional and biomedical paradigms.

In A. J. Schulz & L. Mullings (Eds.), *Gender, race, class and health* (pp. 2–59). San Francisco, CA: John Wiley and Sons.

Wheeler, D., & McClain, A. (2016). *NASW standards for social work practice in health care settings*. Washington, DC: NASW Press.

Wing, A. K. (1997). *Critical race feminism: A reader*. New York, NY: New York University Press.

Witten, T. M., & Eyler, A. E. (2012). Transgender and aging. In T. M. Witten, & A. E. Eyler (Eds.), *Gay, lesbian, bisexual and transgender aging: Challenges in research, practice and policy*. Baltimore, MD: Johns Hopkins University Press.

World Health Organization. (2008). *Final Report of the Commission on Social Determinants of Health. Closing the gap in a generation: Health equity through action on the social determinants of health*. Geneva, Switzerland: Author.

5

Social Work Assessment

Jonathan B. Singer and Ellen Belluomini

Imagine you are sitting in a multi-agency child death review meeting. The person running the meeting might welcome everyone and introduce the meeting by saying something like this:

> Thanks everyone for attending this year's non-homicide Child Death Review panel. We are reviewing deaths for youth 0–21 years that the coroner's office determined to be due to accidental overdose or suicide. As in past years we have representatives from the school district, community mental health, juvenile court, law enforcement, child welfare, emergency shelters, and hospitals/emergency departments. We also have observers from local universities, religious organizations, refugee services, and community athletic organizations. Everyone has signed and returned confidentiality and nondisclosure agreements. Observers are not allowed to speak during the review. The purpose of this meeting is to review deaths, identify possible gaps in service delivery, service coordination or services that might have prevented these deaths. Everyone at this meeting has received the list of decedents. Participating members have completed an informational report about the decedent's involvement with their organization. This year we have 35 child deaths to review in 3 hours. I ask that you keep your remarks focused on the data available. There will be time for discussion of each case after everyone has had the chance to present their reports. The report of child deaths in our city will be submitted to the National Center for Fatality Review and Prevention (www.ncfrp.org/). Any questions? Ok. We'll hear reports in seating order around the room. Our first decedent is an 11-year-old male who died by hanging [details of the investigation omitted in this chapter to preserve confidentiality]. School district, why don't you start . . .

There are several reasons why we started this chapter talking about child death review. First, this group of people is trying to solve the mystery of why these children died. Second, it illustrates that assessments can take many forms. The child death review meeting is a community-level postmortem assessment. For each child there is a review of services used and known risk factors. The review committee identifies any patterns or missed risk factors, recommends system-wide improvements, and then identifies actions that service systems can take to prevent future deaths. The child death review follows the same protocol as an individual biopsychosocial–spiritual (BPSS) assessment, except that instead of relying primarily on the client and a few collateral contacts, detailed information is provided by all relevant parties in person. The single client (individual, couple, or family) assessment provides a context for the presenting problem and guides treatment. Second, it is valuable to consider proximal and distal client outcomes. We cannot predict the future. But thinking beyond this week's crisis is a reasonable perspective for providers. If you knew that the 7-year-old sitting in front of you was going to hang himself at age 11, what information might you want to know? What might you do differently? Finally, it reminds us that effective health care requires both direct services and thoughtful policy. The death review seeks to understand what happened with individuals, but does so with the intention of making systemic change. Data are collected from municipalities across the United States and evaluated to better understand how and why people die. Understanding how health care policies inform practice, and how practitioners can influence policy, is essential for a healthier public.

Health care in the United States is more of a patchwork quilt than a system of care. It is complex, diverse, and rapidly changing. One of the few constants across all health care sectors is assessment. In this chapter we will define the purpose of assessment, briefly describe key concepts in the BPSS assessment, identify and describe visual assessment tools, and introduce a family technology assessment tool. The chapter highlights the intersections among policy, research, and practice. If you are new to the field, this chapter will serve as "headline news" to essential topics. If you are a practitioner, policy maker, or educator, this chapter will augment your understanding of assessment in health care settings.

The *purpose of an assessment* varies based on the type of assessment (e.g., suicide assessment, crisis assessment, family technology assessment, BPSS assessment) and the perceived role of the client and provider. In a system where providers are seen as experts who define and solve clients' problems, the purpose of the assessment is to define the problem (Hall, 2017). In contrast, in a system where clients are seen as the experts and share power with providers, the purpose of the assessment is to explore how the problem will be understood (Hall, 2017). Providers who are trained in a traditional diagnostic or medical approach use assessments to define the problem (e.g., psychopathology or health condition), whereas providers trained in strengths-based systemic thinking use assessments to explore how the problem will be understood. This distinction is not a veiled description of medical doctors versus social workers; many social workers take pride in their mastery of diagnostic assessment and thorough BPSS assessments. Providers should be clear about the purpose of their assessment and how it will be used in their specific practice setting.

BIOPSYCHOSOCIAL–SPIRITUAL ASSESSMENT

Although the components of a traditional BPSS assessment are well documented (see Singer, 2007, for an overview), there are several advances worth reviewing.

Biological and Psychological

The biological domain of an assessment typically includes food, shelter, clothing, medical, health, and physical capabilities in a physical environment. The psychological domain of assessment has traditionally focused on an individual's history, personality styles, intelligence, mental abilities, self-concept and identity, and history of diagnosis, medication, and treatment. Included in the psychological domain is assessment of psychosis (hearing, feeling, smelling, or seeing things that others cannot), and the standard risk assessment, including risk for harm to self (suicide) and others (homicide).

The neurobiological revolution of the past 20 years has led to new understandings of the role of the biological in the psychosocial experience of health and mental health. One of the best developed frameworks for integrating neurobiological assessment and psychosocial intervention in health care settings is Bruce Perry's neurosequential model of therapeutics (NMT; Perry & Szalavitz, 2007). NMT is "an approach to clinical problem solving" that uses neurobiology as a foundation for understanding development and informing clinical intervention (MacKinnon, 2012, p. 2011). NMT is informed by the research on adverse childhood events (ACE), which suggested that physical and mental health problems were related to exposure to abuse, neglect, parental psychopathology, and other family-based interpersonal problems (Larkin, Shields, & Anda, 2012). NMT uses a detailed assessment to inform a specific sequence of therapeutic, educational, and enrichment activities that match the needs and strengths of the individual. What makes NMT well suited for health care settings is that it expands the traditional developmental history so that neurodevelopmental processes can be mapped and connected with current functioning. The human brain has four major developmental and anatomical structures: The NMT assessment looks at neurodevelopment in the brainstem, diencephalon, limbic, and cortical areas to create a picture of how an individual's brain appears to be organized. NMT clinicians determine how well the client is doing with specific domains (e.g., sensory integration, self-regulation, relational, cognitive functioning) that are associated with those four anatomical structures. The clinician compares the client's functioning to what is known about same-age peers. The client-specific neurodevelopmental model helps the clinician decide what types of treatments would be most appropriate.

For example, a 14-year old presents with difficulties paying attention in class, emotion dysregulation, interpersonal problems, and poor academic achievement. A traditional *Diagnostic and Statistical Manual of Mental Disorders (DSM)* diagnosis might find that the youth meets criteria for attention deficit hyperactivity disorder (ADHD), anxiety, or a number of other disorders. *DSM*-informed treatments (e.g., psychostimulants, parent management training) address current symptomology, but do not take into consideration neurodevelopment. If the NMT assessment uncovered neglect (aka an absence of opportunities for the natural developmental process to occur) during key periods of brain development related to emotion regulation (e.g., brainstem development), then treatment recommendations would suggest treatments such as music, dance, yoga, drumming, or play therapies. These therapies would address some of the basic regulation issues that were underdeveloped. After improved brainstem functioning, treatment could move to therapeutics that involve higher-level neurocognitive functions such as insight-oriented or cognitive behavioral therapies (Perry, 2009). It is important to note that NMT is not a treatment model and works in partnership with existing approaches to assessment and intervention.

Sociocultural

Sociocultural assessments have long been the domain of social workers. The psychiatric community officially entered this arena with the publication of the fifth edition of the *DSM* (*DSM-5*; American Psychiatric Association, 2013). The authors of the *DSM-5* note that every diagnostic interview should include a cultural formulation. The *DSM-5* cultural formulation interview is a very basic but user-friendly interview guide and can be downloaded for free (www.psychiatry.org/psychiatrists/practice/dsm/educational-resources/assessment-measures).

The sociocultural assessment gathers information about your client's social network, friends, families, online and offline community characteristics, as well as the social, political, and economic environment. Asking clients to walk you through their online worlds can provide invaluable insight into ways their online and offline sociocultural environments are similar or dissimilar. Assessment can be as basic as "can you tell me about the online communities with which you are involved?" Or it can be as rigorous as using big data to identify trends and patterns in social networks. Scholar Desmond Patton has done groundbreaking work integrating traditional textual analysis with machine learning to better understand the relationship between the online and offline worlds of gang members (Patton, Eschmann, & Butler, 2013). Patton's work is a potent reminder of why we should assess our client's online and offline sociocultural context.

One of the best ways to understanding the sociocultural context of your client's presenting problems is through the use of *visual assessment tools.* The traditional BPSS and *DSM* assessments are verbal assessments. There are several visual assessment tools, including the genogram, family timeline, culturagram, and ecomap, which help providers gather rich data about the client's sociocultural context. *Genograms* (McGoldrick, 2015) are information-rich snapshots of family structure, demographics, and relationships. They do not, however, provide information about changes over time, nor do they provide information about the family's relationships with other systems such as education, medical, religious institutions, immigration status, politics, finances, work, hobbies, and so forth. Other visual assessment tools can provide these missing data, including the *culturagram* (Congress, 2015), *family timeline* to identify milestone events, and the *ecomap* (Hartman, 1978) or sociogram to identify the relationship between a client and other systems. A *family technology ecomap* (Belluomini, 2013) can be used to identify the relationship between family members and personal technology. We summarize and provide examples of the genogram, ecomap, and culturagram visual assessment tools.

Genogram

One of the most well-established and thoroughly described visual assessment tools is the *genogram* (McGoldrick, Gerson, & Petry, 2008). The genogram is an information-rich family tree typically comprising at least three generations. The combination of symbols and relationship lines with narrative information gives providers and family members a quick way to understand complex family dynamics. Genograms are created in collaboration with families. Although genogram software exists, the most practical and easiest way to create a genogram is to draw it by hand while talking with the family. The authors typically use letter-size paper and then scan into the electronic medical record (EMR). Flip boards are larger and can make it easier for family members to see the genogram in progress. Clinicians can take a photo of the flip board and upload that to the EMR. If the clinician has access to a drawing tablet and large screen display, the genogram can be created and saved as an image file and uploaded to the EMR.

Genograms are an essential tool for any family assessment. The process of learning about the family tree, relationships among family members, and key demographic information is often the first time the therapist experiences family dynamics, and simultaneously provides the family with insight into their own family legacy. Genograms place the presenting problems within a family context. Discussion of birth, death, and other family life cycle events often elicit intense emotions, avoidance, or other dynamics that give the therapist insight into family functioning. Therapists should look out for and track family processes during the creation of the genogram. Figure 5.1 illustrates a three-generation family with an opposite sex married couple, their two children (one male and one female) and their spouses, and their grandchildren (including one stillborn male, fraternal twins, and three singletons).

The referred client is identified with double lines. If during the creation of this genogram the parents of the stillborn became visibly upset and said that they feel a deep connection to their dead child, the therapist would indicate that relationship with a line between the parents and stillborn child. Although Figure 5.1 does not depict those relationship lines, a quick web search for "genogram symbols" will return thousands of examples of how to indicate relationships that are strong, weak, abusive, disconnected, as well as symbols for every possible relationship and identity status.

A brief example illustrates the power of hidden loss in families. In a 2013 episode of the Social Work Podcast, Sarah Kye Price told the story of a woman she met while doing hospice work (Singer, 2013). The woman's husband had just died, but her grief reaction appeared to be far more severe than anyone had anticipated given the length of his illness and the amount of closure prior to his death. The woman disclosed to Sarah that she had experienced a stillbirth 64 years earlier. The only other person who knew about the loss was her husband; his death meant that she was alone in her grief. A genogram might have identified the loss prior to the husband's death.

According to McGoldrick (2015), getting data for an assessment is like casting an information net. Questions start with nonthreatening information like family basic structure and end with intimate questions about intergenerational abuse, addiction, and psychopathology. The following broad categories are captured in the information net:

- Presenting problem
- Immediate household
- Current family situation
- Wider family context (including detailed medical histories)
- Ethnic and cultural history
- Informal kinship network

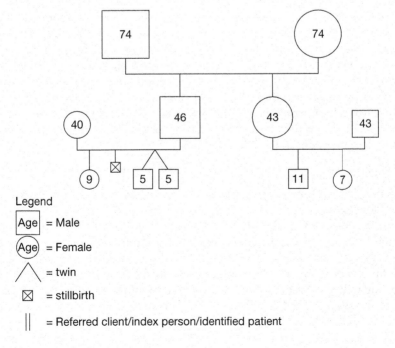

Legend

[Age] = Male

(Age) = Female

/\ = twin

⊠ = stillbirth

‖ = Referred client/index person/identified patient

Figure 5.1 Three-generation genogram.

Although genograms are easier to construct when families are smaller and/or have stable relationships, they are invaluable with larger families or families with more unstable relationships. The genogram prevents clinicians from making assumptions about what constitutes a family, identifies key family relationships that might not be identified through agency paperwork, and provides insight into how much individuals know about their family. It is always a poignant moment when, for example, a family member reveals that they know nothing about an entire part of the family tree, or they didn't know that "Cousin Tara" wasn't a biological relative. For more information about the process of creating and using the genogram in family systems work, see McGoldrick (2015) and McGoldrick et al. (2008).

Culturagram

The *culturagram* (Congress, 2015) lists key categories to assess when gathering information about migrant or refugee status. Congress (2015, p. 1012) identifies 10 areas to assess:

1. Reason for relocation
2. Legal status
3. Time in community
4. Language spoken at home and in the community
5. Health beliefs
6. Impact of trauma and crisis events
7. Contact with cultural and religious institutions, holidays, food, and clothing
8. Oppression, discrimination, bias, and racism
9. Values about education and work`
10. Values about family—structure, power, myths, and rules

Some of the information gathered in these 10 areas will overlap with content gathered for the other visual assessment tool and the *DSM* cultural formulation interview. Although category 5 (health beliefs) is perhaps the category most obviously related to health care settings, all information is relevant to health care. The culturagram will be most useful if the provider is clear on the purpose of the assessment as described previously. If the assessment is intended to define the problem, the provider needs to know how the client defines the problem and how that informs treatment preferences. If, however, the provider is gathering information in order to better understand how the presenting problem is understood by the client, then the assessment areas of the culturagram provide an opportunity for rich information. Given that nearly all people in the United States have a migration story, the culturagram is a useful assessment tool, regardless of the amount of time people have spent in the United States.

Family Timeline

Figure 5.2 illustrates a simple *family timeline* constructed with the "Smart Art" feature in Microsoft Word 2010.

The first task in creating a family timeline is to identify the start and end points (e.g., 2007–present). Next, identify milestone events in the family's history, including important cultural events (including migration history), and history of service use. Because information recall is rarely linear, expect that family members will remember events out of sequence; you will likely redraw the timeline several times. As with all visual assessment tools, clinicians should ask themselves "What information do I need to know in order to better understand the presenting problem?" If the family has already completed other visual assessment tools, clinicians should ask questions that fill in gaps in information. For example, the genogram identifies a stillbirth, but does not convey what happened

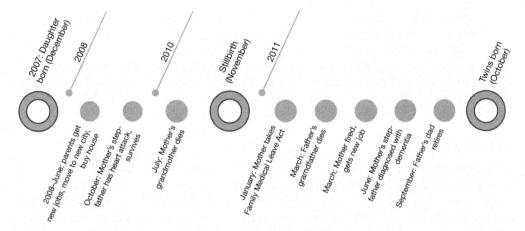

Figure 5.2 Family timeline.

before or after. Clinicians can use the timeline to answer questions such as "Did anything change in the family after the stillbirth?"

Ecomap

An *ecomap* (Hartman, 1978) is a way to visually identify systems that are important to a client (either an individual or a family), the strength of the relationship between the client and systems (strong, weak/tenuous, or stressed), and the direction of energy (one way or reciprocal between client and system). Figure 5.3 shows three different relationship strengths and energy between a client and the primary care provider (PCP):

- Client A: "My PCP is the one person I can trust to have my back. She's known me for years and always has good advice. Not only does she respond when I send her an email but she also checks up on me. Well, sometimes it is her staff that reaches out, but they are a team." [strong, reciprocal]

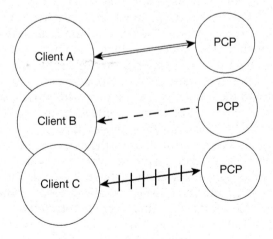

Figure 5.3 Ecomap representing strong, weak, and stressed connections between the client and a single system. PCP, primary care provider.

- Client B: "I know I missed the last couple of appointments, but it just isn't a priority right now. Yes, I got those appointment reminder texts. I don't have a problem with my PCP, I just don't have the time right now." [weak energy from PCP to client]
- Client C: "Bottom line is that my PCP thinks I'm a pill popper and I'm not. She keeps sending me all this information about other ways I can manage pain symptoms, but I know what works for me. Her job is to prescribe medication. My job is to get back to work." [conflictual, reciprocal]

Spiritual

Social workers are expected to include a spiritual assessment in the traditional biopsychosocial assessment. Hodge (2015) synthesizes several existing religious and spiritual assessment models into the acronym ICARING: How *Important* is spirituality or religion? Is there participation in a religious or spiritual *Community*? Are there spiritual beliefs and practices that serve as *Assets* and *Resources*? What is the *Influence* of spirituality and religion on the current situation? Are there spiritual *Needs* that should be addressed? Is incorporating spirituality into treatment one of the client's *Goals*? If so, how?

Technology and Assessment

There are two overlapping spheres in technology and assessment. The first sphere is the use of technology to conduct assessments, including telehealth, mHealth (i.e., mobile devices for health care), and Internet and computer technologies (Berzin, Singer, & Chan, 2015; Singer & Sage, 2015). The traditional biopsychosocial and diagnostic assessments already described, for example, can be conducted remotely using a webcam and through online assessment measures. The second sphere is assessing technology use, including which technologies clients use and how their use is beneficial or detrimental to their well-being. The overlap is that technology can be used to assess technology use, and a person's comfort with technologies can make it easier to use technology to conduct assessments. We will first do a brief review of some of the concepts related to using technology in assessment, and then provide a more extensive overview of assessing technology use.

Using Technology in Assessment

A perennial disconnect between practice and research is that practitioners want to better understand people in their messy environments and researchers want to control for the factors that can make research messy. The proliferation of mobile devices has enabled researchers to use a methodology called "ecological momentary assessment" (EMA) to learn about people's behaviors and experiences in real time (Shiffman, Stone, & Hufford, 2008). EMA uses apps to deliver questions, polls, or other survey formats to participants about their experience in the moment. The responses are sent back immediately to the researchers. For example, in a recent study, people 65 years and older who had cognitive difficulties responded to questions three times a day about clinical issues (Ramsey, Wetherell, Depp, Dixon, & Lenze, 2016). Because the researchers asked older adults what was happening in the moment, their responses were not as likely to reflect recall bias, thereby improving the reliability and validity of the study results and clinical implications.

One of the most vexing assessment issues has always been "How reliable is a suicide assessment?" A recent study used EMA with two groups of adult suicide attempt survivors to identify how much variability there was in suicidal ideation and risk factors over time (Kleiman et al., 2017). The researchers found that the intensity of suicidal ideation varied dramatically over a matter of hours. They also found that even though risk factors correlated with suicidal ideation, they were poor predictors of changes in suicide risk. One implication for clinicians is that the conventional standard that a suicide assessment is "valid" for 72 hours makes little sense. Furthermore, future suicide risk assessment should include the ability to monitor the fluctuations in risk over brief periods of time such as a few hours. One step in that direction is the Suicide Risk Monitoring Tool (Erbacher, Singer, & Poland, 2015). The monitoring tool was designed for school-based mental health professionals, but can be adapted for use in outpatient and inpatient settings to gather data quickly and repeatedly on current suicide risk (Erbacher & Singer, 2017).

Screening

Screening is a process for identifying whether a problem might exist. Screening outcomes are typically dichotomous—either someone screens positive or not. Screening questions have been a standard component in intake assessments to identify which issues need thorough assessments. For example, a standard mental health intake will ask about mood. If the person responds that they have experienced depressed mood more days than not, either the assessor will follow up with more detailed diagnostic questions, or the chart will be flagged that a more thorough assessment of mood disorders is warranted.

Health care settings, particularly primary care, have been identified as ideal locations to screen for mental health problems (Fox, McManus, Irwin, Kelleher, & Peake, 2013; U.S. Department of Health and Human Services Office of the Surgeon General and National Action Alliance for Suicide Prevention, 2012). Computerized screening has the benefit of instantly scoring results, creating personalized reports, and integrating with EMRs (if needed). Since youth, ethnic minorities and men are more likely to seek out physical health care than mental health care (each for different reasons), health care settings provide an opportunity to identify potential emotional, cognitive, or behavioral problems among a group of people who are less likely to be seen in traditional mental health settings. Best practice recommendations encourage universal screening for behavioral health concerns at least at a pediatric well visit, but preferably at all visits (Committee on Adolescence American Academy of Pediatrics, 2008; Shaffer & Pfeffer, 2001; Siu, 2016).

The Behavioral Health Screen (BHS) is one example of a computerized screening tool that has been used and evaluated across service systems, including hospitals, primary care, and schools (Diamond, Herres, et al., 2017; Diamond, Levy, et al., 2010). The BHS screens for depression, anxiety, suicide, and trauma history, as well as several risk behaviors including interpersonal violence, driving while under the influence, and truancy. One benefit of computerized screening is that the program skips follow-up questions when core items are not endorsed and provides additional items to probe more deeply when relevant core items are endorsed. Reports are generated instantly and can be customized to meet the needs of different health care settings. For example, the report in an emergency room might include more psychiatric risk items and fewer behavioral risk items, whereas the report for a primary care office might include all of the items.

Bradford and Rickwood (2014) suggested several usability improvements for electronic screenings:

- Allow the user to identify items (e.g., substance use, sexual behavior) they would like to discuss with providers and items they do not want to discuss.
- Embed informational links and resources within the screen, especially with items they identified as unwilling to discuss.
- Incorporate current user interface technologies for greater accuracy and higher levels of engagement (especially among youth who might have greater facility with computers and expectations around interactivity), including the ability to personalize the assessment with the user's name.

FAMILY TECHNOLOGY ASSESSMENT

An early conceptualization of technology users was Prensky's *digital natives* and *digital immigrants*. Digital natives are born to the digital age, are more fluent in technology, and are more likely to be innovators, early adopters, and early majority (Rogers, 2003). In contrast, digital immigrants were born without the advances of digital learning, and are more likely to be early majority, the late majority, and laggards (Rogers, 2003; Wang, Myers, & Sundaram, 2012). While not prescriptive, these categories can be useful for interns and supervisors as they try to negotiate their different understandings of technology. An additional component to be included which may change digital literacy categories is assessment of socioeconomic status (SES) and educational background. Low SES status and minimal educational attainment can impact information and communication technology (ICT) use negatively not dependent upon age (Wang, Myers, & Sundaram, 2012).

Life-Span Approach to Assessing Technology

The technology assessment described in this section was developed by one of the authors of this chapter, Ellen Belluomini, and first introduced in the *New Social Worker* magazine (Belluomini, 2013). The information gathered from this assessment is part of the more comprehensive assessment discussed in this chapter. We present it as a stand-alone section because, as noted, assessing technology is relatively new in both health and behavioral health care. The categories discussed can be integrated into existing assessment protocols.

Table 5.1 illustrates nine categories of assessment across five common technological platforms. Each area of assessment is followed by a type of digital tool most common with youth. The corresponding questions develop a narrative for a client's technological world. If there is a (G) after a question, this means "General" or ask this question for each type of platform. *Age-/behavior-appropriate* questions need to be assessed by the clinician for the individual. An example of this is dating sites. An 8-year-old playing Club Penguin would not be asked about dating sites, but a 14-year-old should. During this assessment, it is crucial to remember each question can have a positive or negative frame. Utilizing a strengths-based approach to questioning will enable positive engagement and give clues to therapeutic treatment approaches appropriate to the client.

Youth

The initial task for the clinician is to establish rapport and engage the client in honest and productive discussion. Because most youth get excited when discussing their favorite technologies, we recommend starting the discussion asking about *favorite* technologies and *abilities*. Their response to questions about ability will give you some insight into their self-efficacy using digital tools (e.g., "I love Minecraft, but I'm not as good as my cousin"). Even if you do not explicitly ask about problem-solving skills, intelligence, age-appropriate activities, and potential areas of risk, the youth's answer to questions about ability are likely to provide some insight into these categories. Subsequent questions offer a view into youth's constructive or destructive technology interests. Role-playing games (RPGs) can be fun for youth in moderation but when their play begins to interfere in family time, friendships, school performance, self-care, or safety, technology use begins to be a destructive force in their lives. Although it might be tempting to delve into areas of concern, hold off. Questions that tap into potentially shameful or embarrassing

Table 5.1 Technology Assessment Questions

	Social Media	Internet	Gaming	Texting	Apps
Favorites	What are your favorite social media sites? If you had to keep only one which would it be and why?	Which websites interest you the most?	Which games do you play most often? What are your favorite platforms for gaming?	Who texts you the most? Who do you text the most?	Which apps do you most frequently use? Which apps have you started using within the last month?
Ability	How do you use these sites? Do you create memes, blog, have a YouTube channel, etc. Has anyone ever helped you learn how to use technology? Who, what, how?	What is the hardest thing you can do with a computer? Taxes, finances, social, news, etc.	What types of games do you like the most? What are your strongest and weakest skills?	How many texts do you send in a day? (If the client does not text, why?)	Which apps are the most difficult for you to play/use? How often do you download a new app?
Friendships	Number? Define types, family, friends, communities. Online versus face to face? Age range? Has any friend tried contacting you but you felt unsure of if they were your friend?	How do you meet people online? Which social sites do you use? (Match, Meet-up, etc.) Have you ever connected with an old friend online?	Who do you game with? (i.e., face to face, online, family) Do you have a role-playing community? (World of Warcraft)	Who do you text the most? What was the worst text you ever received? Sent?	Which apps help you to interact with your friends? (WhatsApp, Facebook IM, etc.)

(continued)

Table 5.1 Technology Assessment Questions (*continued*)

	Social Media	Internet	Gaming	Texting	Apps
Access	Does anyone else know your passwords? Who do you ask for help with technology?	Where do you have access to the Internet? (work, home, mobile, library, friend's house)	Where do you play your games? (your house, friend's house, gaming store, library)	Which devices/apps do you use for texting? Are any of these hidden?	How do you purchase apps/in-apps?
Emotions	Name a time you felt (happy, sad, angry, hurt, afraid) using social media. (Check for feeling pressured to do something they do not want to do, bullying, and suicidal feelings (G))	Which Internet activities have caused you irritation, anger, joy, being scared?	How do you feel when you cannot play games for a day, week, month? What types of games make you feel scared, happy, nervous, exhilarated?	Has texting ever caused a misunderstanding? Have you ever felt any of these emotions while texting or being texted: anger, sadness, happiness, hurt, bullied, suicidal, vindictive, ashamed, pressured sexually?	Name a time you felt (happy, sad, angry, hurt, afraid) using an app. Which apps have you found frustrating to use?
Behavior	What percentage of posts are positive, negative? (define) Has a post ever taught you something? Has anyone complained about you being on too long? How often do they complain? (G)	What types of sites do you visit? Have you known you shouldn't visit some but do? Have you ever spied/viewed someone else's Internet history? (G) Assess for pornographic use	Have you ever chosen to game vs. going outside? Spending time with a friend? Instead of sleep? Exercising? Eating? Showering? Intimacy?	Have you ever texted something and regretted it? (G) Have you ever bullied someone through texting? (G) Have you ever texted while intoxicated? (age-/behavior-appropriate)	Has an app ever motivated you to do something? (positive or negative) Has an app ever helped you with a life skill? Has an app ever made you regret downloading/using it? Why?

Table 5.1 Technology Assessment Questions (continued)

Time	Which sites do you spend the most time on? Has anyone complained about your use? (G) Check physical issues (G)	How much time do you spend on the Internet?	How much time do you spend gaming? Have you ever played gambling games?	How often do you text? What times of the day? Have you ever been awoken at night because of a text?	Which apps do you spend the most time with?
Supervision (Youth-Specific Category)	Does anyone limit the time you spend online? (G) How? Are your parents "friends" on your accounts? Do your parents know your passwords to your accounts?	Are there any sites you are restricted from? (Do you go on them anyway?) Does your computer have specific restrictions in general?	Are there any types of games your parents do not allow you to play?	Do you share your texts with anyone? Do your parents have access to your texts? Do you ever erase your texts before someone can see them?	Does anyone look at which apps you download? Do you have any apps which have a fake icon?

(continued)

Table 5.1 Technology Assessment Questions (*Continued*)

	Social Media	Internet	Gaming	Texting	Apps
Risk	Have you ever friended a person you do not know?	Does email address include their name?	Do you game with people you don't know?	Do you text friends who are only online friends?	Have you ever hidden apps from your parents/partners?
	Used your real name? (G)	Plan to set up a meeting or met someone you became friends with online? (G)	Have you ever role played with adults? Has your role play ever been sexual?	Have you ever sent any pictures of yourself? (type) Have your texts ever become sexual? Do you text and drive?	Have you ever downloaded a controversial app?
	Given your address/phone number?				Which app do you feel is the most controversial app you have?
	Have you ever wanted to hurt yourself after being on social media? (G)	Have you ever given money to someone in need through an email?	Have you ever felt overly angry or emotional while gaming?	Has a partner/girlfriend/boyfriend ever demanded to see your texts? (check about other areas of tech)	Have you ever tried to hide an app from a partner?
	Have you ever given money to someone you met online? (G)	Have you ever sexted through video?			Have you ever downloaded an app which you give money to on a regular basis? Which ones? Do you spend time exploring the dark web?
	Have you ever bought something online from a site you were unsure of?	Has your computer ever stopped working after opening an email or downloading something from the Internet?	Have you ever become physical during or after playing a game?		
	Have you ever given money to someone you met online? (G)				
	Have women/men flirted with you online (G)				
	Have you ever had sexted or had an affair with someone not your partner/girlfriend/boyfriend?				

Note: (G) = General questions that can be asked of anyone at any age.

information require trust and rapport. You're still in the first 10 minutes of the interview. Your goals are to gather information, note areas that need to be explored in more detail, and most importantly build rapport by demonstrating genuine interest and excitement about the youth's interests and abilities.

Once you have established initial rapport, we recommend assessing *friendships*, access to *technology*, and *emotions*. Questions in these areas continue to build trust, yet add questions on a neutral to probing continuum. Digital natives perceive online friendships no differently than face-to-face friendships (Palfrey & Gasser, 2016). The emotions category begins a deeper probing into the youth's feelings. Clients feel safer disclosing their feelings about prior familiar disclosures in the session when engagement is successful. Paraphrasing, summarization, and clarification encourage clients to share their feelings. Although not intended to be diagnostic, questions about emotions can serve as a first look into possible emotional problems such as depression or anxiety.

The client's evaluation of their *behavior, time,* and *supervision* of technology use offers a client self-reflection on why parents may have concerns and a clinician's understanding of the ability of parents to protect their child in a technological world. The behavior category can identify the youth's perceptions of positive and negative actions with technology. The time category is important to evaluate not only addiction-level behaviors but physical manifestations of intense ICT usage. Sleep disruptions, posture pain, urinary tract infections (from holding urination for long periods of time where bacteria can build), and the like, can be indicators of heavy ICT use or addiction.

Adults/Older Adults

The general approach to assessing technology use is the same for adults as it is for youth. Establish rapport through a discussion of favorite technologies and perceived ability. If the adult is a parent, identify discrepancies between adult/child technology knowledge. A digital immigrant parent with a tech savvy digital native child will not realize when their child has wiped a browser, plugged in the router after they go to bed, or installed an app with a fake icon. Luckily, knowledge discrepancies can be addressed through education. Assess the intersection between ICT and friendship (including social networks). Clarify how and when the parent has access to the Internet. If they have weak or limited Internet access at home this can adversely affect their child's ability to do homework, the likelihood that they will complete assessments from home, or search for health care information online. For older adults, evaluating their use of life-enhancing technologies (e.g., assistive technology, medical apps, social media connecting the older adult to their family or friends) can identify technology use that is rarely discussed in mainstream media. According to a 2017 survey from the Pew Research Center, 67% of adults 65 years and older had access to the Internet and 42% owned a smartphone.

Assessing adults' emotional relationship to ICT can be the first step in evaluating a psychological addiction to ICT, negative reaction patterns, and thoughts of harm to self and others. If, for example, adults say that they go online when they are suicidal, the provider should assess their motivations, intentions, and the connections that they make online. Are they getting support to stay safe (e.g., www.livethroughthis.org) or to kill themselves (e.g., Michelle Carter)? The behavior and time categories address Internet addiction, substance abuse, gambling, pornography, domestic violence, and physical consequences of extended play. Providers can adapt their standard assessments of these domains to include technology-mediated problems. For example, if a 46-year-old male seeks medical attention due to back problems, the provider should ask about how much time he spends sitting in front of his computer.

Assessment of Risk

The digital connection to larger systems is creating risks across the life span not previously experienced by earlier generations. News, only previously available at six and ten at night, appears instantaneously on digital devices. Instead of a few letters by mail a month or interoffice mail, messages take only seconds to transmit through fax and email. An individual's friends' networks consisted of their local, school, work, place of worship, or the block around their house. The digital community goes beyond local community limits. It is not unusual for people to communicate not just across state lines, but across oceans. Parents did not think twice about their children playing Space Invaders on the television in the past. Now children play video games (potentially with video and audio capacity) among people of all ages across the world. The clinician's digital knowledge is often the only barometer for clients in maneuvering through an evolving technology minefield. These technological advancements in connection provide great rewards, but include an exponential amount of risks for individuals and families. The following is an example of assessing for risk related to cell phones:

- Were you using your phone longer than you planned?
- Do you try to manage your use of screen time on your phone but failed?
- Is your performance at work, home, or school impacted by your use of the phone?
- Do you find yourself going back to your phone at inappropriate times?
- Are your relationships either trying to minimize your phone screen time or suffering due to your use?
- Are you unable to spend long periods of time away from your cell phone without emotional consequences? (hours, days, a week)
- Do you use your cell phone while driving? Riding a bike? Walking home at night? With earphones?

The assessment of risk presented by technology requires an understanding of cognitive, moral, ethical, behavioral, and emotional development. Imagine a 6-year-old whose favorite books are about horses. His digital immigrant parents purchase a "horse farm" app for his tablet. The app is free but unbeknownst to his parents the developers make money when the user makes an "in-app purchase." The child does not understand the consequences of clicking a pay icon, only the immediate reward of getting a brand new stable and the most beautiful horse in the app. Risk can increase substantially if the app has a social component. Low risk may be disclosure of the youth's name in an email address, but if a child predator takes that name and develops a friendship online toward a goal of meeting up with the child, then the risk increases exponentially. High risk includes participating and being a victim to online or cyberbullying or searching threads for how to kill themselves (Slovak & Singer, 2014). Each risk should be discussed with youth and parents. High-risk behaviors may include parental or hospital intervention.

Financial abuse is an example of risk with older digital immigrants. A grandparent may understand an immigrant from a foreign country is not really soliciting them for money (which they will pay back as soon as the wire transfer is finished) but willingly give money to a friend stranded in England communicating to them through Facebook IM (which turns out to be a hacked account). People using technology toward ill gains study the art of psychological manipulation. The cure to technological manipulation is education.

All clinicians should familiarize themselves with current technology scams to aid in appropriate assessment of risk. Two federal resources include the Federal Bureau of Investigation's senior fraud site (www.fbi.gov/scams-and-safety/common-fraud-schemes/seniors) and resources from the United States Senate Special Committee on Aging (en.wikipedia.org/wiki/United_States_Senate_Special_Committee_on_Aging).

Risk is relative to the technology being used. The more access the technology facilitates, the greater the risk. Risk areas include privacy, financial and sexual exploitation, emotional contagion, and addiction-like behaviors. The risk increases with vulnerable populations including youth, older generations, people with a mental or physical illness, lower SES, minimal educational background, and immigrants using new technologies. That said, there are no formulas available to assess each risk in a technology assessment. A quality technology assessment consists of knowing and keeping up to date about the risks inherent in technology by age group, building a relationship that facilitates disclosure, the ability to choose which line of probing to follow, and when the risk line is crossed for a specific individual or family system.

CONCLUSION

There are exciting advances in assessment and health care, many of which have emerged from neurobiological advances and technology. As we look to the future, there are several ways to improve assessment in health care. One of the biggest burdens for people entering into service delivery systems is providing the same information multiple times. Rather than expecting the client to repeat information for each department, clients should expect to complete computerized assessments once and have the system generating reports for each department (Morgan, 2010). In addition to reducing survey fatigue and data error, these data can be analyzed to improve services at a local or national level.

An expansion of telehealth services would improve services to people in under-resourced urban and rural environments; provide access to experts; reduce costs associated with brick-and-mortar health care facilities; and improve continuing education for health care providers (Orwat & Key, 2017a, 2017b; Singer & Sage, 2015). On the policy side, social workers should advocate for an expansion of licensure laws to include interstate compacts and more comprehensive reimbursement for psychosocial services delivered using telehealth technologies.

Technology assessments in health care and mental health continue to be an underutilized tool in providing state-of-the-art evaluations. Professional and governmental organizations addressing health and wellness do not assess technology in relation to the proliferation of research into digital behaviors and solutions. Education in technology ethics or use of digital alternatives is not identified in either health care or mental health continuing credit criteria (Young, 2015). Resources like the Social Work Podcast (www.socialworkpodcast.com) should provide regular updates for social workers on current trends in technology and tips for ethical use of technology in social work practice. Further research is needed to form inclusion of client technological literacy self-efficacy standards, opening populations to evidence-based digital interventions and treatment. The development of a technology ecomap provided an example of a visual technology assessment aimed at digital inclusion in family systems evaluation.

CHAPTER DISCUSSION QUESTIONS

1. What education does the social worker need to have in order to conduct a competent technology assessment?

2. How would this session look different using a different practice approach, such as solution-focused, cognitive behavioral, or mindfulness?

3. What ethical dilemmas might arise in the discussion of technology use and families? What resources do social workers have to help them understand ethical dilemmas related to technology?

REFERENCES

American Psychiatric Association. (2013). *Diagnostic and statistical manual of mental disorders* (5th ed.). Arlington, VA: American Psychiatric Publishing.

Belluomini, E. (2013, October 22). Technology assessments for families. *The New Social Worker, 20*(4), 31–32.

Berzin, S. C., Singer, J. B., & Chan, C. (2015). *Practice innovation through technology in the digital age: A grand challenge for social work*. Columbia, SC: American Academy of Social Work and Social Welfare. Retrieved from http://aaswsw.org/wp-content/uploads/2013/10/Practice-Innovation-through-Technology-in-the-Digital-Age-A-Grand-Challenge-for-Social-Work-GC-Working-Paper-No-12.pdf

Bradford, S., & Rickwood, D. (2014). Electronic psychosocial assessment tool: Concept development and identification of barriers to successful implementation. *Journal of Technology in Human Services, 32*(4), 275–296. doi:10.1080/15228835.2014.967906

Committee on Adolescence American Academy of Pediatrics. (2008). Achieving quality health services for adolescents. *Pediatrics, 121*(6), 1263–1270. doi:10.1542/peds.2008-0694

Congress, E. P. (2015). The culturagram. In K. Corcoran & A. R. Roberts (Eds.), *Social workers' desk reference* (3rd ed., pp. 1011–1018). New York, NY: Oxford University Press.

Diamond, G., Levy, S., Bevans, K. B., Fein, J. A., Wintersteen, M. B., Tien, A., & Creed, T. (2010). Development, validation, and utility of internet-based, behavioral health screen for adolescents. *Pediatrics, 126*(1), e163–e170. doi:10.1542/peds.2009-3272

Diamond, G. S., Herres, J. L., Ewing, E. S. K., Atte, T. O., Scott, S. W., Wintersteen, M. B., & Gallop, R. J. (2017). Comprehensive screening for suicide risk in primary care. *American Journal of Preventive Medicine, 53*(1), 48–54. doi:10.1016/j.amepre.2017.02.020

Erbacher, T. A., & Singer, J. B. (2017). Suicide risk monitoring: The missing piece in suicide risk assessment. *Contemporary School Psychology*. Advance online publication. doi:10.1007/s40688-017-0164-8

Erbacher, T. A., Singer, J. B., & Poland, S. (2015). *Suicide in schools: A practitioner's guide to multilevel prevention, assessment, intervention, and postvention*. New York, NY: Routledge Press.

Fox, H. B., McManus, M. A., Irwin, C. E., Jr., Kelleher, K. J., & Peake, K. (2013). A research agenda for adolescent-centered primary care in the United States. *Journal of Adolescent Health, 53*(3), 307–310. doi:10.1016/j.jadohealth.2013.06.025

Hall, J. C. (2017, March). Practice cybernetics. In *Encyclopedia of social work* [Online]. New York, NY: Oxford University Press. doi:10.1093/acrefore/9780199975839.013.1260

Hartman, A. (1978). Diagrammatic assessment of family relationships. *Families in Society, 76,* 465–476.

Hodge, D. R. (2015). *Spiritual assessment in social work and mental health practice.* New York, NY: Columbia University Press.

Kleiman, E. M., Turner, B. J., Fedor, S., Beale, E. E., Huffman, J. C., & Nock, M. K. (2017). Examination of real-time fluctuations in suicidal ideation and its risk factors: Results from two ecological momentary assessment studies. *Journal of Abnormal Psychology, 126*(6), 726–738. doi:10.1037/abn0000273

Larkin, H., Shields, J. J., & Anda, R. F. (2012). The health and social consequences of adverse childhood experiences (ACE) across the lifespan: An introduction to prevention and intervention in the community. *Journal of Prevention & Intervention in the Community, 40*(4), 263–270. doi:10.1080/10852352.2012.707439

MacKinnon, L. (2012). The neurosequential model of therapeutics: An interview with Bruce Perry. *Australian and New Zealand Journal of Family Therapy, 33*(3), 210–218. doi:10.1017/aft.2012.26

McGoldrick, M. (2015). Using genograms to map family patterns. In K. Corcoran, & A. R. Roberts (Eds.), *Social workers' desk reference* (3rd ed., pp. 413–426). New York, NY: Oxford University Press.

McGoldrick, M., Gerson, R., & Petry, S. S. (2008). *Genograms: Assessment and intervention* (3rd ed.). New York, NY: W. W. Norton.

Morgan, G. (2010). Design consideration and experience for multiple assessments. *Journal of Technology in Human Services, 28*(4), 274–281. doi:10.1080/15228835.2011.572610

Orwat, J., & Key, W. (2017a). Analyzing the problem: Disparities in behavioral and mental health for children and youth. In C. Moniz & S. Gorin (Eds.), *Behavioral and mental health care policy and practice: A biopsychosocial perspective.* New York, NY: Routledge Press.

Orwat, J., & Key, W. (2017b). Behavioral health and the Affordable Care Act. In C. Moniz & S. Gorin (Eds.), *Behavioral and mental health care policy and practice: A biopsychosocial perspective.* New York, NY: Routledge Press.

Palfrey, J., & Gasser, U. (2016). *Born digital: How children grow up in a digital age* (revised, expanded edition). New York, NY: Basic Books.

Patton, D. U., Eschmann, R. D., & Butler, D. A. (2013). Internet banging: New trends in social media, gang violence, masculinity and hip hop. *Computers in Human Behavior, 29*(5), A54–A59. doi:10.1016/j.chb.2012.12.035

Perry, B. D. (2009). Examining child maltreatment through a neurodevelopmental lens: Clinical applications of the neurosequential model of therapeutics. *Journal of Loss and Trauma, 14*(4), 240–255. doi:10.1080/15325020903004350

Perry, B. D., & Szalavitz, M. (2007). *The boy who was raised as a dog: And other stories from a child psychiatrist's notebook—What traumatized children can teach us about loss, love, and healing* (Reprint ed.). New York, NY: Basic Books.

Ramsey, A. T., Wetherell, J. L., Depp, C., Dixon, D., & Lenze, E. (2016). Feasibility and acceptability of smartphone assessment in older adults with cognitive and emotional difficulties. *Journal of Technology in Human Services, 34*(2), 209–223. doi:10.1080/15228835.2016.1170649

Rogers, E. M. (2003). *Diffusion of innovations* (5th ed.). New York, NY: Free Press.

Shaffer, D., & Pfeffer, C. R. (2001). Practice parameter for the assessment and treatment of children and adolescents with suicidal behavior. *Journal of the American Academy of Child & Adolescent Psychiatry, 40* (Suppl. 7), 24S–51S.

Shiffman, S., Stone, A. A., & Hufford, M. R. (2008). Ecological momentary assessment. *Annual Review of Clinical Psychology, 4*, 1–32.

Singer, J. B. (Producer). (2007). Bio-psychosocial-Spiritual (BPSS) assessment and Mental Status Exam (MSE). *Social Work Podcast* [Audio podcast]. Retrieved from http://socialworkpodcast .com/2007/02/bio-psychosocial-spiritual-bpss.html

Singer, J. B. (Host). (2013). Perinatal loss: Interview with Sarah Kye Price, Ph.D. *Social Work Podcast*. Retrieved from http://socialworkpodcast.blogspot.com/2013/04/ perinatal-loss-interview-with-sarah-kye.html

Singer, J. B., & Sage, M. (2015). Technology and social work practice: Micro, mezzo, and macro applications. In K. Corcoran & A. R. Roberts (Eds.), *Social workers' desk reference* (3rd ed., pp. 179–188). Oxford, NY: Oxford University Press.

Siu, A. L. (2016). Screening for depression in children and adolescents: US Preventive Services Task Force recommendation statement. *Pediatrics, 137*(3), e20154467. doi:10.1542/ peds.2015-4467

Slovak, K., & Singer, J. B. (2014). School social workers knowledge of and responses to cyberbullying: Results from a national survey. *School Social Work Journal, 39*(1), 1–16.

U.S. Department of Health and Human Services Office of the Surgeon General and National Action Alliance for Suicide Prevention. (2012). *2012 National strategy for suicide prevention: Goals and objectives for action.* Washington, DC: U.S. Department of Health and Human Services Office of the Surgeon General and National Action Alliance for Suicide Prevention. Retrieved from http://www.surgeongeneral.gov/library/ reports/national-strategy-suicide-prevention/full-report.pdf

Wang, E., Myers, M. D., & Sundaram, D. (2012). Digital natives and digital immigrants: Towards a model of digital fluency. *ECIS 2012 Proceedings.* Retrieved from https:// aisel.aisnet.org/ecis2012/39

Young, J. A. (2015). Assessing new media literacies in social work education: The development and validation of a comprehensive assessment instrument. *Journal of Technology in Human Services, 33*(1), 72–86. doi:10.1080/15228835.2014.998577

PART II

Foci of Health Care

6

Health Promotion and Public Health

Robert H. Keefe and Sandra D. Lane

WHAT IS PUBLIC HEALTH?

The field of public health began in the mid-19th century with the sanitary-reform movement to clean the water supply and the development of sanitaria to quarantine and treat tuberculosis patients (Novick, Morrow, & Mays, 2008). Public health's origins shared similar concerns with social work's beginnings in the 19th-century settlement movement, notably concern for the poor and vulnerable. Contemporary public health professionals investigate the spread and distribution of diseases; engage in illness prevention and health promotion endeavors; and participate in activities that foster healthy lives for individuals, families, neighborhoods, and communities. Professor Charles Edward Amory Winslow, a renowned bacteriologist and public health expert, defined public health as,

> *The science and art of preventing disease, prolonging life, and promoting physical health and efficiency through organized community efforts for the sanitation of the environment, the control of community infections, . . . the organization of medical and nursing services for the early diagnosis and preventive treatment of disease, and the development of the social machinery which will ensure to every individual . . . a standard of living adequate for the maintenance of health. (Winslow, 1920, p. 30)*

This definition has been used to guide public health efforts throughout the world. Within the United States, the U.S. Congress in 1798 mandated that merchant seamen be provided with insurance through the Marine Hospital Service. Later, the program was restructured as the United States Public Health Service (USPHS) with the purpose of diagnosing, reporting, and quarantining individuals who were carriers of infectious diseases. Recognizing the possibility that seamen may contract diseases while serving in foreign countries, public health physicians evaluated and treated the seamen upon their return from overseas missions for any illnesses they may have contracted (Keefe & Evans, 2013).

This rather constricted focus was later broadened when the microbial causes of infectious disease were identified by Koch and Pasteur at the end of the 19th century. The early 20th-century influx of impoverished migrants into cities in the United States, combined with greater numbers of people moving from small, rural communities to large, urban areas, led to frequent outbreaks of communicable illnesses. The scientific progress during the 19th century, which included the growth of bacteriology, the introduction of antisepsis, and the discovery of ether (Starr, 1982), helped the field of medicine gain footing in the United States. Twentieth-century advances in antibiotics and vaccines against polio, diphtheria, tetanus, and the eradication of smallpox further established the importance of public health to the health and well-being of all Americans.

Public health views the "community" as the "patient" and much of the focus is on the prevention of illness. Medicine, nursing, and other clinical fields view the individual as the "patient" and focus greater attention on the detection and treatment of disease. Public health divides prevention into *primary* and *secondary*. Primary prevention aims to prevent the spread of communicable diseases and the beginning of chronic disease. Examples of primary prevention include childhood immunizations against measles and chicken pox or school-based programs on exercise and healthy food to prevent childhood obesity. Secondary prevention, which is often undertaken by both public health and clinical health professionals, seeks to reduce the complications of already-established conditions. For example, among individuals infected with HIV, secondary prevention involves taking appropriate medications to prevent the deterioration of the immune system and the onset of AIDS. Among people with hypertension, secondary prevention involves partaking in exercise, eating a healthy diet, and taking appropriate medications to prevent stroke and heart attacks.

Public health and social work share the view that caring for the health and social needs of the population, especially the most vulnerable, benefits society in ways that are worth the public investment. However, frequent backlashes have been directed toward both professions. Social Darwinists, for instance, believed that public funds should not be used to provide services such as vaccinations for childhood illnesses and treatment for sexually transmitted infections, or for establishing clinics for low-income individuals (Keefe & Evans, 2013; Levine & Bashford, 2014). This way of thinking changed when more progressive men and women, known as Social Reformers, advocated for reforms in both public sentiment and legislation geared toward the belief that everyone should receive necessary care and take part in society (Keefe & Evans, 2013; McCoy, 2015).

The Social Reform Movement, begun in the 1890s, was brought about by individuals who were typically from well-educated and privileged backgrounds, who opposed Social Darwinism. Philosophically, the reformers had moved from a "blaming the victim" mind-set of the 19th century to the realization that systemic evolution was necessary for the impoverished to subsist in America. For example, Jane Addams, perhaps the most well-known advocate for social reform, conducted community risk assessments and resources mapping and advocated for access to parks and green space (Schultz, 2007).

The reformers understood that good health was key to longevity, and one way to ensure that people had good health was to impose strict laws so that children remained in school and were not forced to work dangerous jobs that often led to serious illnesses and injuries. In turn, the child labor movement became the means by which additional reforms were to occur. The reformers teamed with union activists to support compulsory education for children and to press industrialists for better wages, unemployment compensation, safety codes/devices, and shorter work hours. They tied child labor to poverty, ill health, and limited opportunities for upward mobility. Social justice became fashionable and disenfranchised groups began to mobilize (Keefe & Evans, 2013) leading to such changes as the ratification of the 19th Amendment to the U.S. Constitution in 1921, which granted women the right to vote. Having achieved legislative success at the local, state, and national levels, the reformers moved to formulate federal programs that would impact poverty, child welfare, disabled persons, and the elderly. Social work and public health professionals helped launch national social policy leading to the passing of the Social Security Act (SSA) in 1935.

WHAT IS HEALTH PROMOTION?

As the public began to realize the limitations of various "curative" measures including antibiotics, professionals interested in health promotion and illness prevention gained favor. Prevention efforts, which began with reducing the spread of communicable diseases, moved to focus on the prevention of chronic conditions and risk factors for those conditions, including diabetes, childhood obesity, and smoking. Professionals working in the area of health promotion and disease prevention seek to help individuals, families, groups, and communities to enact healthy behaviors that promote well-being and prevent premature death. The World Health Organization (WHO), the multinational agency overseeing health promotion policy worldwide, defines health promotion as ". . . the process of enabling people to increase control over, and to improve, their health. It moves beyond a focus on individual behavior towards a wide range of social and environmental interventions" (WHO, n.d.).

Public health and health promotion professionals seek the most effective ways to endorse and protect the health of populations by considering where individuals live, work, go to school, and play (Wallerstein & Duran, 2010). Multi-sector health coalitions have been successful in creating change by organizing around priority health issues. Health promotion experts, including public health social workers, can practice their knowledge and skills by engaging coalitions to build public awareness of particular public health concerns. These coalitions may be organized around reducing food desserts by persuading corner markets to sell fresh fruits and vegetables, encouraging school principals to develop programs to address bullying to help prevent school violence, and motivating business leaders to provide private spaces for mothers to breastfeed newborn infants to promote healthy infant development.

Public health social workers engaged in developing healthy communities play important roles in developing initiatives that bring multiple stakeholders together (e.g., community residents, governmental officials, politicians, and company executives) to enhance the built environment such as housing and sidewalks, and developing parks and other green spaces that will lead to sustained changes in the health of community members (Golden & Earp, 2012). In this regard, community development is critical to health promotion (Marmot, Allen, Bell, & Goldblatt, 2012). Every resource, including faith-based organizations, schools, senior citizens centers, and public markets can become a partner in creating strategies to enhance healthy living.

SOCIAL DETERMINANTS OF HEALTH

Primary prevention efforts have been effective in reducing tobacco use, ensuring people wear seat belts, and preventing polio outbreaks. To be successful, public health professionals must be aware of the effects of societal factors that lead to poor health or impede access to health-promoting resources. Investigating how individuals thrive is therefore not based solely on genetics, but on the individuals' surroundings as well. Although having health care facilities in local communities helps to ensure medical care will be provided during emergencies, the quality of people's surroundings plays a large role. Noise, pollution, dilapidated housing, and community violence are important factors in the length and quality of a person's life. Even more important, discrimination and structural violence in the form of barriers to education, employment, and health insurance profoundly influence health and survival. These conditions, called "social determinants," are critical to consider for public health practice. Poor health can be a product of where people live, work, learn, and play and how they are treated by their society (Williams, McClellan, & Rivlin, 2010), making community-level development and prevention strategies essential for fostering good health and health equity among community residents. The social determinants of health, over and above access to health care services, drive health inequalities (Frieden, 2010) and are shaped both by community conditions (Williams et al., 2010) and by the distribution of money, power, and resources at global, national, and local levels.

Identifying populations at risk of poor health outcomes, providing primary prevention services to reduce illness and disease, as well as providing secondary prevention strategies to decrease the tragic consequences of chronic conditions are rooted in epidemiology. Social epidemiology assumes that diseases, disparities in access to and outcomes of care, as well as poverty are not randomly distributed throughout society but instead affect largely marginalized groups. Therefore, subgroups within a population differ in their frequency of exposure to social problems that lead to poor health. Understanding the social context of an at-risk population is essential for public health social workers to render the most appropriate intervention (Krieger, 2001). Knowledge of the uneven distribution of risk factors as well as awareness of the economic and cultural indicators that can be utilized to formulate programs for health promotion, illness control, and prevention (Mausner & Kramer, 1985, p. 1) are essential for health promotion practitioners to have (see Chapter 3, Social Determinants of Health for further discussion).

WHAT IS PUBLIC HEALTH SOCIAL WORK?

Public health social work recognizes the importance of the interrelationship between individuals, families, groups, and the communities. Public health social workers seek to understand how a person's environment affects his or her adaptation to community surroundings. The social determinants of health call attention to the natural synergies between social work and public health and how each profession views how health and illness are constructed and reinforced by societal conditions. Over the past many decades, public health professionals including public health social workers have grown to rely increasingly on each other's skills (Ruth, Wyatt, Chiasson, Geron, & Bachman, 2006). Public health professionals have become more aware of the psychosocial determinants of health (Awofeso, 2004; Northridge, 2004) and social workers have become more aware of the importance of the effects of illnesses on specific populations (Ruth et al., 2006). Today, public health social work is recognized as a distinct specialization area by the National Association of Social Workers (Ruth, Sisco, & Marshall, 2016), the American Public Health Association with the establishment of the Public Health Social Work Section in 1970 (Keefe & Evans, 2013), and the Health Resources and Services Administration (HRSA) of the U.S. Department of Health and Human Services (USDHHS), which includes public health social workers who practice in all countries and with all populations (HRSA, 2016).

Public health social work emphasizes the identification and reduction or elimination of social stressors associated with poor health (including poverty, discrimination, limited access to care, and fragmented service delivery), and determines the social supports that promote well-being to help protect against poor health outcomes. Public health social workers hold elected office, administer large-scale organizations, conduct research in various settings around the globe, and fill many different roles including educators, case managers, and program evaluators (Sable, Schild, & Hipp, 2012).

Over time, numerous definitions of social work have been offered. For our purposes we will use the following definition:

> *Social work is the professional activity of helping individuals, groups or communities enhance or restore their capacity for social functioning and creating societal conditions favorable to this goal. (National Association of Social Workers, 1973, pp. 3–4)*

Public health social work expands this definition to include:

> *. . . an epidemiological approach to identifying social problems affecting the health status and social functioning of all population groups with an emphasis on intervention at the primary prevention level. (Practice Standards Development Committee, 2005, p. 4)*

These definitions clearly indicate that although public health and social work vary in their methods, their goals are similar: to provide services that enhance the health and well-being of individuals, families, groups, and communities. Both professions share an ecologic perspective for problem solving and have a systemic approach toward intervention that calls upon various sources to bring about change to complex social problems and ameliorate community life (Volland, Berkman, Stein, & Vaughn, 1999). Likewise, each profession shares a core value of "social justice" and targets its interventions at enhancing the lives of disadvantaged members of society (Krieger, 2003; Stover & Bassett, 2003). Both professions use social action and advocacy in numerous domains including community health (Wallerstein, Yen, & Syme, 2011); maternal, child, and adolescent health (Jaffee & Perloff, 2003); substance abuse (Skiba, Monroe, & Wodarski, 2004); immigrant health (Chang-Muy & Congress, 2008); HIV/AIDS (Smith & Bride, 2004); primary prevention (Vourlekis, Ell, & Padgett, 2001); bioterrorism (Mackelprang, Mackelprang, & Thirkill, 2005); and the uniformed services (Wheeler & Bragin, 2007).

PRACTICE

Public health social workers recognize the need to provide culturally relevant services at all levels of intervention (micro, mezzo, and macro; Sable et al., 2012) and acknowledge that there are few interventions that have been tested at each level generalizable across cultural groups (Chin, Walters, Cook, & Huang, 2007).

To provide useful services, public health social workers focus on the three core functions of public health practice that dictate how public health social workers render services: assessment (surveillance of disease/injury), policy development (legislative changes resulting from assessment), and assurance (implementation of policy that in turn leads to service delivery for all citizens; Centers for Disease Control and Prevention, 2017). The professional public health social worker works to identify not only the biomedical (e.g., virus) and psychological aspects of disease (e.g., trauma), but the social determinants (e.g., poverty) as well. By addressing the determinants, public health social workers are better able to render care at the primary and secondary levels.

Practice Assessment

Assessment requires public health social workers to identify population health needs and assets, including social and community-based resources, and apply their knowledge and skills to promote and protect health and foster health equity. Public health social workers engage in dialogues with any number of people including community members, faith leaders, and policy makers. Examples would include research utilizing social surveys, focus groups, and individual interviews to determine risk and protective factors affecting health status. For instance, Nam, Huang, Heflin, and Sherradan (2015) conducted a survey to assess racial/ethnic disparities in food insufficiency. They concluded that African Americans, American Indians, and Hispanics experience food insufficiency at three times the rate as Whites. Lane et al. (2008) studied the effects of food insecurity on birth outcomes and concluded that income level, more than race, predicted greater food insecurity. For community-level assessments (which include community needs, preferences, and local assets), having partnerships with stakeholders across multiple sectors can help address the issues and generate solutions that are tailored to a specific locality (National Association of County and City Health Officials, 2017).

Policy Development

Policy development is concerned with developing, analyzing, and advocating for health policies aimed at improving population health through increasing access to health care and culturally responsive health promotion resources. Examples include community collaborative policy and environmental change work around diabetes prevention and control in specific communities. For several years, Spencer et al. (2011) collaborated with community partners to assess the feasibility of utilizing community health workers to improve the health of people living with diabetes as a matter of local public health policy.

Assurance

Assurance involves conducting research, disseminating findings that enhance evidence-based practices and programs, and engaging in community-based health promotion activities to ensure local conditions and culturally responsive resources that enable healthy living are available. Public health social workers would work with neighborhood watch programs, school boards, and concerned parents to ensure young people were thriving in their home communities. Examples would include disseminating evidence-informed strategies for use in communities that promote positive youth development through prosocial behaviors and thereby reduce risks for substance use and violence, such as those discussed by Hawkins, Shapiro, and Fagan (2010).

To engage in these three practice strategies, public health social workers must strengthen efforts geared toward health promotion by purposeful community organizing across various groups (Marmot et al., 2012). For example, organizing community coalitions to maximize opportunities for citizen participation have been found to be very effective in creating social change (Brathwaite & McKenzie, 2012). Other strategies include local resource development and building community capacity such as enhancing the ability of community-based organizations, faith institutions, schools, cultural institutions, and local small businesses to take on a mission for health through endorsing or providing health promotion activities in neighborhoods (Liberato, Brimblecombe, Ritchie, Ferguson, & Coveney, 2011).

As public health social workers, we must work with the *whole* person. Being able to see the whole person requires time, interest, and analyzing the effects of the social determinants that affect the person's health and well-being. While social workers must have well-developed diagnostic and assessment skills and good clinical judgment, it is important for professionals to recognize the health hazards that come from living in unsafe neighborhoods with dilapidated housing and limited access to healthy food markets and green spaces that hinder residents from moving forward in their lives.

Case Example 6.1

Clifford is a 45-year-old, divorced African American male diagnosed with insulin-dependent diabetes. Clifford is of limited financial means and has had difficulty finding a physician willing to accept Medicaid and provide ongoing care. While living alone in his second floor inner-city apartment, Clifford was unable to participate in secondary prevention efforts that would reduce the likelihood of needing a below-knee amputation. Consequently, Clifford was forced to undergo surgery for a below-knee amputation and a long rehabilitation process. Clifford progressed in physical and occupational therapy and was discharged to his home. While in the rehabilitation hospital, he had been referred to the American Diabetes Association for ongoing diabetes education, the Visiting Nurses Association for dressing changes to his stump, and the city metrocab service for transportation to medical appointments. These referrals were relevant and appropriate given his health care needs. However, they did not take into account the social determinants exacerbating his diabetes. Once discharged, Clifford tried to navigate the labyrinth of the health care system. Since his divorce 3 years earlier, Clifford has lived alone, but has several children and grandchildren who periodically check on him. At the time of discharge Clifford reported that the prosthesis made for him after his amputation fit well and while in physical therapy he learned how to climb stairs so that he could get up to his second floor apartment. However, due to feeling unsafe in his neighborhood, which had a high crime rate, Clifford did not feel safe going out of his apartment to get exercise. There were no grocery stores, so he had to rely on corner markets that did not provide healthy food options, which in turn worsened his diabetes. His apartment was quite old and had lead-based paint that when chipped turned into a powdery substance that caused lead particles to escape into the air. The diabetes literature that pictured happy-looking White families engaging in some outdoor activity, talking about the joys of eating and exercising together, or using recipes that called for whole grains and fresh fruits and vegetables that were not available at the corner markets in neighborhoods.

As illustrated in Case Example 6.1, it was clear that Clifford's diabetes was not his only problem, and in fact was simply a symptom of the health problems that led him into treatment. No matter how much diabetes education he received, there were way too many other health concerns in his life for him to thrive. Despite his improved ambulation, he was not able to walk all the way to a large grocery store so that he could buy healthy foods to make the recipes appropriate to a diabetic diet and carry them back to his second-floor apartment. He also could not get to the drug store to buy new syringes, which meant that he was forced to reuse needles for his insulin two to three times. His neighborhood was not particularly safe, so he was afraid to venture outside to get exercise. Finally, the visiting nurses, convinced that he knew how to self-administer his insulin and that he had no open wounds requiring dressing changes, decided he no longer qualified for skilled care and informed him that his case was closed.

What Clifford received was piecemeal treatment of his pancreas to reduce the free-floating insulin in his blood, dressing changes to his stump, and eyeglasses to correct his vision loss. By focusing only on the individual and not his or her social location, we miss the richness of the many variables that shape the individual's existence and help or hinder the path toward recovery.

POLICY

Policy considerations regarding health care are many. From the Social Security Act (SSA) of 1935 through the Patient Protection and Affordable Care Act (ACA) of 2010, public health social workers have largely focused on the important issues of expanding access to and quality of health care services (Andrews, Darnell, McBride, & Gehlert, 2013). For every health care policy, public health social workers have asked the questions: How do people benefit by the policy? Who will have input on the policy's development and evaluation? Will services be more affordable, accessible, and adequate than they would be if the policy were not enacted? How will the policy be amended as demographics change among groups being served?

The SSA, perhaps the most significant pieces of legislation that arose from the New Deal, was signed by President Franklin D. Roosevelt in 1935. The SSA ensured federal assistance would be provided to people who were unable to work for various reasons including disability. Although the SSA has been amended many times, it remains one of the influential acts affecting social welfare. The SSA resulted from the rise in industrialization in growing and overcrowded cities. Tenement houses sprung up in many cities, which led to overcrowding and poor sanitation (Dobelstein, 2009). Likewise, changes in workplace environments frequently led to catastrophic occupational accidents and an increase in the number of people suffering from disabling conditions (Dobelstein, 2009). Over time, the Act was amended so that funding was given to states to provide services to the elderly (Title I), the uninsured (Title III), maternal and child health (Title V), public health services (Title VI), and Medicare (Title XVIII) and Medicaid (Title XIX). These amendments helped to ensure individuals with various health conditions would not be without health care.

The ever-increasing cost of health care required the federal government to develop cost-saving mechanisms. The Health Maintenance Organization Act of 1973, and the prospective payment systems such as the Diagnostic Related Groups of the 1980s and 1990s, helped to slow the rising cost of health care, but did little to ensure the U.S. population was any healthier than during earlier times. The ACA helped address this concern by expanding access to health care and by recognizing the most effective way to improve population health and achieve health equity is to invest in improving the social contexts within which people live (Frieden, 2010). As we have noted, simply expanding access to health care will not alleviate health disparities as most of the variation in health status is not accounted for by access to health care, but rather by social factors largely outside the control of the individual, including unsafe streets and communities, inadequate housing, low-quality education, limited access to healthy foods, and lack of spaces for physical activity (Rudolph, Caplan, Ben-Moshe, & Dillon, 2013). The ACA has therefore authorized the development of the National Prevention Strategy (NPS) to encourage partnerships among governmental, industry, and private sector (often community-level) entities. The goal of the NPS is to utilize these partnerships to improve the nation's health through four strategic directives: creating healthy and safe communities, expanding clinical and community-based preventive services, empowering people to make healthy choices, and eliminating health disparities (National Prevention Council, 2012).

Today, legislative changes including repealing and replacing the ACA place a spotlight on public health and public health social work practice. To protect the gains made in prior policies, public health social workers must be ready to use their advocacy skills by bringing in stakeholder groups to help advocate for the development of policies that make services affordable, accessible, and adequate. We need to be concerned about policy changes that may risk harm to vulnerable groups including people of low income, the elderly, and the medically frail. Public health social work values and ethics as well as our global responsibilities to help marginalized groups, require us to act in a planful and goal-oriented manner.

RESEARCH

Public health social workers engage in research focused on a plethora of social issues. Of primary importance is research with multiple stakeholders on policy and program evaluation that emphasizes primary prevention and builds local policies, resources, and capacity for health equity (Walters et al., 2016). However, few community development and prevention initiatives focused on population health improvement have been reported in social work journals (Ruth, Marshall, & Valasquez, 2014). Prevention-oriented interventions are needed that develop and deploy local resources for community health improvement in collaboration with governmental and private sector supports (Keefe, 2013). As public health social workers, we must also deploy our findings in ways that will help advocates to maintain the momentum of the ACA's NPS. In the event that the ACA is replaced, public health social workers will be called upon to advocate for public health approaches that enhance primary prevention strategies.

Research studies have focused on many topics. Studies that are of primary importance to public health social workers focus at the neighborhood level where unhealthy and unsafe neighborhoods have created poor health for many residents. Exposure to environmental stressors frequently lead to chronic medical conditions including cardiovascular diseases (Barber et al., 2016; Cox, Boyle, Davey, Feng, & Morris, 2007; Stimpson, Ju, Raji, & Eschbach, 2007), diabetes, and various child health conditions (Gittelsohn, & Trude, 2017; Kim, 2008; Lane et al., 2008; Msall, Avery, Msall, & Hogan, 2007; Riva, Gauvin, & Barnett, 2007). Low-income neighborhoods are unfortunately victim to other risk factors such as poverty, crime, and housing instability (Lindberg et al., 2010; Silverman & Patterson, 2011). Housing instability contributes to adverse health outcomes including school failure, increased asthma and other pulmonary conditions, and developmental delays (Pickard & Ingersoll, 2016). Homes located near major highways often expose residents to toxins that affect pulmonary and cardiac health (Brugge, Durant, & Rioux, 2007; Mazaffarian, 2016). A neighborhood's socioeconomic conditions affect whether its residents have healthy diets (Daniel, 2016), practice safer reproductive behaviors (Frey & Klebanoff, 2016), and smoke cigarettes (Riggs & Pentz, 2015).

Research that highlights the effectiveness of our assessment, intervention, and practice evaluations on all client groups is sorely needed. Public health social workers have various opportunities to collaborate with community and neighborhood groups to conduct their research. For instance, multisector health coalitions exist in many communities and are organized around prioritized health issues (such as preventing and controlling childhood obesity) where social workers can engage residents in strategies that build community awareness and involve community partner organizations in addressing a particular health problem. These organizations might include farmers' markets and schools with the goal of increasing access to healthy food options.

CONCLUSION

This chapter brings together key aspects of the roles for professional public health experts and social workers. The field of public health social work brings together many of the roles of the two professions so as to be of service to various groups. A key focus among both professions is the appreciation of the health and well-being of communities in which individuals, families, and groups live, work, and play. Professionals work on health promotion strategies that enhance the health and well-being and address the social determinants of health. Public health social workers use various interventions to ensure community health and well-being including advocacy efforts to effect change in health policy, which stem from advances made through the SSA and more recently with the ACA. Public health social workers will likely need to continue engaging in advocacy efforts to mitigate the threats to the ACA and the NPS.

As public health social workers, we must be proactive in identifying risks to community health and intervening to reduce those threats so that the communities we work in continue to move forward in a healthy and health-promoting manner.

CHAPTER DISCUSSION QUESTIONS

1. Describe some of the social determinants that negatively affect your home communities. How are these determinants (e.g., poverty, school violence) being addressed and what recommendations would you make to lessen the effects of these determinants?

2. Review one of the sections of the ACA (housedocs.house.gov/energycommerce/ ppacacon.pdf) that represents one of your professional interest areas. For instance, students interested in the elderly might consider Medicaid prescription coverage (Sec. 2501). Review the research that has been done in your interest area, compose a letter to a legislator informing him or her of the importance of the section, and why it is needed in whatever policy may replace the ACA.

3. Review five research articles that have been published in your interest area. Summarize the articles by focusing on what each article says about ensuring health promotion, developing policy change that will help vulnerable groups, and providing recommendations for future research to consider.

4. Think about your interest area in social work. Go to Google Scholar and select five articles that focus on your area. What are some of the best practices in health promotion in your area? What recommendations are being made for health promotion that you would consider putting into practice in your hometown?

5. Select a community other than the city/town where you currently live. Review newspapers or other news sources to inform you about the most pressing public health issues affecting the community. Select one of those issues, such as school bullying or neighborhood violence. What has the community done to address this issue? Where would you begin intervening? Which community stakeholders would you need to develop relationships with to successfully intervene?

CASE EXAMPLE AND DISCUSSION QUESTIONS

Case Example 6.2

Melinda is a 33-year-old, married, African American female who was diagnosed with a chronic back ailment and traumatic brain injury after being struck in a work-related accident in the assembly line at the car manufacturing company where she works. She was admitted to the rehabilitation hospital 3 days ago after being treated at an acute hospital.

(continued)

Case Example 6.2   *(continued)*

She underwent spinal fusion surgery and a craniotomy to release pressure on her brain after the accident. Prior to admission, Melinda and her husband of 8 years, Nathaniel, were living with Nathaniel's parents in the same community. Melinda's parents live nearby and are very supportive. Melinda states that she and her husband moved to her in-laws' home after Nathaniel lost his job at the same company. She states that she feels her in-laws do not want to have her live with them and would like to go to her own parents who live in a two-story home. Melinda's parents state they are worried about Nathaniel, who has not visited Melinda since she was admitted to the rehab hospital, is trying to abandon Melinda, and pursue divorce. They have no children. Melinda is wheelchair dependent, has difficulty controlling her bladder, has uncontrollable tremors, and is unable to speak in coherent sentences. Melinda's case has been referred to workers compensation, which will likely reimburse her medical care. Melinda is the 15th patient admitted to the hospital this year from the same car manufacturing plant for a work-related injury. The administration team has denied any wrongdoing on the factory's part despite a history of citations for unsafe work conditions. While working with Melinda, we need to keep in mind her youth, the possible tenuous relationship with her husband, the burn out her in-laws may be feeling as they try to care for her, and the likelihood that her health will continue to worsen. Although she did not indicate a wish to have children, it is now quite likely that she will be unable to withstand the difficulties carrying a baby throughout the 9-month gestation.

Questions for Discussion

1. As you reflect on the case of Melinda and what you have learned in this chapter, how would you tune into the biopsychosocial–spiritual care needs she has at the micro, mezzo, and macro levels?

2. If Melinda is unable to acknowledge the possibility her husband is trying to move on in his life without her, what resources would you structure for her at the time of discharge?

3. Consider the problem of the prior citations the company has received for unsafe working conditions. How would you go about mobilizing employees to address this issue? Think about coalition building. Start with Melinda, then move on to other patients treated at the rehabilitation hospital.

4. After answering question 3, think about how you would evaluate the success (or failure) of any improvements you recommend?

REFERENCES

Andrews, C. M., Darnell, J. S., McBride, T. D., & Gehlert, S. (2013). Social work and implementation of the Affordable Care Act. *Health & Social Work, 38*(2), 67–71. doi:10.1093/hsw/hlt002

Awofeso, N. (2004). What's new about the "New Public Health"? *American Journal of Public Health, 94*, 705–709.

Barber, S., Hickson, D. A., Wang, X., Sims, M., Nelson, C., & Diez-Roux, A. V. (2016). Neighborhood disadvantage, poor social conditions, and cardiovascular disease incidence among African American adults in the Jackson Heart Study. *American Journal of Public Health, 106*(12), 2219–2226. doi:10.2105/AJPH.2016.303471

Brathwaite, R. L., & McKenzie, R. (2012). The utility of large coalitions for community health programs. *Journal for Health care for the Poor and Underserved, 23*(2 Suppl.), 4–6. doi:10.1353/hpu.2012.0082

Brugge, D., Durant, J. L., & Rioux, C. (2007). Near-highway pollutants in motor vehicle exhaust: A review of epidemiologic evidence of cardiac and pulmonary health risks. *Environmental Health, 6,* 23. doi:10.1186/1476-069X-6-23

Centers for Disease Control and Prevention. (2017). *The public health system and the 10 essential public health services.* Retrieved from https://www.cdc.gov/stltpublichealth/publichealthservices/essentialhealthservices.html

Chang-Muy, F., & Congress, E. (2008). *Social work with immigrants and refugees: Legal issues, clinical skills, and advocacy.* New York, NY: Springer Publishing.

Chin, M. H., Walters, A. E., Cook, S. C., & Huang, E. S. (2007). Interventions to reduce racial and ethnic disparities in health care. *Medical Care Research Review, 64*(5 Suppl.), 7S–28S. doi:10.1177/1077558707305413

Cox, M., Boyle, P. J., Davey, P. G., Feng, Z., & Morris, A. D. (2007). Locality deprivation and type 2 diabetes incidence: A local test of relative inequalities. *Social Service and Medicine, 65,* 1953–1964. doi:10.1016/j.socscimed.2007.05.043

Daniel, C. (2016). Economic constraints on taste formation and the true cost of healthy eating. *Social Science & Medicine, 148,* 34–41. doi:10.1016/j.socscimed.2015.11.025

Dobelstein, A. W. (2009). *Understanding the Social Security Act: The foundation of social welfare for America in the twenty-first century.* New York, NY: Oxford University Press.

Frey, H. A., & Klebanoff, M. A. (2016). The epidemiology, etiology, and costs of preterm birth. *Seminars in Fetal and Neonatal Health, 21*(2), 68–73. doi:10.1016/j.siny.2015.12.011

Frieden, T. R. (2010). A framework for public health action: The health impact pyramid. *American Journal of Public Health, 100*(4), 590–595. doi:10.2105/AJPH.2009.185652

Gittelsohn, J., & Trude, A. (2017). Diabetes and obesity prevention: Changing the food environment in low-income settings. *Nutrition Reviews, 75*(Suppl. 1), 62–69. doi:10.1093/nutrit/nuw038

Golden, S. D., & Earp J. A. (2012). Social ecological approaches to individuals and their contexts: Twenty years of health education & behavior health promotion interventions. *Health Education & Behavior, 39*(3), 364–372. doi:10.1177/1090198111418634

Hawkins, J. D., Shapiro, V. B., & Fagan, A. A. (2010). Disseminating effective community prevention practices: Opportunities for social work education. *Research on Social Work Practice, 20*(5), 518–527. doi:10.1177/1049731509359919

Jaffee, K. D., & Perloff, J. D. (2003). An ecological analysis of racial difference in low birthweight: Implications for maternal and child health in social work. *Health and Social Work, 28,* 9–22. doi:10.1093/hsw/28.1.9

Keefe, R. H. (2013). Neighborhoods and health. In R. H. Keefe & E. T. Jankowski (Eds.), *Handbook for public health social work* (pp. 273–286). New York, NY: Springer Publishing.

Keefe, R. H., & Evans, T. A. (2013). Introduction to public health social work. In R. H. Keefe & E. T. Jankowski (Eds.), *Handbook for public health social work* (pp. 3–20). New York, NY: Springer Publishing.

Kim, D. (2008). Blues from the neighborhood? Neighborhood characteristics and depression. *Epidemiologic Reviews, 30*, 101–117. doi:10.1093/epirev/mxn009

Krieger, N. (2001). A glossary for social epidemiology. *Journal of Epidemiology & Community Health, 55*(10), 693–700. doi:10.1136/jech.55.10.693

Krieger, N. (2003). Latin American social medicine: The quest for social justice and public health. *American Journal of Public Health, 93*, 1989–1991.

Lane, S. D., Keefe, R. H., Rubinstein, R. A., Levandowski, B. A., Webster, N. J., Cibula, D. A., . . . Brill, J. (2008). Structural violence, urban retail food markets, and low birth weight. *Health & Place, 14*(3), 415–423. doi:10.1016/j.healthplace.2007.08.008

Levine, P., & Bashford, A. (2014). Introduction: Eugenics and the modern world. In A. Bashford & P. Levine (Eds.), *The Oxford handbook of the history of eugenics*. Oxford, UK: Oxford University Press.

Liberato, S. C., Brimblecombe, J., Ritchie, J., Ferguson, M., & Coveney, J. (2011). Measuring capacity building in communities: A review of the literature. *BMC Public Health, 11*, 850. doi:10.1186/1471-2458-11-850

Lindberg, R. A., Shenassa, E. D., Acevedo-Garcia, D., Popkin, S. J., Villaveces, A., & Morley, R. L. (2010). Housing interventions at the neighborhood level and health: A review of the evidence. *Journal of Public Health Management Practice, 16*(5, Suppl. E), S44–S52. doi:10.1097/PHH.0b013e3181dfbb72

Mackelprang, R. W., Mackelprang, R. D., & Thirkill, A. D. (2005). Bioterrorism and smallpox: Policies, practices, and implications for social work. *Social Work, 50*, 119–127. doi:10.1093/sw/50.2.119

Marmot, M., Allen, J., Bell, R., & Goldblatt, P. (2012). Building of the global movement for health equity: From Santiago to Rio and beyond. *The Lancet, 379*(9811), 181–188. doi:10.1016/S0140-6736(11)61506-7

Mausner, J. S., & Kramer, S. (1985). *Epidemiology: An introductory text* (2nd ed., p. 1). Philadelphia, PA: Saunders.

Mazaffarian, D. (2016). Dietary and policy priorities for cardiovascular disease, diabetes, and obesity: A comprehensive review. *Circulation, 133*, 187–225. doi:10.1161/CIRCULATIONAHA.115.018585

McCoy, C. A. (2015). The railway switches of history: The development of disease control in Britain and the United States in the 19th and early 20th century. *Journal of Historical Sociology, 30*(3), 650–673. doi:10.1111/johs.12099

Msall, M. E., Avery, R. C., Msall, E. R., & Hogan, D. P. (2007). Distressed neighborhoods and child disability rates: Analyses of 157,000 school-age children. *Developmental Medicine & Child Neurology, 49*, 814–817. doi:10.1111/j.1469-8749.2007.00814.x

Nam, Y., Huang, J., Heflin, C., & Sherraden, M. (2015). Racial and ethnic disparities in food insufficiency: Evidence from a statewide probability sample. *Journal of the Society for Social Work and Research, 6*(2), 201–228. doi:10.1086/681574

National Association of County and City Health Officials. (2017). Mobilizing for Action through Planning and Partnerships (MAPP). Retrieved from https://www.naccho.org/programs/public-health-infrastructure/performance-improvement/community-health-assessment/mapp

National Association of Social Workers. (1973). *Standards for Social Service Manpower*. Washington, DC: Author.

National Prevention Council. (2011). *National prevention strategy*. Retrieved from http://www.surgeongeneral.gov/priorities/prevention/strategy/report.pdf

Northridge, M. E. (2004). Building coalitions for tobacco control and prevention in the 21st century. *American Journal of Public Health, 94*, 178–180.

Novick, L. F., Morrow, C. B., & Mays, G. P. (Eds.). (2008). *Public health administration: Principles for population-based management* (2nd ed.). Sudbury, MA: Jones & Bartlett.

Patient Protection and Affordable Care Act. (2010). 42 U. S. C. § 18001.

Pickard, K. E., & Ingersoll, B. R. (2016). Quality versus quantity: The role of socioeconomic status on parent-reported service knowledge, service use, unmet service needs, and barriers to service use. *Autism, 20*(1), 106–115. doi:10.1177/1362361315569745

Practice Standards Development Committee. (2005). *Public health social work standards and competencies*. Columbus: Ohio Department of Health. Retrieved from http://oce.sph.unc.edu/cetac/phswcompetencies_May05.pdf

Riggs, N. R., & Pentz, M. A. (2015). Inhibitory control and the onset of combustible cigarette, e-cigarette, and hookah use in early adolescence: The moderating role of socioeconomic status. *Child Neuropsychology, 22*(6), 679–691. doi:10.1080/09297049.2015.1053389

Riva, M., Gauvin, L., & Barnett, T. A. (2007). Toward the next generation of research into small area effects on health: A synthesis of multilevel investigations published since July 1998. *Journal of Epidemiology and Community Health, 61*, 853–861. doi:10.1136/jech.2006.050740

Rudolph, L., Caplan, J., Ben-Moshe, K., & Dillon, L. (2013). *Health in all policies: A guide for state and local governments*. Washington, DC: American Public Health Association.

Ruth, B., Marshall, J. W., & Valasquez, E. (2014). Prevention in social work scholarship: A content analysis of Families in Society, 2000–2010. *Families in Society: The Journal of Contemporary Social Services, 94*(3), 182–185. doi:10.1606/1044-3894.4304

Ruth, B. J., Sisco, S., & Marshall, J. W. (2016). Public health social work. In C. Franklin (Ed.), *Encyclopedia of social work* [Online]. Retrieved from http://socialwork.oxfordre.com/view/10.1093/acrefore/9780199975839.001.0001/acrefore-9780199975839-e-324

Ruth, B. J., Wyatt, J., Chiasson, E., Geron, S. M., & Bachman, S. (2006). Social work and public health: Comparing graduates from a dual-degree program. *Journal of Social Work Education, 42*(2), 429–439.

Sable, M. R., Schild, D. R., & Hipp, J. A. (2012). Public health social work. In S. A. Gehlert & T. Browne (Eds.), *Handbook of health social work* (2nd ed., pp. 64–99). Hoboken, NJ: Wiley.

Schultz, R. L. (2007). *Hull House maps and papers: A presentation of the nationalities and wages in a congested district of Chicago, together with comments and essays on problems growing out of the social conditions*. Champaign: University of Illinois Press.

Silverman, R. M., & Patterson, K. L. (2011). The four horsemen of the fair housing apocalypse: A critique of fair housing policy in the USA. *Critical Sociology, 38*(1), 123–140. doi:10.1177/0896920510396385

Skiba, D., Monroe, J., & Wodarski, J. S. (2004). Adolescent substance use: Reviewing the effectiveness of prevention strategies. *Social Work, 49*, 343–353. doi:10.1093/sw/49.3.343

Smith, B. D., & Bride, B. E. (2004). Positive impact: A community-based mental health center for people affected by HIV. *Health and Social Work, 29*, 145–148.

Spencer, M. S., Rosland, A.-M., Kieffer, E. C., Sinco, B. R., Valerio, M., Palmisano, G., . . . Heisler, M. (2011). Effectiveness of a community health worker intervention among

African American and Latino adults with type 2 diabetes: A randomized controlled trial. *American Journal of Public Health, 101*(12), 2253–2260. doi:10.2105/AJPH.2010.300106

Starr, P. (1982). *The social transformation of American medicine: The rise of a sovereign profession and the making of a vast industry.* New York, NY: Basic Books.

Stimpson, J. P., Ju, H., Raji, M. A., & Eschbach, K. (2007). Neighborhood deprivation and health risk behaviors in NHANES III. *American Journal of Health Behavior, 31*(2), 215–222. doi:10.5555/ajhb.2007.31.2.215

Stover, G. N., & Bassett, M. T. (2003). Practice is the purpose of public health. *American Journal of Public Health, 93,* 1799–1801.

Volland, P., Berkman, B., Stein, G., & Vaughn, A. (1999). *Social work education for practice in health care: Final report.* New York: New York Academy of Science.

Vourlekis, B. S., Ell, K., & Padgett, D. (2001). Educating social workers for health care's brave new world. *Journal of Social Work Education, 37,* 177–191.

Wallerstein, N. B., & Duran, B. (2010). Community-based participatory research contributions to intervention research: The intersection of science and practice to improve health equity. *American Journal of Public Health, 100*(Suppl. 1), S40–S46. doi:10.2105/AJPH.2009.184036

Wallerstein, N. B., Yen, I. H., & Syme S. L. (2011). Integration of social epidemiology and community-engaged interventions to improve health equity. *American Journal of Public Health, 101*(5), 822–830. doi:10.2105/AJPH.2008.140988

Walters, K. L., Spencer, M. S., Smukler, M., Allen, H. L., Andrews, C., Browne, T., . . . Uehara, E. (2016). *Health equity: Eradicating health inequalities for future generations* (Grand Challenges for Social Work Initiative Working Paper No. 19). Cleveland, OH: American Academy of Social Work and Social Welfare. Retrieved from http://aaswsw.org/wp-content/uploads/2016/01/WP19-with-cover2.pdf

Wheeler, D. P., & Bragin, M. (2007). Bringing it all back home: Social work and the challenge of returning veterans. *Health and Social Work, 32*(4), 297–300. doi:10.1093/hsw/32.4.297

Williams, D. R., McClellan, M. B., & Rivlin, A. M. (2010). Beyond the Affordable Care Act: Achieving real improvements in Americans' health. *Health Affairs, 29*(8), 1481–1488. doi:10.1377/hlthaff.2010.0071

Winslow, C.-E. A. (1920, January 9). The untilled fields of public health. *Science, 51*(1306), 23–33. doi:10.1126/science.51.1306.23

World Health Organization. (n.d.). *Health promotion.* Retrieved from http://www.who.int/topics/health_promotion/en

7

Integrated Behavioral Health Care

Victoria Stanhope, Janna C. Heyman, James Amarante, and Meredith Doherty

Over the past 10 years, the U.S. health care system has undergone substantial changes, impacted by the Patient Protection and Affordable Care Act (APA; 2010), and motivated by the need to improving health care quality and outcomes, while reducing costs. Health care delivery system changes have included integrating behavioral health care into primary care diverse populations groups, older adults (Alexopoulos et al., 2009; Kaye & Townley, 2013), veterans (Hunter, Goodie, Oordt, & Dobmeyer, 2009), youth (Kang-Yi & Adams, 2017), and other populations.

For many of these population groups, the need for integrated behavioral health care is growing. The United States has seen a sharp increase in the older adult population, with anticipated growth of those age 65 and over nearly doubling by 2050 (Ortman, Velkoff, & Hogan, 2014; U.S. Census Bureau, 2016). As our population ages, there are growing numbers of individuals with complex needs, often impacted by their chronic health conditions, which have led to an increased need for comprehensive behavioral health services (Dangremond, 2015; McClure, Teasell, & Salter, 2015). Currently, an estimated 5 million Americans have Alzheimer's disease, a population that is projected to grow nearly threefold by the year 2050 (Centers for Disease Control and Prevention, 2016). Many of these individuals will have behavioral health care needs.

It is important to recognize the benefits that integrated behavioral health care services may provide for different population groups. For example, with substance abuse on the rise in the United States, particularly with the increase in opioid addiction (Case & Deaton, 2015), behavioral health care can help to screen and treat those in need of services. Veterans may also benefit from integrated behavioral health care to address conditions such as depression and posttraumatic stress disorders (Hunter et al., 2009). For all population groups, addressing prevention is of utmost importance and there is a need to reach the most vulnerable, including individuals living in poverty, those with numerous health problems, and individuals with less access to services.

Integrated behavioral health care has evolved over time. The principles of integrated behavioral health care can be traced back to Engel's biopsychosocial model of the 1960s and the practices of social work, psychology, and medicine, which have used it as a model (Talen & Valeras, 2013). In the 1980s, Spitzer also recognized the need to accurately assess mental health symptoms in primary care settings. His work led to the development of instruments, such as the Patient Health Questionnaire (PHQ-9), that are commonly used in behavioral health settings today (Kroenke & Spitzer, 2002). The Institute of Medicine (IOM; 2001, 2015) reports called for improving the health care delivery system by delivering patient-centered care (PCC), which includes integrating behavioral health care in primary care settings. These efforts have been supported by the Institute for Health care Improvement, which developed the "Triple Aim," a blueprint for reform setting the simultaneous goals of: (a) improving the health of the population; (b) decreasing cost; and (c) enhancing the patient experience (Berwick, Nolan, & Whittington, 2008).

The call for integrated behavioral health care has come from patients, families, and government, in an effort to reshape the way health care is delivered. While there is growing knowledge about how to achieve these goals, there are often challenges, including efforts to repeal the ACA, the lack of access to health insurance throughout the United States, and labor shortages within the health care workforce. Furthermore, only recently have numerous local, regional, and national initiatives promoted practices to start integrating behavioral health in primary care settings (Cohen et al., 2015).

As integrated health care becomes more prevalent, there have been efforts to standardize the terminology. Peek and The National Integration Academy Council (2013) underscore the need for consistent language. They explain that "behavioral health integration also is referred to as 'integrated care,' 'shared care,' 'primary care behavioral health,' or 'integrated primary care'" (p. 11). They developed a lexicon for behavioral health and primary care integration, which is presented in Table 7.1. (For further detail of the clauses, please refer to Peek & The National Integration Academy Council, 2013, pp. 2–9.)

There can be significant variation in the breadth and depth of collaboration among team members in integrated health care. These levels range from minimal collaboration to fully integrated models (Doherty, McDaniel, & Baird, 1996; Heath, Wise Romero, & Reynolds, 2013). Table 7.2 developed by Heath et al. (2013) in their work with SAMHSA-HRSA, described six levels of collaboration/integration with three core categories: (a) Coordinated; (b) Co-located; and (c) Integrated. These different models are defined by the degree to which the interprofessional team functions in terms of location and mode of collaboration.

Within primary care, one of the most common integrated health care models is the IMPACT model (Improving Mood: Promoting Access to Collaborative Treatment), also known as collaborative care. This model was developed by Unützer et al. (2001) to address the depression among seniors and has now been adapted to serve a wide range of populations. By adding a depression care manager to the primary care team, screening for and treating depression using tools, such as the PHQ-9, and coordinating closely with a psychiatrist, the approach demonstrates how behavioral health care can be embedded into the workflow of a primary care clinic. Another key model is the Patient-Centered Medical Home (PCMH), which has been promoted by the ACA. The model places the primary care physician and an interdisciplinary team of providers at the center of a person's care and the entity chiefly responsible for coordinating an individual's care (Vest et al., 2010). Working with a network of providers and using an electronic health record to communicate and implement a shared treatment plan, the PCMH seeks to provide seamless care across different settings.

With these different models and populations, social workers can play a unique role in integrating behavioral health care into primary care settings. They contribute to the interprofessional teams by (a) having an ecological focus; (b) being patient-centered; (c) having knowledge about the biopsychosocial assessment; (d) being able to collaborate both within and across systems, including work with individuals, families, groups, organizations, and communities; (e) overcoming barriers to address access to services; and (f) having an expertise in behavioral health. However, while the integrated health care approach builds on social work values and competencies, there are also new skills for social workers to acquire in order to participate and take leadership roles.

Table 7.1 Lexicon for Behavioral Health and Primary Care Integration: At a Glance

What

The care that results from a practice team of primary care and behavioral health clinicians, working together with patients and families, using a systematic and cost-effective approach to provide patient-centered care for a defined population. This care may address mental health and substance abuse conditions, health behaviors (including their contribution to chronic medical illnesses), life stressors and crises, stress-related physical symptoms, and ineffective patterns of health care utilization.

Defining Clauses	**Corresponding Parameters**
What integrated behavioral health needs to look like in action	*Calibrated acceptable differences between practices*

Parameter numbering at right does not correspond to clause numbering below.

How

1. A practice team tailored to the needs of each patient and situation
   A. With a suitable range of behavioral health and primary care expertise and role functions available to draw from
   B. With shared operations, workflows, and practice culture
   C. Having had formal or on-the-job training
2. With a shared population and mission
   A. A panel of patients in common for total health outcomes
3. Using a systematic clinical approach (and a system that enables the clinical approach to function)
   A. Employing methods to identify those members of the population who need or may benefit
   B. Engaging patients and families in identifying their needs for care and the particular clinicians to provide it
   C. Involving both patients and clinicians in decision-making
   D. Using an explicit, unified, and shared care plan

1. Range of care team function and expertise that can be mobilized
2. Type of spatial arrangement employed for behavioral health and primary care clinicians
3. Type of collaboration employed
4. Method for identifying individuals who need integrated behavioral health and primary care
5. Protocols
   A. Whether protocols are in place or not for engaging patients in integrated care
   B. Level that protocols are followed for initiating integrated care
6. Care plans
   A. Proportion of patients in target groups with shared care plans
   B. Degree to which care plans are implemented and followed
7. Level of systematic follow-up

(continued)

Table 7.1 Lexicon for Behavioral Health and Primary Care Integration: At a Glance (*continued*)

Defining Clauses	Corresponding Parameters
What integrated behavioral health needs to look like in action	*Calibrated acceptable differences between practices*

Parameter numbering at right does not correspond to clause numbering below.

E. With the unified care plan and manner of support to patient and family in a shared electronic health record	
F. With systematic follow-up and adjustment of treatment plans if patients are not improving as expected	

Supported by

4. A community, population, or individuals expecting that behavioral health and primary care will be integrated as a standard of care	8. Level of community expectation for integrated behavioral health as a standard of care
5. Supported by office practice, leadership alignment, and business model	9. Level of office practice reliability and consistency
A. Clinic operational systems and processes	
B. Alignment of purposes, incentives, leadership	10. Level of leadership/administrative alignment and priorities
C. A sustainable business model	11. Level of business model support for integrated behavioral health
6. And continuous quality improvement and measurement of effectiveness	12. Extent that practice data are collected and used to improve the practice
A. Routinely collecting and using practice-based data	
B. Periodically examining and reporting outcomes	

Source: Peek, C. J., & The National Integration Academy Council. (2013). *Lexicon for behavioral health and primary care integration: Concepts and definitions developed by expert consensus.* Rockville, MD: Agency for Health care Research and Quality. Reprinted with permission.

INTEGRATED HEALTH CARE COMPETENCIES

SAMHSA-HRSA Center for Integrated Health Solutions delineated a specific set of competences for Integrated Behavioral Health and Primary Care (Hoge, Morris, Laraia, Pomerantz, & Farley, 2014). These competencies are the following:

1. **Interpersonal Communication.** This refers to using active listening skills and engaging individuals in making decisions about their care and changing health care behaviors. This process is referred to as "patient activation" and stems from building trust and relationships. Interpersonal communication is also exercised among the many providers on a person's team and within the network of care.

Table 7.2 Six Levels of Collaboration/Integration (Core Descriptions)

COORDINATED KEY ELEMENT: COMMUNICATION		CO LOCATED KEY ELEMENT: PHYSICAL PROXIMITY		INTEGRATED KEY ELEMENT: PRACTICE CHANGE	
LEVEL 1 Minimal Collaboration	LEVEL 2 Basic Collaboration at a Distance	LEVEL 3 Basic Collaboration Onsite	LEVEL 4 Close Collaboration Onsite with Some System Integration	LEVEL 5 Close Collaboration Approaching an Integrated Practice	LEVEL 6 Full Collaboration in a Transformed/ Merged Integrated Practice
Behavioral health, primary care and other healthcare providers work:					
In separate facilities, where they:	where they:	In same facility not necessarily same offices, where they:	In same space within the same facility, where they:	In same space within the same facility (some shared space), where they:	In same space within the same facility, sharing all practice space, where they:
>> Have separate systems	>> Have separate systems	>> Have separate systems	>> Share some systems, like scheduling or medical records	>> Actively seek system solutions together or develop work-a-rounds	>> Have resolved most or all system issues, functioning as one integrated system
>> Communicate about cases only rarely and under compelling circumstances	>> Communicate periodically about shared patients	>> Communicate regularly about shared patients, by phone or e-mail	>> Communicate in person as needed	>> Communicate frequently in person	>> Communicate consistently at the system, team and individual levels
>> Communicate, driven by provider need	>> Communicate, driven by specific patient issues	>> Collaborate, driven by need for each other's services and more reliable referral		>> Collaborate, driven by desire to be a member of the care team	>> Collaborate, driven by shared concept of team care
>> May never meet in person	>> May meet as part of larger community				>> Have formal and informal meetings to support integrated model of care

(continued)

Table 7.2 Six Levels of Collaboration/Integration (Core Descriptions) (*continued*)

COORDINATED		CO LOCATED		INTEGRATED	
KEY ELEMENT: COMMUNICATION		**KEY ELEMENT: PHYSICAL PROXIMITY**		**KEY ELEMENT: PRACTICE CHANGE**	
LEVEL 1 **Minimal Collaboration**	**LEVEL 2** **Basic Collaboration at a Distance**	**LEVEL 3** **Basic Collaboration Onsite**	**LEVEL 4** **Close Collaboration Onsite with Some System Integration**	**LEVEL 5** **Close Collaboration Approaching an Integrated Practice**	**LEVEL 6** **Full Collaboration in a Transformed/ Merged Integrated Practice**
Behavioral health, primary care and other healthcare providers work:					
>> Have limited understanding of each other's roles	>> Appreciate each other's roles as resources	>> Meet occasionally to discuss cases due to close proximity >> Feel part of a larger yet non-formal team	>> Collaborate, driven by need for consultation and coordinated plans for difficult patients >> Have regular face-to-face interactions about some patients >> Have a basic understanding of roles and culture	>> Have regular team meetings to discuss overall patient care and specific patient issues >> Have an in-depth understanding of roles and culture	>> Have roles and cultures that blur or blend

Source: Heath, B., Wise Romero, P., & Reynolds, K. (2013). *A review and proposed standard framework for levels of integrated health care.* Washington, DC: SAMHSA-HRSA Center for Integrated Health Solutions. Reprinted with permission.

2. **Collaboration and Teamwork.** The World Health Organization (WHO; 2010) states the importance of teamwork: "In the current global climate, health workers also need to be interprofessional" (p. 36). As discussed in Chapter 1, interprofessional practice is defined as "different health or social care professionals who share a team identity and work together closely in an integrated and interdependent manner to solve problems, deliver services and enhance health outcomes" (Institute of Medicine [IOM], 2015, p. xii). Involvement with the individual and family members is critical for team success. The nature of teamwork requires that each member of the team recognizes and respects the value of each member (Mitchell et al., 2012). Oyama (2016) explains that in order to "work as a team one must think like a team" (p. 9). Often an integrated health care team may need to pull in another perspective, which may in turn change how the team interacts. This additional perspective can be extremely beneficial in both working with the individual and family to develop, refine, or assess care plans. While the team members receive input from others, they can still function to work together to support the shared goals and decisions of the team.

3. **Screening and Assessment.** Social workers need the skills to be able to conduct screenings and assessment across settings, especially for conditions associated with chronic illness. Using standard and structured screening tools, social workers can screen and assess for mental disorders, trauma, substance abuse, activities of daily living, and physical illnesses such as diabetes and asthma.

4. **Care Planning and Care Coordination.** With shared plans, social workers need to be able to coordinate across multiple providers to ensure that plans are patient-centered and calibrated to the person's level of need. This requires constant communication with other health care providers to ensure the flow of information and collaboration.

5. **Intervention.** The integrated health care setting utilizes short-term evidence-based interventions that are effective in less structured fast-moving settings. These interventions include motivational interviewing, cognitive behavioral therapy, relaxation training, psychotropic medications, psychoeducation, and case management. Other key interventions focus on health promotion, wellness self-management, nutrition and weight management, and smoking cessation.

6. **Cultural Competence and Adaptation.** Addressing the persistent health disparities in care requires a culturally responsive health care workforce attuned to cultural and linguistic preferences in how health care is delivered. Understanding the role of social determinants, promoting a diverse workforce, and working closely with communities are also a key part of delivering integrated health care.

7. **Systems-Oriented Practice.** Integrated health care often demands a higher level of coordination so that social workers are intervening at the organizational level as well as the direct practice level. Understanding health care financing and being able to demonstrate how specific services contribute to cost-effectiveness is vital when negotiating the new health care environment. Competencies related to evaluating practice according to quality and implementing health care reform initiatives will help social workers take leadership roles in their settings.

8. **Practice-Based Learning and Quality Improvement Strategies.** Increasingly, social workers must have the skills to keep current with the evidence base and new practices. Related to this knowledge is being able to determine treatment fidelity across the team, adapting interventions when necessary, and using data to inform ongoing practice. While medical centers generally provide access for patient care staff to online libraries and continuing education experiences, not all agencies have the learning infrastructure to provide access to the newest knowledge and intervention technologies.

9. **Informatics.** The electronic health record is the infrastructure that facilitates all aspects of the integrated health care approach. Social workers can utilize the electronic health record to communicate with other health care professionals, receive prompts for screenings or make referrals for behavioral health, track individual and population health outcomes, and document services for quality improvement and reimbursement. Technology with integrated health care settings also includes decision support tools, social media and mobile technologies to manage wellness, and telemedicine for aging and rural populations.

PATIENT-CENTERED CARE

A central organizing principle for the delivery of integrated health services across all settings is that care be patient-centered. The IOM (2001) has defined patient-centered as "care that is respectful of and responsive to individual patient preferences, needs and values and ensuring values guide all clinical decisions" (p. 6). PCC orients around the patient user experience, utilizes techniques such as shared decision making and decision support, and aims to improve patient engagement, patient satisfaction, and clinical outcomes. Although PCC is closely aligned with social work values such as client self-determination, the medical model within which the majority of social workers practice has often placed individuals in a passive role with respect to their own health care. However, beyond the ethical imperative, there is a growing evidence base that has demonstrated that PCC improves outcomes. A systematic review of personalized care planning for people with chronic illnesses found improved self-management capabilities in terms of both self-efficacy and self-care activities, reduced depression, and a moderately positive effect on physical health outcomes (Coulter et al., 2015).

Integrated behavioral health care is patient-centered by actively engaging people in their health care decisions and orienting care plans to an individual's preferences and life goals. The Chronic Care model demonstrates how quality is closely related to how persons feel about their care, communications with their provider, and ownership over treatment decisions, which are often complicated (Wagner, Austin, & Von Korff, 1996). While PCC is an overarching principle that applies both to the organization and delivery of care, specific evidence-based practices that promote PCC include shared decision making (Adams & Drake, 2006), person-centered care planning (Adams & Grieder, 2013), motivational interviewing (Lundahl et al., 2013), and wellness self-management (Goldberg et al., 2012).

PRACTICE

There are a number of issues that relate to direct practice that impact the integration of behavioral health care. These include issues related to identifying patients who may have a need for both medical and behavioral health care, care coordination, and issues related to the complex interplay between medical and behavioral health issues. The ways in which these issues arise may vary depending on the level of integration. The three primary models of integration, as well as the ways in which these practice issues impact care in each model, as well as in nonintegrated systems are described in the following.

As described in Table 7.2, there are three main systems of integrated care, including coordination, co-location, and integration (Heath et al., 2013). Coordinated care represents the more traditional approach to health care in which primary care and behavioral health providers work in separate offices and do not share systems. Co-located systems provide increased opportunity for collaboration. In this approach, providers work in a common facility. This may be in the form of having separate offices in a medical building, working in a shared office space, or the inclusion of a behavioral health provider in a primary care office. A full integrated model transforms practice into a "single health system treating the whole person" (Heath et al., 2013, p. 6) and involves a high level of collaboration between behavioral health and primary care providers.

Identifying patients who may benefit from the integration of behavioral health care is best done through effective screening and assessment. Comprehensive screening may raise additional concerns that were not initially identified, such as depression, anxiety, and other health and mental health risks. Screening and brief assessment tools are now widely utilized and the following are some examples of common tools used in the behavioral health care setting. The PHQ-9 is a validated nine-item screening tool for depressive symptoms (Johnson, Harris, Spitzer, & Williams, 2002; Kroenke, Spitzer, Williams, & Löwe; 2010). It was also adapted for adolescents as the Patient Health Questionnaire-9 Adolescents (PHQ-A). The Beck Depression Inventory for Primary Care is a seven-item instrument that has been used to screen for depression in primary care settings (Steer, Ball, Ranieri, & Beck, 1999). The Generalized Anxiety Disorder 7 Item Scale (GADS-7) has been used to screen for generalized anxiety disorder and is considered a validated brief measure (Spitzer, Kroenke, Williams, & Löwe, 2006). Other instruments, such as the CAGE, a four-item instrument for screening for problems with alcohol (Ewing, 1984), AUDIT, used for alcohol misuse (Saunders, Aasland, Babor, de la Fuente, & Grant, 1993), and DAST, used to screen for drug use other than alcohol (Gavin, Ross, & Skinner, 1989), are validated instruments used when screening for substance abuse. In addition, Curtis and Christian (2012) have written a screening and assessment primer for screening and brief assessment that can flag other risk factors as well. Further assessment may be needed for each individual as his or her risk is identified.

Often an individual may be screened and assessed to address new health concerns. For example, a patient may screen positively for generalized anxiety disorder after the application of the GADS-7. This would indicate that further assessment is needed. Before establishing shared goals and decision making for care, the individual needs to understand what the problem or condition may be. In order to help, the social worker and other members of the interprofessional team may be asked: (a) to provide further information about the diagnosis and what the test(s) revealed; (b) to identify and explore other health-related concerns; and (c) to listen to the life stories regarding concerns about the patient's family, friends, pets, and other complex issues.

If further treatment is needed, integrated systems of care provide opportunities to facilitate the referral process. This process will differ depending on the level of integration. In a coordinated care situation, the primary care provider may refer the patient to a behavioral health provider and these two parties may engage in occasional follow-up communication. A co-located system may involve the scheduling of an appointment with an embedded behavioral health provider. In an integrated practice, the primary care provider may conduct a warm hand-off, introducing the patient to the behavioral health provider, who may be able to further evaluate the patient in the moment, increasing the likelihood that the patient will address the identified behavioral health concerns (Collins, Hewson, Munger, & Wade, 2010).

The complex interplay of the issues that cause patients distress and health problems may be related to complications associated with increasing integration of care. For example, it may not always be evident whether a behavioral health issue or medical issue is at the core of a patient's presenting problem. In many cases, behavioral health and medical issues can be interdependent, potentially creating further complications for patients. This not only underscores the importance of integrating care, but also represents challenges in working with different health care professionals (Carpenter, Schneider, Brandon, & Wolf, 2003).

Further integration of behavioral health may allow providers to uncover the etiology of the symptoms and may present an opportunity to treat the cause of patients' symptoms, potentially improving health outcomes. Many behavioral health disorders contribute to or mimic the symptoms of medical issues and doctors working in nonintegrated systems may be less likely to identify them. For example, internalizing disorders such as depression and anxiety are often accompanied by somatic symptoms (Haftgoli et al., 2010). Medical providers without access to integrated behavioral health may use a purely medical approach to the treatment of such symptoms, allowing the underlying behavioral health disorder to go untreated (Kroenke et al., 2010).

Social workers receiving referrals to see patients who medical providers identify as having behavioral health concerns may work in ways similar to other settings. Medical records, however, may be shared; so, in such cases, the social worker would be able to access the patient's medical treatment history. This may expand the social worker's capacity to conduct a thorough biopsychosocial assessment and understand the complex factors that impact the behavioral health concern. Social workers practicing in settings with patients with interdependent medical and behavioral health concerns may be required to collaborate with medical providers more frequently, rather than just sharing an electronic health record. Similarly, social workers practicing in integrative settings that use a disease management model may work as care managers who monitor patients' adherence to treatment for chronic conditions and provide brief psychotherapy when necessary (Collins et al., 2010).

There are many ways in which social workers can use different approaches to increase treatment compliance because a number of medical disorders require behavioral interventions to ensure effectiveness of treatment. For example, medical providers often struggle to get patients to comply with the dietary changes necessary to effectively treat conditions such as heart disease and diabetes. Motivational interviewing has been found to be particularly effective for such purposes (Christie & Channon, 2014; Creber et al., 2016) and a social worker placed in an integrated practice may be able to use such an approach to increase patient adherence and improve health outcomes.

Case Example 7.1

Leonard is a 59-year-old male who lives in a small city. He worked as a plumber for most of his life but went out on disability last year after having a heart attack. Leonard is overweight and has cardiovascular disease and high blood pressure, which his doctor has had difficulty managing with medication. Leonard's physician has urged him to maintain a strict diet and increase his physical activity but Leonard has had difficulty getting out of his old routines and incorporating a healthy lifestyle. Leonard's physician belongs to a medical group that has made recent attempts to incorporate behavioral health care in the practice. They have hired a part-time social worker and the physicians have begun using quick screening instruments to identify patients who may benefit from behavioral health services. On his most recent visit, Leonard's physician administered the PHQ-9 which suggested he may have moderate depression.

As illustrated in Case Example 7.1, Leonard may benefit from integrative behavioral health care for a number of reasons. Leonard has a life-threatening illness but is having difficulty complying with his physician's treatment recommendations. A social worker can help Leonard explore these difficulties and help him increase his motivation to address his medical concerns. Leonard's depression may be one factor which contributes to his difficulty making lifestyle changes and a social worker may be able to help Leonard work on his depression, so he is more capable of making the lifestyle changes that are so important. Similarly, a social worker may be able to help motivate Leonard to make such lifestyle changes, which may impact both his medical and behavior health issues. In such a case where medical and behavioral health issues affect each other, a social worker can play diverse roles, helping the patient uncover motivations for not properly addressing his health issues and alleviating the symptoms of his behavioral health issue. In working with and establishing a unique relationship with the patient, the social worker may find ways in which the interprofessional team may be able to more effectively address the patient's health needs. This feedback can be provided to the team, increasing the effectiveness of the integrated approach.

Integrated health settings can also be used to deliver supportive counseling within the primary care setting to people coping with the emotional and psychological effects of serious illness. Many cancer survivors return to their primary care providers once active treatment is complete; however, cancer is increasingly considered a chronic illness that requires ongoing monitoring and support.

Case Example 7.2

Sharon is a 49-year-old woman in early remission from breast cancer. After chemotherapy and radiation treatments were completed, she returned to her primary care provider for ongoing care. She expected to feel relieved once the cancer treatment was over, but instead she experienced a persistent fear that the cancer would return. She began making frequent appointments with her primary care doctor with a variety of somatic complaints, like tingling sensations, visual changes, abdominal discomfort, and nausea. Thorough physical examinations and diagnostic testing did not explain these symptoms. Suspecting a mental health issue related to adjustment to cancer diagnosis, the primary care doctor and the social worker met with Sharon together to discuss her health concerns. They were able to conduct screenings for anxiety and depression, provide a prescription for an antidepressant, and offer short-term weekly counseling sessions with the social worker to help her cope with recent life changes.

In Case Example 7.2, Sharon's somatic symptoms had the potential to lead to the overuse of diagnostics. Because a social worker was available to help Sharon to manage her health anxieties, the primary care physician was able to focus on responding to her physical health needs. In this setting, in which the social worker is a team member in the primary care practice, the team has a number of ways to collaborate and coordinate care for each patient. First, an integrated treatment plan that includes mental health diagnoses and goals can be created and reviewed by the entire care team. The electronic medical record should be accessible to all members of the interprofessional care team and documentation can be reviewed from prior visits with other providers. Regular face-to-face case conferences can be used to discuss complex cases, develop a plan of action that addresses medical and psychosocial needs, coordinate care, and make appropriate external referrals.

Social workers are important in integrated health care. They can run support and psychoeducation groups that improve access and engagement in integrated settings. For examples, social workers and other mental health providers can develop groups that teach wellness, support tobacco cessation, and provide chronic illness self-management support. These group interventions can focus on developing peer support, teaching and practicing new health-related skills, and identifying barriers to behavior change (Horevitz & Manoleas, 2013). Support groups that target common mental health conditions like depression and anxiety can also be delivered within these settings. Prevention and health promotion efforts are also part of the social work role in integrated health. Social workers can design health promotion campaigns in and across health care organizations that stress the mind–body connection in common conditions and make resources and referrals readily available. The purpose of these interventions is to increase access and engagement by normalizing mental health and psychosocial issues, reducing the associated stigma, and making resources available and highly visible in traditional health settings.

Macro integrated health efforts aim to track and improve population health. Social workers in these roles may conduct community needs assessments and develop programs that attract underserved populations into care by targeting their needs and concerns (Stanhope, Tondora, Davidson, & Choy-Brown, 2015). Community members can be asked to participate in ongoing feedback forums or advisory councils that guide the development of new health programs that reflect the values and needs of the community. Building formal and informal partnerships with other health and social service agencies are an important aspect of delivering high-quality population level health care. Interagency partnerships can facilitate referrals and access to care, track performance targets and population/community level health outcomes of interest. For example, hospitals, integrated primary care settings, and supported housing/residential treatment facilities can form medical communities that ease transitions from inpatient to outpatient services for people living in the community with multiple health conditions. By collecting outcome and process data on these care transitions, these medical communities can identify gaps in care and work on developing targeted solutions rapidly.

POLICY

The health care delivery system in the United States has often been described as fragmented, with limited integration (Agha, Frandsen, & Rebitzer, 2017; Friedman, Friedman, & Friedman, 2016). This fragmentation may lead to disparities in access to health care across the spectrum (Davis et al., 2015). Integrated behavioral health in primary care has begun to address fragmentation. However, in the coming years it is imperative that further development and expansion of integrated behavioral care include regulatory, legal, operational, and educational improvements.

Ader et al. (2015) highlighted five policy recommendations to improve integration of behavioral health and primary care, which were developed as part of the 2013 Patient-Centered Medical Home Research Conference. These recommendations include: (a) building demonstration projects to test existing approaches and evaluate them using a common central framework; (b) developing interdisciplinary training programs to support critical members of the care team; (c) implementing strategies to improve population health; strengthening relationship between primary care practices and community resources; (d) eliminating carve-outs and aligning innovative payment models; and (e) developing population-based measures to evaluate behavioral health integration.

These recommendations can help to improve practice and expand the health care delivery system. Physicians, nurses, social workers, and other health care professionals need to advocate and advance these recommendations to enhance integrated care.

The comprehensive primary care plus (CPC+) model is another example of innovation in integrating behavioral health into primary care. This model involves a public–private partnership currently made up of 54 payers in 14 regions, supporting 2,866 primary care practices and serving up to 1.76 million patients (Centers for Medicare and Medicaid Services [CMS], 2017a). There are five key functions of the CPC+ model and social workers have key roles in two of these: care management and care coordination. The CPC+ model helps improve services for patients who may benefit from both longitudinal and episodic care management This can include the use of a behavioral health specialist to improve the "management of chronic general medical illnesses, and facilitate specialty care engagement for serious mental illness" (CMS, 2017b). Providers utilize screenings and brief interventions, evidence-based approaches, and support changes in behavior to improve health outcomes. The CPC+ model has still to be widely implemented, highlighting the need for increased advocacy to broaden such policy measures.

Payment for integrated health care varies across states and plans, which often leads to further fragmentation (Kathol et al., 2014). Allocation of Medicaid dollars and whether "managed behavioral health organizations are 'carved-in' (owned by medical insurer but sold as an independent insurance product) or 'carved out' (owned by a standalone behavioral health insurance vendor) segregate[s] benefit management by states" (Miller, Ross, Davis, Melek, & Kathol, 2017, p. 57) may influence the way services are delivered. Reimbursement practices also have unintended consequences in clinical delivery of integrated care (Kathol et al., 2010). Miller et al. (2017) suggest that "global payment structures provide the best fit to enable and sustain integrated behavioral health clinicians in ways that align with the Triple Aim" (p. 55).

Because there are clear advantages to integration, it is important that social workers have the necessary skills to advocate for and practice integrative behavioral health care. Part of this begins early in educating social workers to practice holistically. The Council of Social Work Education "recognizes a holistic view of competence; that is, the demonstration of competence is informed by knowledge, values, skills, and cognitive and affective processes that include the social worker's critical thinking, affective reactions, and exercise of judgment in regard to unique practice situations" (Council of Social Work Education, 2015, p. 6). It is essential to prepare students to work in an integrated care environment that requires specialized skills (Hunter et al., 2009). Ensuring that educational policy emphasizes this holistic competency is essential to preparing social workers for both working in and advocating for individuals in integrative health care settings.

Recent workforce initiatives by the federal agency Health Resources and Services Administration (HRSA) have focused on preparing providers for integrated behavioral health care. Collaborating with SAMHSA and the National Council on Behavioral Health, the agency has created the Center for Integrated Health Solutions (www.integration. samhsa.gov), a comprehensive website, which disseminates information on best practices, financing, and research related to integrated health care. HRSA has also provided grants to schools of social work to train social workers in integrated health care through specialized placements and enhanced curriculum. The Council on Social Work Education has supported these initiatives by developing curriculum focused on integrated health care (www.cswe.org/Centers-Initiatives/Initiatives/Social-Work-and-Integrated -Behavioral-Healthcare-P) and advocating for social workers to be included in national interprofessional education initiatives.

RESEARCH

There are several integrated behavioral health care models that have been assessed. One of the seminal works is the IMPACT research, which is viewed as a collaborative care chronic disease management model for older adults with depression (Unützer et al., 2001, 2002). This model is built on a team-based approach to health care, which included a case manager, often a social worker, primary care provider, and psychiatrist. Routine screening for depression is conducted. A range of treatment options includes brief psychotherapy and medication. Research has indicated that the IMPACT model reduced depression and had lower health care costs (Unützer et al, 2008).

Other research with older adults and integrated care is the Prevention of Suicide in Primary Care Elderly Collaborative Trial (PROSPECT). This research examined the effectiveness of using case managers, social workers, nurses, and psychologists working with physicians to monitor and assess depression among older adults. Using a randomized controlled trial, the PROSPECT study found that, compared to usual care, the intervention led to improved access to care and declines in suicidal ideation, earlier treatment response, and higher rates of remission (Alexopoulos et al., 2009).

More research is needed to understand the processes and outcomes of interprofessional practice (Reeves, Boet, Zierler, & Kitto, 2015). Reeves, Perrier, Goldman, Freeth, and Zwarenstein (2013) documented a growing number of studies in the field, but recognized that further studies are needed on program-specific interventions, and other practice areas.

Research conducted by the New York State Department of Health (2013) compared PCMH sites to non-PCMH sites. They concluded that "PCMH providers have outperformed non-PCMH providers in several domains of care, in particular, management of chronic disease which is essential to improving outcomes, quality of life and lowering costs" (p. 3). This research advances knowledge about the impact of a statewide PCMH initiative on patient outcomes and quality of care.

There is also a need to increase our understanding of PCC, namely how integrated behavioral health models can embed patient-centered approaches and their potential to improve both the processes and outcomes of care. Overall, we know that having people more actively involved in their care in terms of decision making promotes adherence to both medical and mental health treatment (Davidson et al., 2012). One study of PCC planning among low-income African American and Latino adults found increased involvement in planning related to health, housing, education, and employment (Tondora et al., 2010). In a randomized controlled study within a community mental health setting, clinics that practiced PCC planning showed a significant increase in medication adherence over time and a significant decrease in missed appointments compared to those delivering treatment-as-usual (Stanhope, Ingoglia, Schmelter, & Marcus, 2013). As patient care approaches are increasingly promoted in primary care settings, further implementation research is needed to understand how organizational factors and provider behavior influence the adoption and effectiveness of PCC in real-world settings.

CONCLUSION

The need for integrated health care driven by the poor outcomes and high costs prevalent throughout the U.S. health care system has led to significant changes in service delivery, particularly in primary care settings. In order to meet the Triple Aim of improving the quality of care and population health while reducing costs, many have focused on primary care as a key site for health care reform. The strategy of making primary care the "hub" of each person's care has been realized by innovative models such as the IMPACT model and PCMHs. These models build on the fundamental components of integrated behavioral care which are the delivery of holistic PCC, the use of interprofessional teams focused on both medical and behavioral care, and ensuring care coordination across systems to provide a seamless experience for the individual. Settings with integrated behavioral health care can take many forms, from having close communications or networks with other providers to co-location of facilities or being a fully integrated self-contained system.

Social work as a profession is now in the process of adapting to these profound changes in the health care environment that will likely continue irrespective of the current political climate. This adaptation means being able to demonstrate the contribution of social workers to integrated health approaches, particularly through our role on interprofessional teams, our strengths in engaging and activating patients in their own care, addressing health disparities, delivering holistic PCC and our ability to coordinate care across systems. Primary care will increasingly provide opportunities for social workers, particularly as these settings employ more people with behavioral health expertise. But these changes also put the onus on social workers developing a more robust knowledge of health conditions, screening tools, brief interventions, and informatics. In addition to broadening the profession's practice repertoire, social workers must also continue to advocate for health care policies that improve people's access to health care and fund innovative models that integrate care. The continuing opposition to health care reform demands that social workers be constantly vigilant in fighting for policies that improve the health and mental health of vulnerable populations.

CHAPTER DISCUSSION QUESTIONS

1. Review Peek's Lexicon for Behavioral Health and Primary Care Integration and discuss how a practice team might tailor the needs of each patient and situation.

2. Select one of the SAMHSA-HRSA Center for Integrated Health Solutions competences for Integrated Behavioral Health and Primary Care and reflect on the core elements that may comprise the competency.

3. Discuss the unique contributions of patient-centered care.

4. Discuss the current federal policies that have shaped integrated behavioral health care.

CASE EXAMPLE AND DISCUSSION QUESTIONS

Case Example 7.3

Sam is a 68-year-old woman with a history of depression and anxiety. Blood tests from her annual physical examination revealed she had very high blood sugar and she was diagnosed with type 2 diabetes. The physician wrote a prescription for metformin and home blood sugar testing supplies, and recommended she return for a follow-up appointment in 1 month. Sam did not present for her 1 month follow-up and was not reachable by phone. It was unclear how she was managing her dangerously high blood sugar. As part of the clinic intake process, every patient completes a HIPAA consent form to involve family or friends in their care. The social worker on staff was able to locate this information

(continued)

Case Example 7.3   *(continued)*

and reach out to Sam's daughter Isabelle. Isabelle was aware of her mother's diabetes diagnosis and informed the team that she had refused to fill her prescriptions and was not testing her sugar levels at home. She frequently complained of fatigue, tingling in arms and legs, hot flashes, and seemed to be more forgetful than usual.

Questions for Discussion

1. What steps should the social worker take first to make sure Sam gets the care she needs?

2. Which interventions could be helpful in engaging Sam in care? Describe how social work competencies and practices can be used to improve patient access and engagement.

3. Discuss the ethical implications of family involvement in medical decision making and adherence. How should the social worker negotiate these concerns?

REFERENCES

Adams, J. R., & Drake, R. E. (2006). Shared decision-making and evidence-based practice. *Community Mental Health Journal, 42*(1), 87–105.

Adams, N., & Grieder, D. (2013). *Treatment planning for person-centered care: Shared decision making for whole health* (2nd ed.). Boston, MA: Academic Press.

Ader, J., Stille, C. J., Keller, D., Miller, B. F., Barr, M. S., & Perrin, J. M. (2015). The medical home and integrated behavioral health: Advancing the policy agenda. *Pediatrics, 135*(5), 909–917.

Agha, L., Frandsen, B., & Rebitzer, J. B. (2017). *Causes and consequences of fragmented care delivery: Theory, evidence, and public policy.* NBER Working Papers from National Bureau of Economic Research.

Alexopoulos, G. S., Reynolds, C. F., Bruce, M. L., Katz, I. R., Raue, P. J., Mulsant, B. H., . . . Ten Have, T. (2009). Reducing suicidal ideation and depression in older primary care patients: 24 month outcome of the PROSPECT study. *The American Journal of Psychiatry, 166*(8), 882–890. doi:10.1176/appi.ajp.2009.08121779

Berwick, D. M., Nolan, T. W., & Whittington, J. (2008). The triple aim: Care, health, and cost. *Health Affairs, 27*, 759–769. doi:10.1377/hlthaff.27.3.759

Carpenter, J., Schneider, J., Brandon, T., & Wolf, D. (2003). Working in multidisciplinary community mental health team: The impact on social workers and health care professionals of integrated mental health care. *British Journal of Social Work, 33*(8), 1081–1103.

Case, A., & Deaton, A. (2015). Rising morbidity and mortality in midlife among white non-Hispanic Americans in the 21st century. *Proceedings of the National Academy of Sciences of the United States of America, 112*(49), 15078.

Centers for Disease Control and Prevention. (2016). *Preventive health care.* Retrieved from http://www.cdc.gov/healthcommunication/ToolsTemplates/EntertainmentEd/Tips/PreventiveHealth.html

Centers for Medicare and Medicaid Services. (2017a). Comprehensive primary care plus. *Innovation models.* Retrieved from https://innovation.cms.gov/initiatives/comprehensive-primary-care-plus

Centers for Medicare and Medicaid Services. (2017b). CPC+ behavioral health integration menu of options. *Comprehensive primary care plus.* Retrieved from https://innovation.cms.gov/Files/x/cpcplus-bhinteg-options.pdf

Christie, D., & Channon, S. (2014). The potential for motivational interviewing to improve outcomes in the management of diabetes and obesity in paediatric and adult populations: A clinical review. *Diabetes, Obesity and Metabolism, 16*(5), 381–387. doi:10.1111/dom.12195

Cohen, D. J., Balasubramanian, B. A., Davis, M., Hall, J., Gunn, R., Stange, K. C., . . . Miller, B. F. (2015). Understanding care integration from the ground up: Five organizing constructs that shape integrated practices. *Journal of the American Board of Family Medicine, 28*(Suppl. 1), S7–S20. doi:10.3122/jabfm.2015.S1.150050

Collins, C., Hewson, D. L., Munger, R., & Wade, T. (2010*). Evolving models of behavioral health integration in primary care.* New York, NY: Millbrook Memorial Fund.

Coulter, A., Entwistle, V. A., Eccles, A., Ryan, S., Shepperd, S., & Perera, R. (2015). Personalised care planning for adults with chronic or long-term health conditions. *Cochrane Database Systematic Review,* (3), CD010523. doi:10.1002/14651858.CD010523.pub2

Council of Social Work Education. (2015). *2015 Educational policy and accreditation standards educational policy and accreditation standards for Baccalaureate and Master's Social Work programs.* Alexandria, VA: Author.

Creber, R. M., Patey, M., Lee, C. S., Kuan, A., Jurgens, C., & Riegel, B. (2016). Motivational interviewing to improve self-care for patients with chronic heart failure: MITI-HF randomized controlled trial. *Patient Education and Counseling, 99*(2), 256–264. doi:10.1016/j.pec.2015.08.031

Cuijpers, P., Sijbrandij, M., Koole, S. L., Andersson, G., Beekman, A. T., & Reynolds, C. F. (2014). Adding psychotherapy to antidepressant medication in depression and anxiety disorders: A meta-analysis. *World Psychiatry, 13*(1), 56–67. doi:10.1002/wps.20089

Curtis, R., & Christian, E. (2012) A screening and assessment primer. In R. Curtis & E. Christian (Eds.), *Integrated care: Applying theory to practice* (pp. 35–57). New York, NY: Routledge.

Dangremond, C. K. (2015) A visual overview of health care delivery in the United States. In J. R. Knickman & A. R. Kovner, (Eds.), *Jonas and Kovner's health care delivery in the United States* (11th ed., pp. 13–28). New York, NY: Springer Publishing.

Davidson, L., Roe, D., Stern, E., Zisman-Ilani, Y., O'Connell, M., & Corrigan, P. (2012). If I choose it, am I more likely to use it? *International Journal of Person Centered Medicine, 2*(3), 577–592.

Davis, T. S., Guada, J., Reno, R., Peck, A., Evans, S., Sigal, L. M., & Swenson, S. (2015). Integrated and culturally relevant care: A model to prepare social workers for primary care behavioral health practice. *Social Work in Health Care, 54*(10), 909–938. doi:10.1080/00981389.2015.1062456

Doherty, W. J., McDaniel, S. H., & Baird, M. A. (1996). Five levels of primary care/behavioral health collaboration. *Behavioral Health care Tomorrow, 5,* 25–27.

Ewing, J. A. (1984). Detecting alcoholism. The CAGE questionnaire. *Journal of the American Medical Association, 252*(14), 1905–1907.

Friedman, D., Friedman, H. H., & Friedman, L. W. (2016). US health care: A system in need of a cure. *American Journal of Medical Research, 3*(1), 125.

Gavin, D. R., Ross, H. E., & Skinner, H. A. (1989). Diagnostic validity of the drug abuse screening test in the assessment of DSM-III drug disorders. *Addiction, 84*(3), 301–307.

Goldberg, R. W., Dickerson, F., Lucksted, A., Brown, C. H., Weber, E., Tenhula, W. N., Kreyenbuhl, J., & Dixon, L. B. (2012). Living well: An intervention to improve self-management of medical illness for individuals with serious mental illness. *Psychiatric Services, 64,* 51–57.

Haftgoli, N., Favrat, B., Verdon, F., Vaucher, P., Bischoff, T., Burnand, B., & Herzig, L. (2010). Patients presenting with somatic complaints in general practice: Depression, anxiety and somatoform disorders are frequent and associated with psychosocial stressors. *BMC Family Practice, 11*(1), 67. doi:10.1186/1471-2296-11-67

Heath, B., Wise Romero, P., & Reynolds, K. (2013). *A review and proposed standard framework for levels of integrated health care.* Washington, DC: SAMHSA-HRSA Center for Integrated Health Solutions.

Hoge, M. A., Morris, J. A., Laraia, M., Pomerantz, A., & Farley, T. (2014). *Core competencies for integrated behavioral health and primary care.* Washington, DC: SAMHSA-HRSA Center for Integrated Health Solutions.

Horevitz, E., & Manoleas, P. (2013). Professional competencies and training needs of professional social workers in integrated behavioral health in primary care. *Social Work in Health Care, 52*(8), 752–787.

Hunter, C. L., Goodie, J. L., Oordt, M. S., & Dobmeyer, A. C. (2009). *Integrated behavioral health in primary care; Step-by-step guidance for assessment and intervention.* Washington, DC: American Psychological Association.

Institute of Medicine. (2001). *Crossing the quality chasm: A new health system for the 21st century.* Washington, DC: National Academies Press.

Institute of Medicine. (2015). *Measuring the impact of interprofessional education on collaborative practice and patient outcomes.* Washington, DC: National Academies Press.

Johnson, J. G., Harris, E. S., Spitzer, R. L., & Williams, J. B. W. (2002). The patient health questionnaire for adolescents: Validation of an instrument for the assessment of mental disorders among adolescent primary care patients. *Journal of Adolescent Health, 30*(3), 196–220.

Kang-Yi, C. D., & Adams, D. R. (2017). Youth with behavioral health disorders aging out of foster care: A systematic review and implications for policy, research, and practice. *Journal of Behavioral Health Service Research, 44*(1), 25–51. doi:10.1007/s11414-015-9480-9

Kathol, R. G., Degruy, F., & Rollman, B. L. (2014). Value-based financially stable behavioral health components in patient-centered medical homes. *Annual of Family Medicine, 12,* 172–175. doi:10.1370/afm.1619

Kathol, R. G., Butler, M., McAlpine, D. D, & Kane, R. L. (2010). Barriers to physical and mental conditions integrated service delivery. *Psychometric Medicine, 72*(6), 511–518. doi:10.1097/PSY.0b013e3181e2c4a0

Kaye, N., & Townley, C. (2013). Medical and health homes provide enhanced care coordination for elders with complex conditions. *Generations, Journal of the American Society on Aging, 37*(2) 39–46.

Kroenke, K., & Spitzer, R. (2002). The PHQ-9: A new depression and diagnostic severity measure. *Psychiatric Annals, 32,* 509–521.

Kroenke, K., Spitzer, R. L., Williams, J. B., & Löwe, B. (2010). The patient health questionnaire somatic, anxiety, and depressive symptom scales: A systematic review. *General Hospital Psychiatry, 32*(4), 345–359. doi:10.1016/j.genhosppsych.2010.03.006

Lundahl, B., Moleni, T., Burke, B. L., Butters, R., Tollefson, D., Butler, C., & Rollnick, S. (2013). Motivational interviewing in medical care settings: A systematic review and meta-analysis of randomized controlled trials. *Patient Education Counseling, 93*(2), 157–168. doi:10.1016/j.pec.2013.07.012

McClure, A., Teasell, R., & Salter, K. (2015). Psychosocial issues educational supplement. In R. Teasell, N. Foley, K. Salter, M. Richardson, L. Allen, N. Hussein, . . . M. Speechley (Eds.), *Evidence based review of stroke rehabilitation* (16th ed.). London, ON, Canada: Heart and Stroke Foundation, Canadian Partnership for Stroke Recovery. Retrieved from http://www.ebrsr.com/sites/default/files/F_Psychosocial_Issues_(Questions_and_Answers).pdf

Miller, B., Ross, K. M., Davis, M. M., Melek, S. P., & Kathol, R. (2017). Payment reform in the Patient-centered Medical Home: Enabling and sustaining integrated behavioral health care. *American Psychologist, 72*(1), 55–68.

Mitchell, P., Wynia, M., Golden, R., McNellis, B., Okun, S., Webb, C. E., . . . Von Kohorn, I. (2012). Core principles & values of effective team-based health care [Discussion paper]. Washington, DC: Institute of Medicine. Retrieved from https://www.nationalahec.org/pdfs/vsrt-team-based-care-principles-values.pdf

New York State Department of Health. (2013). *The patient-centered medical home initiative in New York State Medicaid.* Albany, NY: Author.

Ortman, J. M., Velkoff, V., & Hogan, H. (2014). *An aging nation: The older population in the United States.* Current Population Reports, P25-1140. U.S. Census Bureau, Washington, DC.

Oyama, O. (2016). Introduction in the integrated primary care health. In M. A. Burg & O. Oyama (Eds.), *The behavioral health specialists in primary care* (pp. 1–20). New York, NY: Springer Publishing.

Peek, C. J., & The National Integration Academy Council. (2013). Lexicon for behavioral health and primary care integration: Concepts and definitions developed by expert consensus. Rockville, MD: Agency for Health care Research and Quality.

Reeves, S., Boet, S., Zierler, B., & Kitto, S. (2015). Interprofessional education and practice guide no. 3: Evaluating interprofessional education. *Journal of Interprofessional Care, 29*(4), 305–312. doi:10.3109/13561820.2014

Reeves, S., Perrier, L., Goldman, J., Freeth, D., & Zwarenstein, M. (2013). Interprofessional education: Effects on professional practice and health care outcomes (update). *Cochrane Database of Systematic Reviews,* (3), CD002213. doi:10.1002/14651858.CD002213.pub3

Saunders, J. B., Aasland, O. G., Babor, T., de la Fuente, J. R., & Grant, M. (1993). Development of the alcohol use disorders identification test (AUDIT): WHO collaborative project on early detection of persons with harmful alcohol consumption, II. *Addiction, 88,* 791–804.

Spitzer, R. L., Kroenke, K., Williams, J. B. W., & Löwe, B. (2006). A brief measure for assessing generalized anxiety disorder: The GAD-7. *Archives of Internal Medicine, 166*(10), 1092–1097.

Stanhope, V., Ingoglia, C., Schmelter, B., & Marcus, S. C. (2013). Impact of person-centered planning and collaborative documentation on treatment adherence. *Psychiatric Services, 64*(1), 76–79. doi:10.1176/appi.ps.201100489

Stanhope, V., Tondora, J., Davidson, L., & Choy-Brown, M. (2015). Person-centered care planning and service engagement: A study protocol for a randomized controlled trial. *Trial, 16,* 180. doi:10.1186/s13063-015-0715-0

Steer, R. A., Ball, R., Ranieri, W. F., & Beck, A. T. (1999). Dimensions of the Beck Depression inventory-II in clinical depressed outpatient. *Journal of Clinical Psychology, 55,* 117–128.

Talen, M. R., & Valeras, A. B. (2013). *Integrated behavioral health in primary care: Evaluating the evidence, identifying the essentials.* New York, NY: Springer.

Tondora, J., O'Connell, M., Miller, R., Dinzeo, T., Bellamy, C., Andres-Hyman, R., & Davidson, L. (2010). A clinical trial of peer-based culturally responsive person-centered care for psychosis for African Americans and Latinos. *Clinical Trials, 7*(4), 368–379. doi:10.1177/1740774510369847

Unützer, J., Katon, W., Callahan, C. M., Williams, J. W., Jr., Hunkeler, E., Harpole, L., . . . Langston, C. (2002). Collaborative care management of late-life depression in the primary care setting: A randomized controlled trial. *Journal of the American Medical Association, 288*(22), 2836–2845.

Unützer, J., Katon, W. J., Fan, M. Y., Schoenbaum, M. C., Lin, E. H. B., Della Penna, R. D., & Powers, D. (2008). Long-term cost effects of collaborative care for late-life depression. *The American Journal of Managed Care, 14*(2), 95–100.

Unützer, J., Katon, W., Williams, J. W., Callahan, C. M., Harpole, L., Hunkeler, E. M., . . . Langston C. A. (2001) Improving primary care for depression in later life: The design of a multicenter randomized trial. *Medical Care, 39*(8), 785–799.

U.S. Census Bureau. (2016). U.S. Population Aging Slower than Other Countries, Census Bureau Reports. Retrieved from https://www.census.gov/newsroom/press-releases/2016/cb16-54.html

Vest, J. R., Bolin, J. N., Miller, T. R., Gamm, L. D., Siegrist, T. E., & Martinez, L. E. (2010). Medical homes: Where you stand depends on where you sit. *Medical Care Research and Review, 67*(4), 393–411. doi:10.1177/1077558710367794.

Wagner, E. H., Austin, B. T., & Von Korff, M. (1996). Organizing care for patients with chronic illness. *Millbank Quarterly, 74*(4), 511–544.

World Health Organization. (2010). *Framework for action on interprofessional education and collaborative practice. Health professions networks, Nursing and Midwifery, Human Resources for Health.* Geneva, Switzerland: Author.

8

Substance Misuse, Abuse, and Substance-Related Disorders

Linda White-Ryan

Substance misuse, abuse, and substance-related disorders constitute a major public health crisis in the United States. This places a tremendous strain on the nation's health care system. The statistics are disheartening, with approximately 20.8 million people meeting the criteria for a substance use disorder in 2015 (Center for Behavioral Health Statistics and Quality, 2016). However, only 2.2 million people received any type of treatment (Substance Abuse and Mental Health Services Administration [SAMHSA], 2016). According to the SAMHSA, the numbers are even larger with 40 million Americans ages 12 and older abusing mood altering substances or are addicted to nicotine, alcohol, or other drugs. This is more than the number of Americans with heart conditions (27 million), diabetes (26 million), or cancer (19 million; SAMHSA, 2015a, 2015b). The widespread misuse, abuse, and addiction to mood altering substances include alcohol, illicit drugs, and prescription medications. There is considerable scientific evidence that treatment for substance use disorders is cost effective when compared to the mounting costs of no treatment. Yet only about a small percentage of persons with a substance-related disorder receive any type of treatment.

Currently, there is a widespread problem among youth and young adults abusing both alcohol and other drugs (Volkow, Koob, & McLellan, 2016). According to SAMHSA (2015a), "in 2014 there were 139.7 million current alcohol users aged 12 or older, with 23% classified as binge drinkers and 6.2% as heavy drinkers" (p. 1). Substance abuse and addiction has increased dramatically and this has resulted in many deaths across the nation. In young people ages 12 through 19, illicit drug use and abuse presents a devastating societal dilemma (Spoth, Redmond, Shin, Greenberg, & Feinberg, 2007). The adolescent brain is especially vulnerable to exposure to substance abuse due to the neurocognitive and psychosocial stage of development (Siegel, 2013). The number of those affected is rapidly expanding and poses a grave threat to society as a whole (Camchong, Lim, & Kumra, 2017; Case & Deaton, 2015; Jacobus, Squeglia, Bava, & Tapert, 2013; Lubman, Cheetham, & Yücel, 2015; National Institute on Drug Abuse [NIDA], 2015). Alcohol and other mood altering drugs such as cannabis (marijuana) frequently abused by American youth can have a harmful effect on the brain (Camchong et al., 2017). According to experts on public health, the abuse and addiction to opioids has reached epidemic proportions resulting in a severe increase in morbidity and mortality (Kolodny et al., 2015). The health and well-being of many individuals, families, and communities of all races, ethnicities, cultures, and socioeconomic status depend on scientific research, evidence-based practices, and policies that address this health care crisis. It is especially important to note that addiction is considered to be a family disease. Every member of the family system is affected when there is a family member suffering from a substance use disorder.

Not only are the youth in American society affected but there is evidence of a growing epidemic among older adults reported to abuse alcohol, illicit drugs, and prescription and over-the-counter medications (Blow, Oslin, & Barry, 2002). Along with the rapid growth of the older adult population, adults aged 50 and older with alcohol and substance abuse problems are projected to double from 2.8 million to 5.7 million by the year 2020 (Briggs, Magnus, Lassiter, Patterson, & Smith, 2011; Colliver, Compton, Gfroerer, & Condon, 2006; Han, Gfroerer, Colliver, & Penne, 2009).

The problem of alcohol and drug abuse in older adults is often "invisible" to health care providers and family members (Han et al., 2009; Hanson & Gutheil, 2004; Klein & Jess, 2002; Oslin, 2006; Sorocco & Ferrel, 2006). In addition, older adults may "take prescribed medication (sometimes not as prescribed) for physical and psychiatric ailments, buy over the counter medication (which they may not take according to instructions), drink alcohol, smoke cigarettes, and use illicit drugs" (Crome & Crome, 2005, p. 343). The older adult cohort may experience feelings of shame about the abuse of alcohol and other drugs such as prescription and over-the-counter medications (Conner & Rosen, 2008). Older adults may be especially sensitive to feelings of despair and shame (Briggs et al., 2011). Shame may lead older adults to disguise misuse or abuse of alcohol or medications, which creates a barrier to obtaining assistance (Han et al., 2009).

The United States prison system is overwhelmed with inmates with substance use disorders. A study conducted by the National Center on Addiction and Substance Abuse (2010) reported that 65% of all national prison inmates meet the criteria for a substance use disorder. Joseph A. Califano, Jr., Chairman of the National Center on Addiction and Substance Abuse and former President of United States Secretary of Health, Education, and Welfare, called the nation's current prison policies "inane and inhuman." Between 1996 and 2006, the number of adults incarcerated increased by 33% due to alcohol or other drug problems (National Center on Addiction and Substance Abuse, 2010).

The profession of social work can be instrumental in addressing the public health problem of substance abuse and addiction on many levels. Throughout history, social workers such as Mary Richmond in her use of social casework have played a significant role in working with individuals and their families facing the consequences of substance abuse. Currently, social workers are on the cutting edge of conducting research and developing best practices for use in addiction treatment programs. Social workers, as agents of change, are advocating for policy changes aimed at preventing and reducing the serious adverse consequences of substance abuse disorders. This chapter will underscore the importance of addressing prevention and treatment with various population groups and will include the following three subsections: Practice, Research, and Policy for substance misuse, abuse, and addiction.

HISTORY

Throughout history, substance abuse and addiction treatment has changed in a variety of ways. There have been many attempts made at different points to treat the deleterious health and social consequences of substance abuse (Henninger & Sung, 2014). Frequently, these efforts have shifted between moralistic and positive ways to address the negative outcomes associated with substance abuse. The pendulum has swung from moderation to complete abstinence and back again (Saah, 2005). Prohibition, beginning with the Eighteenth Amendment in 1920, banned the manufacture, distribution, sale, and transportation of alcohol, and made it illegal throughout the United States. This was an attempt to extinguish the problems and ills associated with the abuse of alcohol (Lemanski, 2001). Throughout the middle to late 1920s the public showed opposition to Prohibition and frequently disregarded the sanction completely. The ban remained in place until 1933 when the Eighteenth Amendment was repealed. This opened the door to developing alternative means of treatment.

Critical contributions toward identifying the negative physical consequences of alcohol addiction were developed by physicians in the early 19th century, most notably Dr. Benjamin Rush (Henninger & Sung, 2014; Lemanski, 2001; White, 1998). Initially, treatment focused only on alcohol abuse and not on other mood altering drugs. Most psychotropic substances were legal until the institution of the Harrison Act of 1914, which then made certain substances such as opiates illegal. By criminalizing addiction to these drugs, the jails were crowded with people who had substance use disorders who had violated the Harrison Act. To this day, a large percentage of those in prison have problems with substance abuse. This was the beginning of the use of disease terminology for addiction by medical professionals instead of addressing it as a moral problem (White, 1998). As the pendulum once again swung, "treatment options for alcoholics all but disappeared by 1930. In 1935, Bill Wilson and Dr. Robert Smith developed a self-help recovery group called Alcoholics Anonymous (A.A.) in an effort to fill this treatment void" (Lemanski, 2001, p. 2262). The 12-step recovery program of A.A. has provided support and played an important role in the process of recovery from addiction to millions worldwide.

By the 1950s, many advances were made in the treatment of substance abuse and addiction. Most notable was the advent of the Minnesota Model, which advocated the 28-day inpatient stay in rehabilitation units (White, 1998). The 1970s brought the beginning of federal funding for methadone treatment programs to address heroin addiction (White, 1998). Following deinstitutionalization in the early 1980s, a growing awareness and concern emerged regarding large numbers of individuals with dual diagnoses of both mental health and substance use disorders. Since that time, a great deal of change has occurred in the treatment field. An emphasis on integrated treatment has been found to be most effective for the needs of this particular population (Drake, O'Neal, & Wallach, 2008).

PRACTICE

Social workers frequently work with individuals with problems associated with substance use, misuse, and abuse leading to the development of substance use disorders. In addition, the family members of those with substance use disorders are included in assessment, diagnosis, intervention, and treatment plans. It is critical to use a strengths-based approach when addressing substance use disorders with individuals, families, and communities (Van Wormer & Davis, 2008). Social workers provide services in hospitals, community agencies, mental health clinics, schools, homeless shelters, missions, and other health care settings. All of these settings perform screening, assessment, and diagnosis for substance use disorders. Assessment and diagnosis leading to effective interventions and treatment are critical to positive outcomes when dealing with substance abuse and substance use disorders (Dziegielewski, 2005). It is important that social workers and other health care professionals keep in mind that no individual looks forward to the future with a desire to develop a problem with the drug alcohol or other mood altering substances. Substance abuse problems carry tremendous stigma creating a barrier to obtaining treatment. The stigma surrounding substance abuse contributes to negative attitudes of communities, institutions, and health care professionals (Eliason, 2007). Feelings of shame are linked to the stigma associated with problems associated with alcohol or other drugs.

Psychoeducation regarding the effects of addiction is an important early intervention for both individuals and families. Providing accurate definitions and information for clients and their families is critical in order to initiate the process of understanding the complexities involved in substance use problems. Substance abuse entails the use of any mood altering substance in a way that can cause harm. Addiction is the most severe use of a substance that is compulsive, and can prove life-threatening. A standard alcoholic drink is equivalent to 12 ounces of beer, 5 ounces of wine, or 1.5 ounces of 80 proof alcohol. Heavy drinking is drinking eight or more alcoholic beverages per week for women, and 15 or more per week for men (SAMHSA, 2015a, 2015b). Binge drinking is the consumption within about 2 hours of four or more drinks for women and five or more drinks for men (National Institute on Alcohol Abuse and Alcoholism [NIAAA], 2015).

Only through education regarding the disease of addiction can people begin to understand what happens to the brain in substance abuse and substance use disorders. Mood altering substances including alcohol and other addictive drugs affect the reward system of the brain. Transmitters known as neurotransmitters serve as the chemical messengers of the human brain. The neurotransmitter dopamine is one of the major agents in the development of addiction (SAMHSA, 2015a, 2015b). When the human brain receives positive reinforcement, the reward or pleasure pathway is activated. "All behaviors and substances that are addictive involve the release of dopamine" (Siegel, 2013, p. 68). It also influences thinking, decision making, and behaviors. It is important for health care professionals to understand that addictive disorders are a disease involving the brain; therefore, when the pleasure centers of the brain are affected, it sets up a vicious cycle that may have death as a possible outcome. The American Society of Addiction Medicine (2005) describes addiction as a chronic disease with genetic, psychosocial, and environmental factors influencing its development and manifestations. The disease is progressive and often fatal. It is characterized by (a) impaired control over drinking or use of other mood altering drugs (AODs), (b) preoccupation with alcohol and other mood altering drugs, (c) use of alcohol and other mood altering drugs despite adverse consequences, and (d) distortions in thinking, most notably denial (American Society of Addiction Medicine, 2005). It is critical for social workers to understand that addiction is a lifelong chronic illness like heart disease, diabetes, and other chronic diseases.

Assessment by social workers begins with systematically collecting data and interpretation of the information collected. The first task of a comprehensive assessment for substance abuse or a substance use disorder is to identify the individual's need for treatment. The severity of the condition is then evaluated. The evaluation and diagnosis is based on the formal criteria outlined in the *Diagnostic and Statistical Manual of Mental Disorders*, Fifth Edition (*DSM-5*) as well as on screening. Many levels of gathering information are used by social workers in a comprehensive biopsychosocial assessment (Shulman, 2012). The use of interviews with individuals and family members as well as standardized instruments is important. This includes asking clients about the presenting problem and getting a complete developmental, family, and medical history. Special emphasis is placed on obtaining a substance use history, specifically on the onset, pattern, and type of mood altering drugs involved in use, frequency, progression, and duration of substance use (Dziegielewski, 2005; Straussner, 2004). Questions regarding the condition of health, financial and legal status, and employment history are important. It is vital for social workers to take an extremely thorough mental health history. Substance use disorders are frequently co-occurring with other mental health disorders. In addition, other relevant issues should be noted, including spiritual assessment and nutritional issues and other possible medical or health concerns.

Co-occurring substance use disorders and mental health disorders present special challenges for social workers and other health care professionals. Research has informed the behavioral health field that integration of services is paramount in treating both types of disorders (DiClemente, Nidecker, & Bellack, 2008; Drake et al., 2008; Mueser, Noordsy, Drake, & Fox, 2003).

Screening

The initial steps in effective assessment of substance use disorders may involve screening for substance use and addictive disorders. In the 1980s, the World Health Organization (WHO) introduced a model of Screening, Brief Intervention, and Referral to Treatment known as SBIRT. This was an attempt to address the widespread public health problem of the abuse of alcohol and other mood altering drugs (Ong-Flaherty, 2012). The most important aspect of this universal screening tool is that it offers a means of screening and brief intervention that is flexible and feasible for use by health care providers. It also provides information that can result in appropriate referrals for substance abusers. A strong positive is that it is efficient to use and can screen large numbers of people that otherwise might slip through the cracks of health care assessment (Mitchell, Gryczynski, O'Grady, & Schwartz, 2013). According to Johnston, O'Malley, Bachman, and Schulenberg (2012), SBIRT is effective with adolescents whose substance use may place them at risk of developing serious addictive disorders.

Adolescence is a time of many physical and emotional changes making adolescents vulnerable to peer pressure and substance use. SBIRT may be used for screening in schools, universities, mental health treatment centers, emergency rooms, trauma centers, physician's offices, and any setting where there is potential for intervention and referral. There is also mounting evidence that SBIRT is also effective with older adults when screening for alcohol and medication misuse (Schonfeld et al., 2010). Assessment instruments that are reliable and valid are critical to making an accurate diagnosis for substance use disorders.

One of the most commonly used screening tools for alcohol use problems is called the CAGE instrument. The CAGE is the simplest screening instrument for alcohol problems consisting of four questions: (1) Have you ever felt you should cut down on your drinking? (2) Have people annoyed you by criticizing your drinking? (3) Have you ever felt bad or guilty about your drinking? (4) Have you ever had a drink first thing in the morning to get rid of your hangover or to steady your nerves? (Ewing, 1984; Mayfield, McLeod, & Hall, 1974). The typical cutoff for a positive score is two positive answers (Ewing, 1984). This instrument is integrated into the information gathering process without difficulty and has well-documented validity and reliability.

NIAAA suggests a one-item prescreen question to screen for alcohol problems, which is "Do you sometimes drink beer, wine, or other alcoholic beverages?" If the person being screened answers no, then the screen is complete. If the person answers yes, then questions about heavy drinking days are asked. For men, the question is "How many times this past year have you had five or more drinks in one day?" For women, the question is "How many times this past year have you had four or more drinks in one day?" According to the responses, it is recommended that the Alcohol Use Disorders Identification Test (AUDIT) screen be completed. The AUDIT is a 10-item questionnaire designed by the WHO to screen for problem drinking and is a more sensitive instrument than the one-question approach. The AUDIT is a 10-item questionnaire that takes a few minutes to complete. It has a maximum score of 40 and a score of 8 or above may indicate problematic drinking (Fujii et al., 2016).

The Drug Abuse Screening Test (DAST) developed by Dr. Harvey Skinner (1982) is a 28-item self-report measure of problematic substance use for clinical screening. Reponses to the DAST are yes/no items, each with a value of 1 point. The total score ranges from 0 to 28. A score of 6 has been found to provide excellent sensitivity for identifying patients with substance use disorders as well as satisfactory specificity (i.e., identification of patients who do not have substance use disorders). A score of more than 12 indicates a substance abuse or dependence problem (Yudko, Lozhkina, & Fouts, 2007).

The CRAFFT is a behavioral health-screening tool for use with individuals under age 21. It consists of a series of six questions developed to screen adolescents for alcohol risk and other drug use disorders simultaneously. It is a short, effective screening tool meant to assess whether a longer conversation about the context of use, frequency, and other risks and consequences of alcohol and other drug use is warranted. Knight, Sherritt, Shrier, Harris, and Chang (2002) conducted a study in 538 adolescent participants ranging from age 14 to18 and found the CRAFFT instrument to be a valuable tool for identifying substance use problems for this population.

The Michigan Alcoholism Screening Test (MAST), developed in 1971, is a 24-item alcohol-screening test shown to be effective in identifying problem drinkers with excellent validity and reliability. It has a cutoff score of 5 for middle problem drinking and 6 or more for severe or dependent problem drinking. The Michigan Alcoholism Screening Test–Geriatric Version (MAST-G) is a 24-item test developed to screen older adults for alcohol problems (Blow et al., 1992). The cutoff is five affirmative responses and studies have found comparable sensitivity and specificity to the CAGE for identifying alcohol problems in older adults (Menninger, 2002). The short version, SMAST-G, is a 10-item instrument, has a cutoff score of 2 with a possible range of scores of 0 to 10 and is valid and reliable. Two or more positive responses is indicative of an alcohol problem. According to Blow et al. (1992), the SMAST-G is more appropriate and sensitive for use with older adults.

The Substance Abuse Treatment Scale, developed in 1988, is used to assess individuals with severe mental illness for co-occurring substance abuse problems (Conners, Donovan, & DiClemente, 2001). The questions refer to the past 6 months of the individual's use of substances and is considered reliable and found useful in monitoring progress throughout treatment. The Substance Abuse Treatment Scale–Revised (SATS-R) was developed to accurately assess a client's level of motivation and readiness to change substance use behavior (McHugo, Drake, Burton, & Ackerson, 1995; Mueser et al., 1995). The SATS-R is an 8-item scale that focuses on asking about engagement, persuasion, active treatment, and relapse prevention, and has good validity and reliability (Mueser et al., 2003).

Diagnosis

Following the completion of a comprehensive history, substance abuse screening, and creating a tentative formulation of the problem, the social worker, in collaboration with the client, makes a diagnosis and develops a treatment plan. It is important to consider culture, gender, sexual orientation, and socioeconomic status when evaluating an individual for a substance use problem or disorder (Corcoran & Walsh, 2006; DiNitto & McNeece, 2007).

The *DSM-5* is the classification system used for all mental disorders and provides health care professionals a common clinical language and reimbursement determinations (Hasin et al., 2013). According to the American Psychiatric Association (APA, 2013), the *DSM-5* provides criteria that can be used to inform not only making an accurate diagnosis, but also assists in developing an effective intervention plan. The *DSM-5* allows the social worker to form a hypothesis about the mental health problems of the client by looking at pathological patterns of use that are common to the diagnosis of substance use disorders. Those individuals with substance use disorders have the compulsion to use their drug of choice and devote a great deal of time and energy thinking about and obtaining the substance. The *DSM-5* chapter on Substance Related and Addictive Disorders includes problems with 10 classes of drugs: alcohol; caffeine; cannabis; hallucinogens; inhalants; opioids; sedatives, hypnotics, and anxiolytics; stimulants (amphetamine-type substances, cocaine, and other stimulants); tobacco; and other (or unknown), and gambling (APA, 2013). The diagnosis of substance-related disorders is based on patterns of use as well as continued use despite adverse negative consequences related to the substance use (Sharfstein, 2016).

According to the National Association of Social Workers (2013), "consistent with a change in conceptualization in the *Diagnostic and Statistical Manual of Mental Disorders* (5th edition) (*DSM-5*) . . . addiction is no longer viewed as an 'either/or' phenomenon" (p. 7).

Treatment

There has been considerable progress in the addiction field over the past 20 years regarding effective treatment models. However, there continues to be a pressing need for the use of evidence-based practices to treat the serious problem of alcohol and substance abuse. Much of the research has contributed to the development of evidence-based treatments such as motivational interviewing (MI), cognitive behavioral therapy (CBT), and harm reduction (Marlatt, Larimer, & Witkiewitz, 2011; Miller & Rollnick, 2013).

MI was developed in 1983 by William Miller to address his concerns over the poor outcomes of counseling individuals experiencing substance abuse problems. MI is "a client-centered, directive method for enhancing intrinsic motivation to change by exploring and resolving ambivalence" (Miller & Rollnick, 2002, p. 25). It involves collaboration, exploration, and shared decision making between the clinician and the client. MI is based on the Transtheoretical Model of the Stages of Change (Prochaska, Norcross, & DiClemente, 1994). The stages of change are the following: (a) pre-contemplation, the individual sees no perceived need to change; (b) contemplation, the individual begins to have an awareness that there may be a problem but experiences ambivalence about change; (c) preparation, there is movement toward change but there may be backward sliding; (d) action, the individual takes steps to change, and uses change talk; (e) maintenance, the individual is able to maintain the changes made and develops a plan for long-term maintenance to prevent relapse (Prochaska et al., 1994). The model assumes that motivation is fluid and can be influenced in the context of a relationship between the individual and the clinician. The principle tasks are to work with the client's ambivalence and resistance. The major goal is to encourage change in the direction of health.

The techniques involved in MI are an effective treatment model for social workers to encourage positive change in the health behaviors of individuals with substance use disorders (Cummings, Cooper, & Cassie, 2009). MI is a client-centered technique that operationalizes the concept of starting where the client is and has the potential to empower individuals with alcohol and/or substance abuse issues to resolve ambivalence and increase their motivation to change. The process of MI involves listening, reflecting to check understanding, and clarification. A manualized protocol is used and has had greater success than other long-term, confrontational treatment interventions. There are five important principles involved in MI—to express empathy, develop discrepancy, avoid argumentation, roll with resistance, and support self-efficacy (Miller & Rollnick, 2002). Change talk is encouraged and elicited from the client and the client is encouraged to present an argument for or against change (Magill et al., 2014; Miller & Rollnick, 2013).

MI is not only considered an evidence-based treatment but an outstanding clinical approach to working with substance abusers. Research indicates that MI-based interventions are as effective as treatment approaches that are longer in duration and have greater intensity (Burke, Arkowitz, & Dunn, 2002; Project MATCH Research Group, 1997).

Case Example 8.1

Rosa is a 77-year-old, Hispanic female who lives alone in an apartment in a suburban area. Eighteen months ago, her husband died after a lengthy illness. Rosa's three children are all on good terms with her but all of them reside in other states. All of her children express a strong desire to support their mother in any way possible. Two months ago, a neighbor found Rosa on the floor after a bad fall and called for help and she immediately was transported to the local hospital emergency room by ambulance. The fall resulted in a broken hip that required surgery and intensive ongoing physical therapy followed by a long period of being homebound. During her assessment, conducted by a social worker in the hospital emergency room, it was determined that Rosa had been increasing her usage of alcohol to two to three glasses of wine per day. Rosa also takes seven prescription medications for high blood pressure, high cholesterol, heart issues, and insomnia, as well as two to three over-the-counter medications for back pain and allergies. She sometimes takes more of her prescribed insomnia medications in combination with alcohol in the evenings when she feels lonely and cannot fall asleep.

When considering possible approaches to engaging Rosa, MI as an approach provides an excellent option. Substance abuse problems in the older adult population often create a great deal of shameful feelings. The older adult cohort presents unique challenges for health care professionals regarding the stigma of substance abuse and such a nonjudgmental and nonconfrontational approach can be effective in addressing Rosa's barriers to changing her behaviors regarding her use of alcohol. The social worker's use of MI with Rosa may work to develop a discrepancy between her current alcohol use behaviors and her stated values and interest in the improvement in her health. The social worker can elicit change talk keeping in mind the stages of change and let Rosa present an argument for change. The social worker must emphasize Rosa's strengths, including her strong family ties. It is also critical to acknowledge both the positive and negative aspects of behavioral change including what she would perceive she might gain and lose if she chooses to change her use of alcohol and prescription medications.

Cognitive behavioral therapy (CBT) is an evidence-based, effective approach for working with individuals with substance use disorders. A grounding principle of CBT is that individuals abuse substances to reinforce certain behaviors. Used in combination with MI, CBT has been found to be especially efficacious (Burke, Arkowits, & Menchola, 2003; McHugh, Hearon, & Otto, 2010). There are specific interventions and techniques that can be used alone or in combination with other treatment approaches such as group therapy and family therapy. The treatment protocols for CBT may vary. However, all CBT interventions use a learning-based approach that may include agenda and goal setting, and substance-specific homework assignments regarding maladaptive thoughts and beliefs. The exploration of reinforcement of both positive and negative behaviors is involved in the discussion of the adverse consequences experienced by the individual due to his or her drug use. Examination of underlying beliefs about expectancies of substance use provides material used toward initiating new patterns and behaviors for recovery.

The targeting of specific cues and triggers are involved in developing a plan to prevent relapse (McHugh et al., 2010).

Traditional treatment approaches usually involve complete abstinence from all mood altering substances (Willenbring, Schneekloth, Gupta, & Pankratz, 2010). Harm reduction, in direct contrast, consists of strategies to address the gap for many who never receive treatment services. This approach engages individuals not yet ready to actively participate in any type of treatment. Harm reduction is a set of strategies that encourage drug users and others to reduce the harm done by licit and illicit drugs and behaviors associated with substance abuse. In supporting drug users in gaining access to the tools to improve their health, the harm reduction model recognizes the right for comprehensive, nonjudgmental medical and social service and the fulfillment of basic needs of all individuals and communities, including users, their loved ones, and the communities affected by drug use (Marlatt, Larimer, & Witkiewitz, 2011). Harmful consequences of substance abuse are part of a continuum with the goal being to move along the continuum taking steps to reduce harm. The continuum includes excess use, moderate use, and abstinence. There is a direct focus on reducing harm by increasing safety and reducing dependence on drugs. All steps made toward decreased risk are considered positive and moving in the right direction. Some of the important strategies include needle/syringe exchange programs that reduce HIV, Hepatitis C, and other infectious diseases as well as overdose education programs about potentially dangerous substances and access to naloxone to reverse potentially fatal consequences of opioid overdose (Hawk, Vaca, & D'Onofrio, 2015; Volkow, 2015). Harm reduction does not judge substance use as good or bad. Rather, it examines the individual's relationship to drugs, emphasizing the reduction of substance-related harm and the encouragement of safer drug use. There is no moral stance involved. However, it does explore what the individual feels about his or her use of substances. Ultimately, it recognizes the competency of the individual to make choices to change his or her life and substance use (Ritter, & Cameron, 2006). Harm reduction is a public health approach that is evidence-based and presents strategies to support substance abusers who are not ready to stop using to keep them safe from harm.

Medications and Medication-Assisted Treatment

An important aspect of treatment for substance abuse disorders is pharmacology. Some of the symptoms of withdrawal can be relieved through medications, which increases the chance that an individual with a substance use disorder completes the detoxification process. Most critical is determining if an individual requires medication for safe detoxification to stabilize his or her condition. Social workers should always keep in mind that medical safety is the primary consideration when conducting an assessment and developing a treatment plan for an individual with a substance use disorder. Medications to assist in withdrawal from alcohol and anxiolytic anti-anxiety drugs must be prescribed and monitored by a physician. Medical detoxification is frequently conducted on an inpatient basis but in some cases, a physician will monitor the individual in an outpatient setting (Volkow, 2015). Medications used in the detoxification/stabilization of alcohol, anxiolytic drugs, and barbiturates all act on the same chemical pathway in the brain as the addictive substance. Agonist medications are used to assist with withdrawal symptoms and cravings. Agonist drugs attach to receptors in the brain and then produce a chemical reaction. The best example of this is the use of the medication Librium or Valium, both of which are central nervous system depressants. There are also medications called antagonists. These drugs block addictive drugs from activating the brain's receptors (Urschel, 2009).

There are medications approved to treat alcohol and opioid substance use disorders. Currently, there are no medications approved to treat substance use disorders involving the drugs marijuana, cocaine, or amphetamines. Medications used to assist in the treatment of alcohol use disorder are: (a) naltrexone (ReVia) blocks craving and is an antagonist drug; (b) acamprosate (Campral) repairs the neurotransmitter system; (c) Vivitrol (an injectable form of naltrexone), injected only once a month reduces craving and the pleasurable sensation of feeling high, and is an antagonist drug; (d) Antabuse (disulfiram) makes persons extremely sick if the individual drinks alcohol and is an antagonist drug. For addiction to heroin and other opiates, the medications available are: (a) methadone, which is an agonist drug; (b) naltrexone (ReVia), an antagonist drug; (c) buprenorphine (Suboxone), which decreases opioid cravings and blocks effects of other opioids, is a partial agonist drug; and (d) Vivitrol, injected only once a month to reduce craving and the pleasurable sense of feeling high, is an agonist drug (Volkow, 2014). A medication that has saved numerous lives of people who would otherwise have died is Narcan (naloxone). Narcan has been administered in emergency rooms by physicians, nurses, and paramedics for more than 40 years as an antidote for opiate overdoses. It is an opiate antagonist, which reverses opiate overdoses. Currently, there is a public health initiative sweeping the nation to train police officers and firefighters as well the general public to administer Narcan due to the opioid crisis the United States is facing. Recent medical advances have made available medications to assist with withdrawal symptoms, to help individuals deal with the cravings, and begin to heal the damaged brain (Urchel, 2009).

Treatment needs are determined using a varied number of approaches and interventions. Initially, it is critical to identify if medical detoxification/stabilization is indicated to safely withdraw the individual from the drug to which he or she is addicted. However, treatment does not stop there. Medical management of withdrawal is only the first step. Next is referral for further treatment. Types of treatment may include Intensive Inpatient Care Programs which are 28 days the most restrictive, or outpatient treatment that can be intensive outpatient which meets 3 to 5 days per week for about 4 hours, or outpatient individual or group patient. Group therapy is extremely effective for those with substance use disorders (McNeece & DiNitto, 2012). In addition, other types of treatment consist of Therapeutic Communities (TC), which are generally residential and long term, lasting 12 or more months with the focus on resocialization, 12-Step Programs such as A.A. that provide peer support and are an important adjunct support to treatment, and Extended Care, which is offered in residential settings when further treatment is needed following 28-day inpatient rehabilitation programs (Volkow, 2015). What has become clear is that integrated treatment services produce the best results for individuals and families suffering from substance abuse and substance use disorders. The combination of education that includes a focus on prevention and integration of available resources is imperative going forward. Interprofessional collaboration of social workers with other health care professionals contributes to the successful treatment outcomes for the major public health crisis of addiction.

POLICY

Substance misuse, abuse, and substance use disorders are serious public health problems and require treatment funding through local, state, and federal governments. Private insurance provided by employers also funds treatment for substance use disorders. However, funding has always been an issue for many reasons including stigma. Managed care plans provide health coverage for the medical problems that are the consequences of addiction. However, there has been a ~~tremendous gap in~~ the funding of substance use disorders in comparison to other chronic medical diseases such as diabetes and asthma (McLellan & Woodworth, 2014; Volkow, 2015).

The Mental Health Parity and Addiction Equity Act ~~(Parity Act~~, 2008) and the Patient Protection and Affordable Care Act of 2010 ~~(ACA)~~ constitute groundbreaking legislation that mandates insurance coverage to include screening as well as brief interventions for the treatment of all substance abuse issues and not only for severe alcohol and substance dependence (McLellan & Woodworth, 2014; Volkow, 2015). Both of these acts increase the opportunity for individuals suffering from substance abuse and addiction to have access to quality health care.

The current opioid crisis in the United States is a priority health concern. In 2014, the Centers for Disease Control and Prevention (CDC) declared the problem to be so serious that it determined opioid prevention to be one of the top five public health challenges in the United States. This epidemic requires multifaceted opioid prevention and treatment strategies (Kolodny et al., 2015). In 2016, there were 20,101 overdose deaths related to prescription pain relievers, and 12,990 overdose deaths related to the use of heroin (Dahlman, Kral, Wenger, Hakansson, & Novak, 2017). Four out of five people addicted to heroin started out by misusing prescription pain medications to address chronic pain (Jones, Logan, Gladden, & Bohm, 2015). In 2014, a survey of people in treatment for opioid addiction reported that they chose to use heroin because prescription opioids were far more expensive and harder to obtain than heroin (NIDA, 2015).

The Comprehensive Addiction and Recovery Act of 2016 increases the availability of naloxone (Narcan), an opioid antagonist. It also strengthens prescription drug monitoring programs (PDMPs) by assisting states with monitoring and tracking prescription drug diversion, and expands prevention and educational efforts with teens and adult populations. Although progress has been made to address policy reform, further work needs to be done.

In March 2011, the CDC developed new guidelines regarding prescribing opioid medications for chronic pain. The guidelines informed clinicians to consider opioid therapy only if the benefits outweigh the risks for medical conditions involving chronic pain. Before starting opioid therapy for chronic pain, clinicians should establish treatment goals and consider discontinuation of opioid therapy if benefits do not outweigh risks. In addition, prior to starting opioid therapy and periodically during the medication use, clinicians should discuss with patients known risks and realistic benefits of opioid therapy. There are additional guidelines developed by the CDC that improve recommendations for prescribing opioid pain medication for patients in primary care settings.

In 2009, New York was one of 36 states that developed a child endangerment law with stronger sanctions to protect children who were at risk of driving with an adult impaired from any mood altering substance. Titled the Child Passenger Protection Act or Leandra's Law, the law was named after the death of a 11-year-old child due a highway car crash caused by an impaired driver. The law mandates that any age limits on drinking alcohol are a measure aimed at preventing drinking in adolescents at risk of alcohol and substance abuse. There has been a great deal of policy-oriented research dealing with minimum drinking age limitations. It consistently shows that it has decreased fatal car accidents. Policies lowering the legal intoxication limits as well as zero-tolerance laws have proved useful in decreasing the number of intoxicated drivers. As mentioned previously, it is important for adolescents to delay the age of onset of use of alcohol because the brain of a young person is more vulnerable to developing substance use problems with regular use and abuse (Siegel, 2013).

RESEARCH

Many years of research have informed health care professionals that substance misuse and abuse can lead to the development of the brain disease of addiction. In 1989, the NIAAA conducted the landmark study, Project MATCH. The purpose was to provide clinicians with critical information about which treatment was most efficacious. This study lasted 8 years and investigated the importance of matching patients with specific treatments for substance abuse. Three psychosocial treatments were tested: (a) cognitive behavioral therapy, (b) motivational enhancement therapy, and (c) 12-step facilitation therapy (TST; NIAAA, 1998). The results were interesting and showed that all of the treatments produced favorable and very similar outcomes (Donovan & Matteson, 1994). The study found none of the three treatments to be superior to the other. Miller, Forcehimes, and Zweben (2011) made an important point when discussing research in addiction treatment. They stated that a critical aspect of treatment is the relationship between the clinician and the client. The approach used in this stigmatized illness may not be the most important feature of the treatment process, but rather the clinician–client relationship.

The past 20 years of research has proved enlightening for understanding evidence-based practices for the treatment of substance abuse. For example, CBT has demonstrated efficacy in treating substance use disorders in various populations with addiction when using computer-based modality (Kiluk et al., 2016). The researchers conducted this study to determine if individuals with no computer skills that were experiencing alcohol use disorder could benefit from CBT as treatment alone (TAU), or by computer in combination with TAU, or by computer only (Kiluk et al., 2016). The findings showed that there was an increase in completion of treatment in individuals receiving CBT treatment as TAU in combination with virtual treatment, and computer only as compared with TAU only. This study points to creating innovative, new methods of engaging people with alcohol use disorder in treatment. As a method of treatment, CBT provides the clinician with tools for assisting the client with learning that supports and opens the door for behavior change. In the treatment of problems with addiction, behavior change is critical in assisting individuals to enter recovery and maintain the gains made in treatment.

There is a great deal of research evidence supporting the use of MI for the treatment of substance abuse and substance use disorders. Madson et al. (2016) systematically reviewed the effectiveness of MI with various populations. The researchers found that MI has been very effective and widely implemented in working with adolescents. A number of studies of at-risk college students have found that MI addresses the ambivalence of young adults regarding heavy and binge drinking by effectively exploring with the youth the positives and negatives about the use of alcohol and other mood altering substances (Naar-King & Suarez, 2010). Comparison studies between using a harm reduction approach versus an abstinence-only approach have found that both perspectives can be utilized providing a continuum of care with positive outcomes (Logan & Marlatt, 2010).

Additional studies show that harm reduction strategies have produced promising results in working with college students regarding the risks of binge drinking (NIAAA, 2002). Research regarding alternative therapies such as Mindfulness Based Relapse Prevention (MBRP) used in combination with relapse prevention approaches and 12-step programs increased the likelihood of achieving and maintaining gains made in the process of recovery (Bowen et al., 2014). Future research is critical to ensure best practices to address the treatment of the serious public health problem of substance abuse and substance use disorders.

CONCLUSION

The current public health crisis of substance abuse and substance-related disorders presents all health care professionals with the challenge of finding ways to address the problems of individuals, families, and communities. The stigma attached to this serious brain disease creates a barrier to individuals, families, and communities accessing services to address this serious illness. Current statistics indicate that there are more persons with substance abuse problems than other chronic illnesses such as diabetes and heart disease. The widespread misuse, abuse, and addiction to mood altering substances include alcohol, illicit drugs, and prescription medications.

Advances made in scientific research demonstrate that treatment for substance use disorders is cost effective when compared to the mounting costs and adverse consequences associated with no treatment. However, only a small number of individuals receive any type of treatment. There are evidence-based treatment approaches such as MI and CBT that have been effective in addressing addiction. Medication is an important component of treatment and is frequently included as part of a comprehensive plan of treatment.

As we move forward into the future, it is crucial that research emphasizes approaches to prevent relapse and improve outcomes. The development of policies that support health care reform and treatment is vital for addressing the major public health crisis of substance use disorders. Social workers have played an important role throughout history in working with the complex problems of addictive disorders. The education and training of social workers and all health care professionals about the issues associated with addiction are critical to reducing stigma and providing competent and quality treatment services.

CHAPTER DISCUSSION QUESTIONS

1. What are the most important components of biopsychosocial assessment of individuals who may have a substance-related disorder?

2. What are some screening instruments that are effective for evaluating whether an individual is at risk of a substance-related disorder?

3. What are the criteria for the diagnosis of a substance-related disorder according to the *DSM-5*?

4. What are some evidence-based approaches and best practices for the treatment of substance abuse problems?

5. What are some current policies that have been developed over the past 5 years that address substance abuse?

6. Discuss the ways in which social workers are well-positioned to collaborate with individuals, families, and communities to address the problems associated with substance-related disorders by using the approach of motivational interviewing.

CASE EXAMPLE AND DISCUSSION QUESTIONS

Case Example 8.2

Charles is a 45-year-old African American man. He works in the high-stress, high-powered world of corporate finance. Charles presents himself as a no-nonsense business professional. He has come to the clinic where you are presently working as a social worker for an assessment because his wife and two teenage children are very concerned about his drinking. His wife has insisted that he seek professional help. Charles tells you that although he tells himself that he will only have one or two glasses of wine per day, he lately finds himself finishing the whole bottle and sometimes half or more of a second bottle. He does not see this as a huge issue but he has missed a few important business meetings lately. This has made him feel quite upset with himself and guilty because he has lied to his boss about the absences. About 3 years ago, following the death of his father, Charles began to have trouble sleeping and the doctor prescribed Xanax (an anti-anxiety drug and central nervous system depressant). During the past year, he has increased his use of alcohol and Xanax. He often takes five or six times the prescribed dose of Xanax and when questioned by his physician he began to search for other physicians in order to obtain more pills. Charles reports that he was recently in an automobile accident. His children have told him that they feel embarrassed in front of their friends when his speech becomes slurred and he appears unsteady on his feet.

Questions for Discussion

1. When conducting an assessment, what are some possible screening instruments regarding Charles's use of alcohol and other mood altering substances?

2. Does Charles need to be referred to a physician to be assessed for possible medical detoxification/stabilization and if so why?

3. Should Charles's family be involved in his treatment plan?

REFERENCES

American Psychiatric Association. (2013). *Diagnostic and statistical manual of mental disorders* (5th ed.). Arlington, VA: Author.

American Society of Addiction Medicine. (2005). *Public policy statement on definition of alcoholism.* Retrieved from https://www.asam.org/docs/default-source/public-policy-statements/1definition-of-alcoholism-2-902.pdf?sfvrsn=0

Blow, F. C., Brower, K. J., Schulenberg, J. E., Demo-Dananberg, L. M., Young, K. J., & Beresford, T. P. (1992). The Michigan Alcoholism Screening Test, Geriatric Version (MAST-G): A new elderly specific screening instrument [Abstract] *Alcoholism: Clinical and Experimental Research, 16,* 172.

Blow, F. C., Oslin, D. W., & Barry, K. L. (2002). Misuse and abuse of alcohol, illicit drugs and psychoactive medication among older people. *Generations, 26*(1), 50–54.

Bowen, S., Witkiewitz, K., Clifasefi, S. L., Grow, J., Chawla, N., Hsu, S. H., . . . Larimer, M. E. (2014). Relative efficacy of mindfulness-based relapse prevention, standard relapse prevention, and treatment as usual for substance use disorders: A randomized clinical trial. *JAMA Psychiatry, 71*(5), 547–556.

Briggs, W., Magnus, V., Lassiter, P., Patterson, A., & Smith, L. (2011). Substance use, misuse, and abuse among older adults: Implications for clinical mental health counselors. *Journal of Mental Health Counseling, 33*(2), 112–127.

Burke, B. L., Arkowitz, H., & Dunn, C. (2002). The efficacy of motivational interviewing and its adaptations: What we know so far. *Motivational Interviewing: Preparing People for Change, 2*, 217–250.

Burke, B. L., Arkowitz, H., & Menchola, M. (2003). The efficacy of motivational interviewing: A meta-analysis of controlled clinical trials. *Journal of Consulting and Clinical Psychology, 71*(5), 843–861.

Camchong, J., Lim, K. O., & Kumra, S. (2017). Adverse effects of cannabis on adolescent brain development: A longitudinal study. *Cerebral Cortex, 27*(3), 1922–1930.

Case, A., & Deaton, A. (2015). Rising morbidity and mortality in midlife among white non-Hispanic Americans in the 21st century. *Proceedings of the National Academy of Sciences, 112*(49), 15078–15083. doi:10.1073/pnas.1518393112

Center for Behavioral Health Statistics and Quality. (2016). *Key substance use and mental health indicators in the United States: Results from the 2015 National Survey on Drug Use and Health* (HHS Publication No. SMA 16-4974, NSDUH Series H-051). Retrieved from http://www.samhsa.gov/data

Colliver, J. D., Compton, W. M., Gfroerer, J. C., & Condon, T. (2006). Projecting drug use among aging baby boomers in 2020. *Annals of Epidemiology, 16*(4), 257–265.

Conner, K. O., & Rosen, D. (2008). "You're nothing but a junkie": Multiple experiences of stigma in an aging methadone maintenance population. *Journal of Social Work Practice in the Addictions, 8*(2), 244–264.

Conners, G. J., Donovan, D. M., & DiClemente, C. C. (2001). *Substance abuse treatment and the stages of change.* New York, NY: Guilford Press.

Corcoran, J., & Walsh, J. (2006). *Clinical assessment and diagnosis in social work practice.* New York, NY: Oxford University Press.

Crome, I., & Crome, P. (2005). "At your age what does it matter": Myths and realities about older people who use substances. *Drug Education, Prevention & Policy, 12*(5), 343–347.

Cummings, S. M., Cooper, R. L., & Cassie, K. M. (2009). Motivational interviewing to affect behavioral change in older adults. *Research on Social Work Practice, 19*(2), 195–204.

Dahlman, D., Kral, A. H., Wenger, L., Hakansson, A., & Novak, S. P. (2017). Physical pain is common and associated with nonmedical prescription opioid use among people who inject drugs. *Substance Abuse Treatment, Prevention & Policy, 12*, 1–11. doi:10.1186/s13011-017-0112-7

DiClemente, C. C., Nidecker, M., & Bellack, A. S. (2008). Motivation and the stages of change among individuals with severe mental illness and substance abuse disorders. *Journal of Substance Abuse Treatment, 34*(1), 25–35.

DiNitto, D. M., & McNeece, C. A. (2007). Addictions and social work practice. *Social work issues and opportunities in a challenging profession* (pp. 171–193). Oxford, UK: Oxford University Press.

Donovan, D. M., & Matteson, M. E. (1994). Alcoholism treatment matching research: Methodological and clinical approaches. *Journal of Studies on Alcohol, Suppl. 12*, 5–14.

Drake, R. E., O'Neal, E. L., & Wallach, M. A. (2008). A systematic review of psychosocial research on psychosocial interventions for people with co-occurring severe mental and substance use disorders. *Journal of Substance Abuse Treatment, 34*(1), 123–138.

Dziegielewski, S. (2005). *Understanding substance addictions.* Chicago, IL: Lyceum Books.

Eliason, M. J. (2007). *Improving substance abuse treatment: An introduction to the evidence-based practice movement.* Thousand Oaks, CA: Sage.

Ewing, J. A. (1984). Detecting alcoholism: The CAGE questionnaire. *JAMA,* 252, 1905–1907.

Fujii, H., Nishimoto, N., Yamaguchi, S., Kurai, O., Miyano, M., Ueda, W., . . . Okawa, K. (2016). The Alcohol Use Disorders Identification Test for Consumption (AUDIT-C) is more useful than pre-existing laboratory tests for predicting hazardous drinking: A cross-sectional study. *BMC Public Health, 16*(1), 379. doi:10.1186/s12889-016-3053-6

Han, B., Gfroerer, J. C., Colliver, J. D., & Penne, M. A. (2009). Substance use disorder among older adults in the United States in 2020. *Addiction, 104*(1), 88–96. doi:10.1111/j.1360-0443.2008.02411.x

Hanson, M., & Gutheil, I. (2004). Motivational strategies with alcohol-involved older adults: Implications for social work practice. *Social Work, 49*(3), 364–372.

Hasin, D., O'Brien, C. P., Auriacombe, M., Borges, G., Bucholz, K., Budney, A., . . . Grant, B. F., (2013). DSM-5 criteria for substance use disorders: Recommendations and rationale. *The American Journal of Psychiatry, 170*(8), 834–851. doi:10.1176/appi.ajp.2013.12060782

Hawk, K. F., Vaca, F. E., & D'Onofrio, G. (2015). Reducing fatal opioid overdose: Prevention, treatment and harm reduction strategies. *The Yale Journal of Biology and Medicine, 88*(3), 235–245.

Henninger, A., & Sung, H. E. (2014). History of substance abuse treatment. In *Encyclopedia of criminology and criminal justice* (pp. 2257–2269). New York, NY: Springer.

Jacobus, J., Squeglia, L. M., Bava, S., & Tapert, S. F. (2013). White matter characterization of adolescent binge drinking with and without co-occurring marijuana use: A 3-year investigation. *Psychiatry Research: Neuroimaging, 214*(3), 374–381. doi:10.1016/j.pscychresns.2013.07.014

Johnston, L. D., O'Malley, P. M., Bachman, J. G., & Schulenberg, J. E. (2012). *Monitoring the Future national results on adolescent drug use: Overview of key findings, 2011.* Ann Arbor, MI: Institute for Social Research.

Jones, C. M., Logan, J., Gladden, R. M., & Bohm, M. K. (2015). Vital signs: Demographic and substance use trends among heroin users—United States, 2002–2013. *Morbidity and Mortality Weekly Report, 64*(26), 719–725.

Kiluk, B. D., Devore, K. A., Buck, M. B., Nich, C., Frankforter, T. L., LaPaglia, D. M., . . . Carroll, K. M. (2016). Randomized trial of computerized cognitive behavioral therapy for alcohol use disorders: Efficacy as a virtual stand-alone and treatment add-on compared with standard outpatient treatment. *Alcoholism: Clinical and Experimental Research, 40*(9), 1991–2000. doi:10.1111/acer.13162

Klein, W. C., & Jess, C. (2002). One last pleasure: Alcohol use among elderly people in nursing homes. *Health and Social Work, 27*(3), 193–203.

Knight, J. R., Sherritt, L., Shrier, L. A., Harris, S. K., & Chang, G. (2002). Validity of the CRAFFT substance abuse screening test among adolescent clinic patients. *Pediatric Adolescent Medicine, 156,* 607–613.

Kolodny, A., Courtwright, D. T., Hwang, C. S., Kreiner, P., Eadie, J. L., Clark, T. W., & Alexander, G. C. (2015). The prescription opioid heroin crisis: A public health approach to an epidemic of addiction. *Annual Review of Public Health, 36,* 559–574. doi:10.1146/annurev-publhealth-031914-122957

Lemanski, M. (2001). *History of addiction and recovery in the United States.* Tucson, AZ: See Sharp Press.

Logan, D. E., & Marlatt, G. A. (2010). Harm reduction therapy: A practice-friendly review of research. *Journal of Clinical Psychology, 66*(2), 201–214. doi:10.1002/jclp.20669

Lubman, D. I., Cheetham, A., & Yücel, M. (2015). Cannabis and adolescent brain development. *Pharmacology & Therapeutics, 148,* 1–16. doi:10.1016/j.pharmthera.2014.11.009

Madson, M. B., Schumacher, J. A., Baer, J. S., & Martino, S. (2016). Motivational interviewing for substance use: Mapping out the next generation of research. *Journal of Substance Abuse Treatment, 65,* 1–5. doi:10.1016/j.jsat.2016.02.003

Magill, M., Gaume, J., Apodaca, T. R., Walthers, J., Mastroleo, N. R., Borsari, B., & Longabaugh, R. (2014). The technical hypothesis of motivational interviewing: A meta-analysis of MI's key causal model. *Journal of Consulting and Clinical Psychology, 82*(6), 973–983. doi:10.1037/a0036833

Marlatt, G. A., Larimer, M. E., & Witkiewitz, K. (Eds.). (2011). *Harm reduction: Pragmatic strategies for managing high-risk behaviors.* New York, NY: Guilford Press.

Mayfield, G., McLeod, P., & Hall, C. (1974). The CAGE questionnaire: Validation of a new screening instrument. *American Journal of Psychiatry, 131,* 1121–1123. doi:10.1176/ajp.131.10.1121

McHugh, R. K., Hearon, B. A., & Otto, M. W. (2010). Cognitive behavioral therapy for substance use disorders. *Psychiatric Clinics of North America, 33*(3), 511–525. doi:10.1016/j.psc.2010.04.012

McHugo, G. J., Drake, R. E., Burton, H. L., & Ackerson, T. H. (1995). A scale for assessing the stage of substance abuse treatment in persons with severe mental illness. *The Journal of Nervous and Mental, 183*(12):762–767.

McLellan, A. T., & Woodworth, A. M. (2014). The Affordable Care Act and treatment for "substance use disorders": Implications of ending segregated behavioral health care. *Journal of Substance Abuse Treatment, 46*(5), 541–545. doi:10.1016/j.jsat.2014.02.001

McNeece, C. A., & DiNitto, D. M. (2012). *Chemical dependency: A systems approach* (4th ed.). Boston: Allyn & Bacon.

Menninger, J. A. (2002). Assessment and treatment of alcoholism and substance related disorders in the elderly. *Bulletin of the Menninger Clinic, 66*(2), 166–184.

Mental Health Parity and Addiction Equity Act. (2008). H.R. 1424, 117th Cong. Retrieved from ProQuest Congressional.

Miller, W. R., Forcehimes, A. A., & Zweben, A. (2011). *Treating addiction: A guide for professionals.* New York, NY: Guilford Press.

Miller, W. R., & Rollnick, S. (2002). *Motivational interviewing: Preparing people for change* (2nd ed.). New York, NY: Guilford Press.

Miller, W. R., & Rollnick, S. (2013). *Applications of motivational interviewing.* New York, NY: Guilford Press.

Mitchell, S. G., Gryczynski, J., O'Grady, K. E., & Schwartz, R. P. (2013). SBIRT for adolescent drug and alcohol use: Current status and future directions. *Journal of Substance Abuse Treatment, 44*(5), 463–472. doi:10.1016/j.jsat.2012.11.005

Mueser, K. T., Drake, R. E., Clark, R. E., McHugo, G. J., Mercer-McFadden, C., & Ackerson, T. H. (1995). *Toolkit on evaluating substance abuse in persons with severe mental illness*. Cambridge, MA: Human Services Research Institute.

Mueser, K. T., Noordsy, D. L., Drake, R. E., & Fox, L. (2003). *Integrated treatment for dual disorders: A guide to effective practice*. New York, NY: Guilford Press.

Naar-King, S., & Suarez, M. (2011). *Motivational interviewing with adolescents and young adults*. New York, NY: Guilford Press.

National Association of Social Workers. (2013). *NASW standards for social work practice with clients with substance use disorders*. Washington, DC: Author.

National Center on Addiction and Substance Abuse. (2010). *Behind bars II*. Retrieved from https://www.centeronaddiction.org/newsroom/press-releases/2010-behind-bars-II

National Institute on Alcohol Abuse and Alcoholism. (1998). Matching patients with alcohol disorders to treatments: Clinical implications from Project MATCH. *Journal of Mental Health, 7*(6), 589–602.

National Institute on Alcohol Abuse and Alcoholism. (2002). *A call to action: Changing culture of drinking at U.S. colleges*. NIH Publication No. 02-5010. Rockville, MD: Author.

National Institute on Alcohol Abuse and Alcoholism. (2015). *College drinking*. Retrieved from https://pubs.niaaa.nih.gov/publications/CollegeFactSheet/CollegeFact.htm

National Institute on Drug Abuse. (2015). *Monitoring the future: 2015 survey results*. Retrieved from https://www.drugabuse.gov/related-topics/trends-statistics/infographics/monitoring-future-2015-survey-results

Ong-Flaherty, C. (2012). Screening, brief intervention, and referral to treatment: A nursing perspective. *Journal of Emergency Nursing, 38*(1), 54–56. doi:10.1016/j.jen.2011.09

Oslin, D. W. (2006). The changing face of substance misuse in older adults. *Psychiatric Times, 23*(13), 41–48.

Prochaska, J. O., Norcross, J. C., & DiClemente, C. C. (1994). *Changing for good: A revolutionary six-stage program for overcoming bad habits and moving your life positively forward*. New York, NY: Avon Books.

Project MATCH Research Group. (1997). Matching alcoholism treatments to client heterogeneity: Project MATCH posttreatment drinking outcomes. *Journal of Studies on Alcohol, 58*, 7–29.

Ritter, A., & Cameron, J. (2006). A review of the efficacy and effectiveness of harm reduction strategies for alcohol, tobacco and illicit drugs. *Drug and Alcohol Review, 25*(6), 611–624.

Saah, T. (2005). The evolutionary origins and significance of drug addiction. *Harm Reduction Journal, 2*(1), 8.

Schonfeld, L., King-Kallimanis, B. L., Duchene, D. M., Etheridge, R. L., Herrera, J. R., Barry, K. L., & Lynn, N. (2010). Screening and brief intervention for substance misuse among older adults: The Florida BRITE project. *American Journal of Public Health, 100*(1), 108–114. doi:10.2105/AJPH.2008.149534

Sharfstein, S. S. (2016). Understanding mental disorders: Your guide to *DSM-5. Journal of Psychiatric Practice, 22*(2), 163. doi:10.1080/02763869.2016.1220766

Shulman, L. (2012). *The skills of helping individuals, families and communities* (6th ed.). Belmont, CA: Brooks/Cole.

Siegel, D. (2013). *Brainstorm: The power and purpose of the teenage brain*. New York, NY: Penguin Publishing.

Skinner, H. A. (1982). The drug abuse screening test. *Addictive Behaviors, 7*(4), 363–371.

Sorocco, K. H., & Ferrell, S. W. (2006). Alcohol use among older adults. *The Journal of General Psychology, 133*(4), 453–467.

Spoth, R., Redmond, C., Shin, C., Greenberg, M., Clair, S., & Feinberg, M. (2007). Substance use outcomes at 18 months past baseline: The PROSPER community-university partnership trial. *American Journal of Preventive Medicine, 32*(5), 395–402. doi:10.1016/j.amepre.2007.01.014

Straussner, S. L. A. (2004). *Clinical social work with substance abusing clients* (2nd ed.). New York, NY: Guilford Press.

Substance Abuse and Mental Health Services Administration. (2015a). *Alcohol.* Retrieved from https://www.samhsa.gov/atod/alcohol

Substance Abuse and Mental Health Services Administration. (2015b). *Other drugs.* Retrieved from https://www.samhsa.gov/atod/other-drugs

Urschel, H. (2009). *Healing the addicted brain: The revolutionary, science-based alcoholism and addiction recovery program.* Naperville, IL: Sourcebooks, Inc.

Van Wormer, K., & Davis, D. R. (2008). *Addiction treatment.* Belmont, CA: Cengage Learning.

Volkow, N. (2015). *Principles of drug addiction treatment: A research based guide* (3rd ed.). Bethesda, MD: National Institute on Drug Abuse, National Institutes of Health.

Volkow, N. D., Koob, G. F., & McLellan, A. T. (2016). Neurobiologic advances from the brain disease model of addiction. *New England Journal of Medicine, 374*(4), 363–371. doi:10.1056/NEJMra1511480

White, W. L. (1998). *Slaying the dragon: The history of addiction treatment and recovery in America* (p. xvi). Bloomington, IL: Chestnut Health Systems/Lighthouse Institute.

Willenbring, M., Schneekloth, T., Gupta, L., & Pankratz, V. S. (2010, July). Anxiety and depressive symptoms in alcoholics: Correlation with urge to drink during early abstinence. *American Journal on Addictions, 19*(4), 380.

Yudko, E., Lozhkina, O., & Fouts, A. (2007). A comprehensive review of the psychometric properties of the Drug Abuse Screening Test. *Journal of Substance Abuse Treatment, 32*(2), 189–198. doi:10.1016/j.jsat.2006.08.002

9

Palliative and End-of-Life Care

Cathy Berkman, Gary L. Stein, and Myra Glajchen

The vast majority of Americans want to die at home, surrounded by family, free of pain and other distressing symptoms, and treated with respect, so they can die with dignity. The reality is often very different. The majority of American die in institutions, including hospitals and nursing homes (Institute of Medicine [IOM], 2014). Those in hospitals may spend days or weeks isolated in an intensive care unit. The cost of caring for patients at the end of life is financially and emotionally costly for families. Palliative care provides an alternative to this reality. In this chapter, we present the benefits of palliative care and the role of palliative social workers.

DEFINITION OF PALLIATIVE CARE

Palliative care is specialized care for persons with serious illness. The World Health Organization (WHO) provides a comprehensive definition of palliative care:

> *Palliative care is an approach that improves the quality of life of patients and their families facing the problem associated with life-threatening illness, through the prevention and relief of suffering by means of early identification and impeccable assessment and treatment of pain and other problems, physical, psychosocial and spiritual. (WHO, 2017)*

The aim of palliative care is to improve quality of life for the patient and family. Palliative care specialists facilitate communication among the patient, health care providers, and family members to better understand the illness and goals of care. They manage complex physical and emotional symptoms, including pain, depression, and fatigue, and coordinate care transitions across health care settings. The purpose of these interventions is to help patients and family members make informed decisions about their care in a timely manner, manage symptoms, and maximize functional ability (Center to Advance Palliative Care, 2017). Palliative care provides support to help families cope during the patient's illness and after the patient's death. It is appropriate for any life-limiting diagnosis, including cancer, cardiovascular disease, respiratory illness, neurological illness, or dementia. Eight domains of palliative care were established by the National Consensus Project for Quality Palliative Care (NCP): Structure and Processes of Care,

Physical, Psychological, Social, Spiritual, Cultural, End-of-Life Care, and Ethical and Legal (National Quality Forum, 2006).

PALLIATIVE CARE CONTINUUM

Palliative care is beneficial and appropriate at all stages of a serious illness. Figure 9.1 illustrates the palliative care continuum (adapted from Lynn, 2005; Mudigonda & Mudigonda, 2010). Ideally, palliative care is initiated at the time of diagnosis and is delivered simultaneously with curative care. As the illness progresses, the amount and scope of palliative care services increases. In the final stage of the disease, when curative care is no longer wanted by the patient or no longer beneficial, hospice care should be considered.

Hospice care is provided in the final stage of a terminal illness. The philosophy of hospice is that death is a natural process and individuals have the right to die free of pain and with dignity (National Hospice and Palliative Care Organization, 2017). While hospice incorporates palliative care practices, the timing, setting, and payment mechanism of hospice differs from palliative care. Currently, the Medicare Hospice Benefit, which pays for almost 90% of hospice care in the United States, stipulates that death is expected within 6 months and that curative care must be discontinued. Curative treatment is allowed only for potentially curable conditions, such as bladder infections, if the patient chooses, with brief hospital stays if necessary. A current trial allows Medicare beneficiaries to receive hospice-like support services from hospice providers while receiving curative treatment (Centers for Medicare and Medicaid Services [CMS], 2017). The CMS is evaluating whether this improves quality of life and care, increases patient satisfaction, and reduces expenditures.

The Medicare Hospice Benefit covers services provided by physicians, nurses, social workers, chaplains, and aides, and medications, equipment, grief support following a death, and other services deemed appropriate by the hospice provider. In 2014, 1.6 to 1.7 million patients received hospice services (National Hospice and Palliative Care Organization, 2016). The median length of stay in hospice was 17.4 days, with 35.5% staying less than a week.

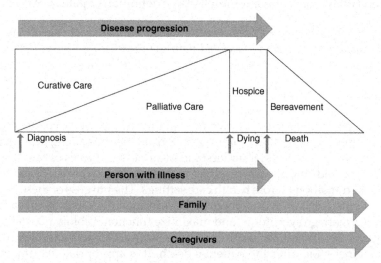

Figure 9.1 Continuum of palliative care.
Source: Adapted from Lynn, J. (2005). Living long in fragile health: The new demographics shape end of life care. *The Hastings Center Report, Spec No*, S14–S18; Mudigonda, P., & Mudigonda, T. (2010). Palliative cancer care ethics: Principles and challenges in the Indian setting. *Indian Journal of Palliative Care, 16*(3), 107–110.

PALLIATIVE CARE SETTINGS AND MODELS

Palliative care is delivered in a wide range of settings and with different models of care. These settings include: inpatient facilities, including intensive care units (ICUs) and emergency departments, outpatient settings, community-based settings, long-term care facilities, and home-based settings. In 2015, 56.0% of days of hospice care were received at a private residence, 41.3% in a nursing facility, 1.3% in a hospice inpatient facility, 0.5% in an acute care hospital, and 0.9% in another location (National Hospice and Palliative Care Organization, 2017). Palliative and hospice care may also be delivered by telehealth (Bishop, Flick, & Wildman, 2015). Regardless of the setting, hospice services are available 24 hours a day, 7 days a week.

There are many models for delivering palliative care. Palliative care is best delivered by an interdisciplinary team that integrates the physical, psychological, social, and spiritual aspects of care. The core team includes a physician, nurse, social worker, and chaplain. In many settings, the team may be augmented by pharmacists, physical therapists, occupational therapists, arts therapists, massage therapists, and other complementary and alternative care practitioners. Embedded programs are a newer model, in which a palliative care specialist or team is employed by a primary specialty, such as oncology, to provide palliative care. Volunteers may play an important role in supporting the patient and family, particularly in hospice care. In smaller facilities or those with fewer resources, palliative care may be delivered by only a palliative care physician or nurse, or by generalist-level palliative care practitioners.

ADVANCE DIRECTIVES

An advance directive may be one of several types of legally executed documents that contain an individual's instructions for the provision, withholding, or withdrawal of life-sustaining treatment. Every adult, regardless of health status, should have a health care agent (HCA) and a living will because it is often not predictable when these will be needed. Making decisions in a medical crisis is stressful and may not be in accordance with the patient's preferences. The different types of advance directives are as follows.

Living Will

This is a legal document that states the medical treatments that the individual would, and would not, want if the individual is unable to make or communicate such decisions. These treatments might be used to prolong life or to bring symptom relief, and may include resuscitation, mechanical ventilation, nutrition and hydration, tube feeding, dialysis, antibiotics or antiviral medication, diagnostic tests, surgery, transfusions, and comfort care.

Health Care Agent (aka Health Care Proxy, Health Care Surrogate, Health Care Power of Attorney, Durable Power of Attorney)

This is a person named by the patient to make medical decisions, according to the patient's wishes, when the patient is no longer able to communicate. The HCA may be authorized to consent or withhold consent for medical treatment, hire or fire medical personnel, and make decisions about medical facilities. The HCA cannot override the patient's preferences if the patient is able to make and communicate treatment decisions.

Do Not Resuscitate (DNR), Do Not Attempt Resuscitation (DNAR) or Do Not Intubate (DNI) Order

These may be noted in the medical record apart from a living will, or these preferences may be included in the living will. Increasingly, Allow Natural Death (AND) is being used instead of DNR.

Medical Orders for Life-Sustaining Treatment

Medical Orders for Life-Sustaining Treatment (MOLST) is a medical order in which the physician records patient preferences for medical treatment wanted and not wanted. MOLST is appropriate for persons likely to be in their final year of life. It is portable and stays with patients as they move through different care settings. MOLST differs from a living will because it is a medical order that is actionable and can be followed by doctors and first responders (e.g., emergency medical technicians, police, and fire departments; Hickman, Sabatino, Moss, & Nester, 2008). In some states, this is called Physician Orders for Life-Sustaining Treatment (POLST).

Social workers can help facilitate conversations about preferences for treatment at end of life between patients and health care agents. Advance directives should be reviewed and revised as needed when there is a new diagnosis, change in prognosis, the patient's wishes change, or a new HCA is appointed.

PRACTICE

Competencies and Certification

The National Association of Social Workers (NASW) established standards for palliative social work in 2004 (NASW, 2004), but core social work competencies in the eight domains of palliative care have not been developed. The Clinical Practice Guidelines for Quality Palliative Care were published by the National Quality Forum (National Quality Forum, 2006). This report identifies the skills required to manage symptoms and needs of seriously and terminally ill patients.

NASW Advanced Certified Hospice and Palliative Social Worker (ACHP-SW)

This credential captures the knowledge, skills, and abilities of specialist-level social workers in hospice and palliative care settings, using a standardized measurement process (NASW, 2015). Eligibility requirements include: masters of social work (MSW) degree, at least 2 years of supervised post-MSW practice in hospice or palliative care, weekly supervision by a social worker, positive ratings of knowledge applied to practice and performance, and at least 20 hours of continuing education in hospice and palliative care.

Social Work Hospice and Palliative Network (SWHPN) Palliative Care Certification

In 2016, SWHPN initiated development of a certification for specialist-level palliative social workers that parallels medicine and nursing. The certification will include an examination assessing knowledge and skills required for specialty practice. Specialty certification in palliative social work will raise the standard of practice and contribute to professional and public confidence in certified palliative social workers.

Generalist-Level Palliative Social Work Core Competencies

Not all seriously and terminally ill individuals will need, or have access to, specialty palliative care. This means that social workers in all health care settings, as well as in social service settings, need generalist-level palliative care skills. The knowledge, skills, and competencies that reflect best practices in generalist-level palliative social work have not been established, nor have core competencies been defined. The goal of the National Consensus Project to Define Generalist-Level Core Competencies, led by the MJHS Institute for Innovation in Palliative Care, is to define generalist-level palliative social work competencies in the eight domains of palliative care.

Education

Widely accepted palliative care curricula tied to competency acquisition in MSW programs do not exist. Few MSW programs have specialty palliative social work electives or content on palliative care in required or elective courses (Berkman & Stein, 2017). The SWHPN initiative will develop specialty-level curricula and the National Consensus Project to Define Generalist-Level Core Competencies will develop curricula for post-MSW social workers in generalist palliative care.

Role of the Social Worker on the Interdisciplinary Team

Palliative care is usually delivered by an interdisciplinary palliative care team for patients requiring specialist expertise. Physicians have primary responsibility for pain and symptom management. They assist the primary health care providers, patient, and/or family in decision making and medical management. Nurses focus on pain and symptom control, and may also address psychological, social, and spiritual well-being. Chaplains assess the spiritual needs of the patient and family and discuss spiritual and emotional distress, while advocating for care that fits the patient's spiritual values and beliefs.

Social workers are most likely to view the patient and family in the context of their micro and macro environment, taking into account their psychosocial history, family dynamics, and culture. Their responsibilities include: completing a biopsychosocial–spiritual (BPSS) assessment; assisting with advance care planning, goals of care, and completion of advance directives; developing and implementing a comprehensive social care plan; educating the patient and family; providing support and counseling; enhancing communication within and between the family, the interdisciplinary team, primary caregivers, and the health care system; advocating for the patient and family with the palliative care team and primary caregivers; assisting the patient and family in navigating medical and social service systems; and assisting in securing benefits and services (Stark, 2011). Social workers participate in, and may lead, the family meeting. The social worker has a role in pain and symptom management and in resolving ethical issues. An important role of the palliative social worker is providing support and counseling to patients and family members. Patients and families facing life-threatening illness often experience psychological, social, physical, spiritual, and/or financial problems. Attention to social networks, culture, finances, communication, and access to services is enhanced by the social work focus and expertise in patient, family, and social systems (Altilio, Otis-Green, & Dahlin, 2008).

Clinical Skills

Palliative social workers are specialized in assisting patients and families with the complex and challenging tasks encountered in advanced and terminal illness.

Assessment

Assessment is often the first step in working with a client and/or family members. Palliative social workers are trained in conducting a BPSS assessment. In addition to assessing the social, psychological, financial, and legal domains, social workers also assess the physical and spiritual domains. Physicians or nurses should conduct a detailed physical assessment, and chaplains a spiritual assessment, but social workers should also include these domains. This facilitates a holistic view of the patient and family, and a comprehensive approach to care planning. Social workers play an important role in pain and symptom management, and in responding to spiritual needs. Risk and protective factors are identified during the assessment process. Risk factors may include lack of social support, financial strain, depression, or declining health. Protective factors may include strong social support, adequate health insurance, a health care agent who understands the patient's preferences, or stable health.

The *physical* domain includes: functional limitations; physical symptoms, such as pain, fatigue, and dyspnea; mental status; and sexual health. The *psychological* domain includes: level of distress; depression, anxiety, and other syndromes; internal resources; problem-solving skills; and quality of life. The *social* domain includes: external resources; adequacy and availability of support; employment history; and family functioning. The *spiritual* domain includes: religious affiliation; spiritual values and beliefs; spiritual history and behavior; and spiritual well-being. The *financial* domain includes: insurance status; income; access to other financial resources; and debt burden. The *legal* domain includes: will and estate planning; advance care planning; and durable power of attorney.

There are tools available for conducting a comprehensive assessment (Reese et al., 2006) and for assessing specific domains, such as spirituality (Nelson-Becker, Nakashima, & Canda, 2006) or symptoms within a domain, such as depression (Kroenke & Spitzer, 2002). Most providers of palliative care have an assessment tool or protocol for social workers to use. The assessment tool should not be used as a checklist, but rather as a guide for a comprehensive assessment of patient risk and protective factors. A proper assessment process requires a high skill level.

Communication

Good communication skills are particularly important in palliative care, where anxiety, fear, and low health literacy may make comprehension by clients more challenging. Social work communication skills include listening empathically; tailoring information to the level of patients and caregivers; assessing, organizing, and interpreting patient and family data; and more (Glajchen & Gerbino, 2016). Physicians are most likely to inform patients of a serious diagnosis, but social workers have an important role in helping patients understand and cope with the diagnosis, prognosis, and treatment. Patients may not understand their disease, the prognosis, expected symptoms, side effects of treatment, and how this may affect their life. Social workers allow patients time to process difficult information and to connect with the emotional aspect of this information. Often, the patient or family does not fully comprehend what was said due to the overwhelming emotions that they experience upon receiving this information.

Palliative social workers can help clarify the issues for the patient and family. This requires that social workers understand the patient's medical condition and prescribed treatments. The social worker often starts by asking the patient and family about their understanding of what the physician has told them. This is a good starting point for correcting misunderstandings, discussing the meaning of the information, answering questions, addressing concerns, and offering support, benefits, and services. Patients are sometimes labeled by health care providers as non-adherent or difficult. Social workers often play the role of eliciting the patient's or family's concerns, communicating these to the team, and advocating for the patient and family when appropriate.

Advance Care Planning

Advance care planning involves making decisions about the care that is preferred by the patient. This allows the HCA and health care providers to understand the patient's wishes if the time comes when the patient can no longer communicate. Advance care planning is not limited to completing a living will, MOLST, or DNR. It is a process of understanding the patient's values, what gives his or her life meaning, and the types of treatment the patient would, and would not, want under different circumstances (Berlinger, Jennings, & Wolf, 2013). This requires multiple in-depth conversations with the patient and the family, allowing time for questions and discussing whether the treatment options are aligned with their goals of care, values, and preferences. These conversations should be repeated when necessary, and always when the medical condition or treatment options change.

Shared decision making is a patient-centered approach often used by palliative care specialists. It is a process in which patients, family members, and health care providers determine the most appropriate treatment or care choices together (Barry & Edgman-Levitan 2012). Shared decision making is respectful of patient preferences, needs, and values (Committee on Improving the Quality of Cancer Care: Addressing the Challenges of an Aging Population, Board on Health Care Services, and IOM, 2013). It is particularly important when there is more than one treatment option and no one option is clearly advantageous (National Learning Consortium, 2013).

The physician is most qualified to discuss prognosis and treatment, and therefore typically initiates the advance care planning discussion. These discussions may involve the primary caregivers and/or the palliative care physician. Social workers and other members of the palliative care team often participate in these discussions.

Family Meeting

The purpose of the family meeting is to address the patient's diagnosis and prognosis, the goals of care, and patient and family needs and preferences. It is a forum to assess the family's strengths and needs, make joint medical decisions, and develop a plan of care. Some or all of the interdisciplinary team attends the family meeting. The patient should participate whenever possible, either in person or by phone. The family meeting facilitates communication and strengthens the therapeutic alliance between the team and the family. It is a safe space to process emotions and can provide validation for the caregiver's concerns and roles. Technology, including videoconferencing and Skype, can be used to allow participation from family members who are not able to be in the room.

A family meeting should be held under any of these circumstances: change in medical status; major decline in functional status; transition in care; patient aged 80 years or older; two or more life-threatening comorbidities; mortality risk greater than 25%; when tracheotomy, ventilator, or feeding tube are being considered; within 72 hours of admission to the ICU; to introduce hospice; when there is family conflict, distress, or crisis; extended hospital stay; lack of a HCA; new prognostic information; advance care planning or discharge planning is necessary; or when there is an ethical dilemma (Billings, 2011; Hudson, Quinn, O'Hanlon, & Aranda, 2008). The family meeting should not be a one-time intervention. Changes in prognosis or goals of care require additional meetings.

There are three phases to the family meeting: preparation, the talk, follow-up. In the *preparation* phase, some or all of the team plans the meeting, reviews the medical chart, contacts current and former care providers for useful information and invites them to the meeting when appropriate, and arranges the meeting space to foster participation. Decisions made at this phase include who will lead the meeting, who will speak for the family, whose agenda will be followed, and who will summarize the meeting.

The *talk* portion of the meeting begins by reviewing the purpose of the meeting and the participants. The agenda is reviewed and revised as necessary (Hannon, O'Reilly, Bennett, Breen, & Lawlor, 2012). The providers assess family resiliency, vulnerability, social support, cultural beliefs, risk factors, and decision-making style. Support and validation of caregivers is provided. Recommendations for care are made. Providers make sure that the patient and family have a clear understanding of treatment choices and are included in decision making.

The *follow-up* phase entails offering support services (including social work, patient advocacy, ethics consultation, or palliative care), summarizing the meeting and action plan, and developing a follow-up plan. Providers check in with the patient and family about whether the meeting achieved their goals and whether anything important was omitted. Providers debrief after the meeting.

Psychosocial Interventions and Supportive Counseling

One of the most important roles of the palliative social worker is providing support and counseling to patients and family members (NASW, 2004). Among the most widely used approaches in palliative care are meaning-based therapy (Breitbart et al., 2012) and dignity therapy (Chochinov, 2012). Meaning-based therapy is rooted in the work of Viktor Frankl (2006) and posits that life has meaning, even in the most difficult circumstances. Dignity therapy is a brief intervention with the goal of helping terminally ill patients and family members maintain a sense of dignity by addressing psychological, spiritual, and existential challenges.

Social Work Role in Pain and Symptom Management

Social workers have an important role to play in pain and symptom management (Blacker & Christ, 2011). The dimensions of the pain experience and suffering affect more than physical suffering. They also include the emotional, cultural, social, familial, and spiritual domains. A holistic approach to pain and symptom management requires that all of these domains be addressed in treating distressing symptoms, and that each member of the interdisciplinary team contributes to the assessment and management of these symptoms (Otis-Green, Sherman, Perez, & Baird, 2002). In addition to pain, distressing symptoms include fatigue, agitation, anxiety, depression, dyspnea, nausea, and insomnia.

Pain assessment is based on patient report, clinician evaluation, nonverbal pain behaviors, responses of the family and social network, and the impact on self: self-concept, mood, sleep, social roles and isolation, and sexuality. Barriers to optimal pain management include: inadequate education about communicating pain and treatment effects; stigma associated with pain medications; concerns related to fears of addiction; concerns about adverse effects; fear of developing tolerance; and fear of overdose. These fears may be experienced by the patient and family, and also by clinicians.

The social work role in pain management is rooted in the values of respect for dignity of individuals and social justice (Altilio & Otis-Green, 2005). Populations that are undertreated for pain include persons of color, older adults, women, children, cognitively impaired persons, low-income persons, persons with lower educational attainment, and persons with limited fluency in English (Altilio & Colón, 2007). Social work interventions for pain and symptom management include education of the patient and family, relaxation techniques, and cognitive therapies. Palliative social work requires becoming knowledgeable and experienced about pain and symptom management in order to assess, treat, and advocate for the treatment that patients need and deserve.

Bereavement Support

Grief is a normal response to the death of a loved one. Each person grieves in his or her own way. Grief may be expressed emotionally, physically, cognitively, behaviorally, and/or spiritually. The Dual Process Model of grief posits that there are two tasks of bereavement: (a) separating from the deceased person; and (b) building a new life and identity in the absence of the deceased (Stroebe & Schut, 1999). According to this theory, part of the healthy grief process involves oscillating between loss-oriented and restoration-oriented coping in a dynamic process of confronting the loss and avoiding the loss. The Medicare Hospice Benefit includes bereavement services for up to 1 year after the death. Bereavement services are often provided by bereavement specialists, rather than by the palliative or hospice social worker.

The type and duration of grief reaction is based on many factors, including the quality of the relationship to the deceased, the duration of the illness, and the coping mechanisms and supports available to the bereaved (Sormanti, 2015). Grief counseling may be helpful for loved ones who are experiencing uncomplicated grief that is within the typical range of reactions and duration. This usually includes normalizing the grief process and facilitating normal grieving.

Complicated grief is diagnosed when the bereaved individual is unable to resume normal activities and responsibilities within 6 months and experiences persistent maladaptive thoughts and behaviors. Grief therapy is recommended in these cases (Worden, 2008). Risk factors for complicated grief include cause of death, such as suicide or traumatic death, loss of a child or spouse, preexisting psychological disorder, an ambivalent or conflicted relationship with the deceased, and a high level of dependency in the relationship. Professionals disagree about delineating normal grief from complicated grief. There are cultural differences in the expression of grief that may result in misdiagnosis (Sormanti, 2015).

Palliative Care Across the Lifespan

Children and Adolescents

Palliative social work with children and adolescents involves treating the family unit of parents, siblings, and possibly other relatives, as the client (Orloff, 2015). Children coping with life-threatening illness and death, and their family, need a lot of support. Very young children may have issues of trust, fear of strangers, changing health care providers, fear of pain, and fear of separation from family. School age children often have concerns about accomplishing goals and feeling inferior to peers. Adolescents and young adults experience confusion about how the illness affects roles and relationships, concerns about intimacy, and the ability to form long-term relationships and to have a family (Block, 2015). Children and adolescents may feel guilty about getting sick and requiring so much family time and resources. They may feel responsible for their illness. They often understand the seriousness of their illness and their chance of dying and seek clear, honest, communication, which the social worker can help provide (Cincotta, 2004). The autonomy of older adolescents who are still minors may cause conflict with parents and providers. Parents often experience emotional and financial stress, feel inadequate to meet the caregiving needs of their sick child, their other children, and job demands. Siblings may be scared, confused, challenged by changing roles in the family, feel guilty for being healthy, neglected, and/or angry that their sibling is receiving so much attention (Wiener & Sansom-Daly, 2015).

The role of the pediatric palliative social worker is psychosocial assessment, support and counseling for the child, education of and supportive counseling with family members, advocacy, and bereavement counseling (Jones, 2005). They help convey medical information to children and adolescents and educate them about their illness, appropriate to their developmental stage. The pediatric palliative social worker may also guide the family in broaching topics about difficult transitions in care and planning for death (Remke, 2015).

Older Adults

Serious illness may present differently in older adults than in younger age groups. Older adults approaching the end of life often have multiple comorbidities and more functional decline than younger adults (Bakitas, Kryworuchko, Matlock, & Volandes, 2011). Palliative care services may be needed for a longer time period of time (Hall, Petkova, Tsouros, Constantini, & Higginson, 2011). Better palliative care for older adults is a public health priority (Hall et al., 2011). There are not enough health care providers trained in geriatrics (Amella, 2003), which often results in overlooking the markers for needing palliative care in older adults. These include frailty, functional dependence, comorbidity, cognitive impairment, symptom distress, and family support needs. Pain is often undertreated in older adults. Health care providers must be able to diagnose and manage geriatric syndromes and understand complex long-term care settings in order to provide high-quality palliative care to older adult patients (Kapo, Morrison, & Liao, 2007). Models of palliative care services for older adults must take into consideration increased psychosocial vulnerability and altered physiology (Kapo et al., 2007; Kite, 2006). Treating older adults often necessitates cooperation between geriatric and palliative care specialists in order to provide excellent geriatric and palliative care simultaneously.

Cultural Dimensions in Palliative Care

The diversity of cultures throughout the United States and globally demands awareness of differences in perceptions and preferences related to serious illness and its treatment. While it is not possible to become culturally competent in all the cultural groups encountered, aiming to be culturally sensitive, open-minded, and respectful of other cultures will result in more appropriate care. Working in multicultural settings requires learning more about other cultures in order to minimize cultural misunderstandings (Del Rio, 2004). Cultural humility and cultural sensitivity should begin with self-awareness of one's values, beliefs, and how these affect the way we work with patients, families, and colleagues.

A comprehensive cultural assessment should include: race; language; gender identity; sexual orientation; ethnicity; religious beliefs and spirituality; socioeconomic status; important customs, rituals, and traditions; degree of acculturation; importance of traditions and health beliefs; whether the decision-making approach is individual or includes family and friends; and preferences regarding written or oral advance directives (Brangman & Periyakoil, 2014; Stein & Bonuck, 2001). Asking the patient what he or she wants to know about the illness, in what detail, and when, is important to document and respect. Some cultural groups are more likely to prefer full disclosure as soon as the health care providers know something, while others prefer minimal, indirect, or euphemistically couched information and to have it delivered later in the course of illness (Barclay, Blackhall, & Tulsky, 2007; Berkman & Ko, 2009, 2010; Mystakidou, Parpa, Tsilila, Katsouda, & Vlahos, 2004). It is important to avoid cultural stereotypes and assumptions based on the cultural group to which the patient belongs. There are likely to be as many differences within as between cultural groups.

Cultural sensitivity includes understanding the patient's explanatory model of illness and how this affects advance care planning and resolving conflicts between the patient, family, and health care providers (Fadiman, 2012; Kleinman, 1988). Cultural differences in the interpretation and response to pain and other symptoms are important for palliative social workers to assess and address (Lasch, 2002).

Language barriers may result in misunderstandings and misguided treatment choices (Del Rio, 2004). Choosing appropriate translators, preferably trained in a medical setting, is the best practice. Having a family member translate is often fraught with mistranslation, both intentional and unintentional. Choosing a minor who is bilingual should be avoided when possible because hearing the content and being put in this situation may be very upsetting. Checking the patient's understanding of what has been communicated is especially critical when there is a cultural or language difference.

Spirituality in Palliative Care

Spiritual care is an essential component of palliative care (Puchalski et al., 2009). A diagnosis of life-threatening illness often triggers thoughts about the meaning of one's life, and raises religious, spiritual, or existential questions (Scott, Thiel, & Dahlin, 2008; Sulmasy, 2002). Patients may question why they have become ill, whether it is a punishment, why they are suffering, and what their legacy will be. Studies have found that many patients have spiritual needs, experience spiritual pain, are searching for forgiveness, or feel abandoned by God (Astrow, Wexler, Texeira, He, & Sulmasy, 2007; Delgado-Guay, 2014; Delgado-Guay et al., 2016; Moadel et al., 1999). The prevalence of spiritual pain among caregivers may also be high (Delgado-Guay et al., 2013). Spiritual pain in patients (Winkelman et al., 2011) and caregivers (Delgado-Guay et al., 2013) is associated with lower psychological distress and quality of life. This supports the importance of spiritual assessment of, and spiritual support for, patients and caregivers at the end of life (Daaleman, Williams, Hamilton, & Zimmerman, 2008).

The chaplain is the team member with primary responsibility for religious and/or spiritual concerns, but other members of the team, especially the social worker, should be competent in this area. Palliative social workers need to be comfortable discussing religion and spirituality with patients, regardless of their own beliefs and faith tradition. They should be competent in conducting a spirituality assessment as part of a comprehensive assessment and to incorporate spirituality into their work with the patient and family when appropriate. In addition to the importance of relieving religious, spiritual, and existential pain, many patients view their illness as an opportunity for spiritual growth (Delgado-Guay, 2014). Social workers can facilitate this connection with spirituality.

Ethical Issues in Palliative Care

There are many ethical issues related to palliative care, including withholding and withdrawing medical treatment or nutrition and hydration, determination of decision-making capacity, informed consent, decision making by minors, decision making by persons with limited decisional capacity, surrogate decision making, pain management, futile medical care, terminal sedation, and aid in dying (Hickey, 2007; McCabe & Coyle, 2014; University of Minnesota Center for Bioethics, 2005). The ethical principles that guide decisions in health care, including palliative care, are: autonomy, beneficence, non-maleficence, and justice (Beauchamp & Childress, 2012). Veracity, confidentiality, and fidelity are also frequently included in ethical principles guiding palliative care (Taylor, 2015). Ethical dilemmas in practice can be referred to an ethics committee in the institution or agency.

An important social justice issue is access to palliative and hospice care. As Jennings, Ryndes, D'Onofrio, and Baily (2003) note, care of terminally ill patients and their families is a question of values, rather than of the technical details and means. Reasons for lack of access to palliative care in the United States include a shortage of palliative care professionals, limits on the availability of palliative care in outpatient and long-term care settings, eligibility requirements for hospice services under the Medicare Hospice Benefit, delay in referral to hospice until close to death, access to pharmacies that stock commonly prescribed pain medicines, and disparities in access to palliative care for non-White and poor persons (American Academy of Hospice and Palliative Medicine, 2008; Del Rio, 2004; IOM, 2014; Meier, 2011). Social workers are involved in advocating for increased access to palliative care within health care institutions and at the state and federal levels of government, and need to continue these efforts as long as necessary to achieve full access to palliative and hospice care for all.

Self-Care

Palliative social work is a rich and fulfilling area of practice. However, it exposes social workers to a higher degree of loss and places them at risk of burnout and vicarious trauma (Clark, 2011; Remke, 2015). The positive impact of working with clients who experience difficulties, such as life-threatening illness, has been recognized. This concept, named vicarious resilience, is based on the professional satisfaction and growth that derives from observing clients coping with their illness and the challenges they face (Hernandez, Gangsei, & Engstrom, 2007). This instills great professional resilience and increased confidence and hope in the social worker.

Experienced palliative social workers develop self-awareness and mechanisms for professional, organizational, and personal self-care (Mathieu, 2012). Personal self-care may include a social support system, taking time for relaxation and enjoying activities, time to process emotions, and being aware of one's core values (Neenan, 2009). Professional self-care may include: maintaining and strengthening the interdisciplinary palliative care team; clinical supervision, increasing knowledge and skills by attending conferences and continuing education; and becoming involved in ethics practice in the workplace (Cincotta, 2004; Clark, 2011; Joubert, Hocking, & Hampson, 2013; Simon, Pryce, Roff, & Klemmack, 2005). Organizational self-care is based on the resources and working conditions at the workplace. This may involve the choice of workplace, as well as advocating for resources needed for patients and providers in the workplace (Lipsky & Burk, 2009; Neenan, 2009).

Case Example 9.1

Presenting problem: Mr. C is a 69-year-old man in relatively good health. During his annual visit to his primary care provider (PCP), he complains of persistent cough, fatigue, loss of appetite, and breathlessness. He has significant weight loss, pain in his left chest, and diminished breath sounds in the left lung. A chest CT scan reveals a left pleural-based mass with lymphadenopathy.

(continued)

(continued)

Social history: Mr. C has been married for 25 years. One son lives nearby in New York City and the other in California. He has good relationships with family and close friends. He works full time for a lighting company. He is a nonobservant Protestant. He smokes half a pack a day and drinks four to five beers on the weekend. Ten years ago, Mr. C was treated for moderate depression after his mother died of lung cancer. The episode resolved with brief psychotherapy and SSRI medication.

Medical history: A biopsy confirms stage IIIB non-resectable non-small cell lung cancer. The oncologist tells the PCP the disease is incurable with an average 5-year survival of 5% to 10%. Mr. C starts chemotherapy but has strong side effects, including insomnia, anxiety, and debilitating fatigue. He can no longer work and applies for long-term disability. After 3 months, his tumor has shrunk by 75% and his cough has resolved. He is optimistic, but still functioning poorly. One year later, he develops chest wall pain, increased dyspnea on exertion, fatigue, and anorexia. New imaging shows the pleural mass growing and eroding into the chest wall, and metastases to the liver and bone. The oncologist recommends second-line chemotherapy, but the PCP is concerned about toxicity. Mr. and Mrs. C and their sons are divided about whether Mr. C should opt for the chemo. The PCP prescribes opioids (for pain) and oxygen (for shortness of breath). Mr. C is never able to return to work. Two years after his diagnosis, Mr. C lapses into a coma and dies at home. Mrs. C and her sons are distraught because they did not realize that Mr. C was terminal, and they did not have the opportunity to say goodbye.

Case 9.1 illustrates a number of missed opportunities for introducing palliative care. Palliative care from the time of diagnosis would have provided better management of distressing physical and psychological symptoms. Family meetings could have improved communication and advance care planning among the providers, Mr. C, and his family. Goals of care should have been discussed at the time of diagnosis and revised throughout the course of the illness. Mr. C's preference for curative treatment to increase survival or a shift to supportive care to increase comfort and quality of life may have changed over the course of the illness and treatment trajectory.

The palliative social worker could have provided support and counseling to Mr. C and his family as they coped with the diagnosis of lung cancer and the stress of chemotherapy. The social worker could have helped the patient and his family better understand the prognosis and the pros and cons of undergoing another round of chemotherapy. This would have included the medical issues, but also the social and psychological consequences. The social worker could have facilitated appointment of a HCA and completion of a living will. Hospice would likely have been suggested for Mr. C in the final months of his life. The hospice benefit would also have provided the C family with bereavement support and counseling as needed.

POLICY

As in most social work arenas, hospice and palliative care practice is shaped by law and public policy. This section reviews key trends for future practice and policy, as determined by the federal and state legislatures and courts. These policy trends include challenges to health care decision making and advance care planning, aid in dying, alternative payment models (APMs) for care, and professional training.

Challenges to Health Care Decision Making and Advance Care Planning

The gold standard for advance care planning includes thoughtful advance directives—including appointment of a health care agent for decision making when one is incapacitated, declaring one's preferred choices regarding specific life-sustaining medical interventions through living wills, and doctor's orders incorporating preferences regarding resuscitation, specific interventions, and choice of surrogate through MOLST/POLST. While a majority of Americans think it is important to educate patients and families about options for end-of-life care, most Americans do not complete advance directives, often due to lack of information, denial of need, cultural preferences, and difficulties in making thoughtful decisions before the onset of illness (IOM, 2014; The Regence Foundation, 2011). Several strategies have been advanced to address these shortcomings.

Absence of Advance Directives

A majority of states (38) have default health care surrogate laws that provide the hierarchy of family members (and sometimes close friends) who can make decisions in the absence of an appointed health care agent. For example, New York State's surrogate hierarchy lists a court-appointed guardian, the spouse or domestic partner, an adult child, a parent, a sibling, or a close friend (N.Y. Public Health Law, §2994-d.1, 2010). Conflicts can occur among surrogates at the same level, such as among adult children, parents, or siblings, requiring health care teams and ethics committees to seek consensus or other means for reaching decisions. Future state policies may be required to address these dilemmas.

Unrepresented Patients

How to make decisions for incapacitated patients who lack advance directives and families or friends to serve as surrogates—sometimes referred to as unbefriended or unrepresented patients, or adult orphans—is a significant challenge in hospitals and nursing homes. This is likely to be a growing concern as the baby boomer generation ages: More than 10 million of this group live alone, and 20% are childless (Redfoot, Feinberg, & Houser, 2013). The American Geriatrics Society published a revised position statement calling for uniform legal standards on unbefriended individuals to be adopted by all states; safeguards against ad hoc approaches to decision making; and institutional committees, such as ethics committees, to synthesize all available evidence about patients, including cultural and ethnic factors, before decisions are made (Farrell et al., 2016). Thoughtful policymaking will be needed to address this serious and growing problem.

Social Work Reimbursement for Advance Care Planning

To encourage health care providers to engage patients and their families in advance care planning discussions, the CMS amended its Physician Fee Schedule in 2016 to allow reimbursement for 30-minute planning discussions by physicians, nurse practitioners, and physician assistants (CMS, 2015). Social workers are not included as eligible for reimbursement, despite evidence that the majority of palliative social workers conduct and lead advance care planning discussions (Stein, Cagle, & Christ, 2016). The federal Patient Choice and Quality Care Act 2017 addresses these reimbursement shortcomings (Patient Choice and Quality Care Act, 2017). If this bill is enacted, licensed clinical social workers could receive payment for advance care planning discussions.

Innovative Approaches to Advance Care Planning

In addition to reimbursing social workers for advance care planning services, the Patient Choice and Quality Care Act promotes a range of innovative strategies to support advance care planning. These interventions include: enhanced information on advance care planning for Medicare beneficiaries; national standards for electronic medical records; a national public awareness and education campaign; a study on policy barriers to advance directives; and enhanced portability of advance directives across state lines (i.e., directives executed in one state would be given full effect in other states where patients may require care).

Advocacy for Aid in Dying

Patient autonomy advocates have promoted aid-in-dying laws (also known as physician-assisted suicide) that allow physicians to legally assist terminally ill patients to end their lives by prescribing lethal medications that the patient self-ingests. Advocates of this practice suggest that this allows patients for whom death is imminent to maintain as much dignity as possible and avoid intolerable pain and suffering at the end of their life. While the U.S. Supreme Court rejected claims by patients with AIDS and cancer that assisted suicide is a fundamental right protected by the U.S. Constitution (*Vacco v. Quill*, 1997; *Washington v. Glucksberg*, 1997), aid in dying is a growing movement with increasing support (Span, 2017).

As of 2017, six states (Oregon, Washington, Vermont, California, Montana, and Colorado) and Washington, DC, have enacted Death with Dignity Acts. Modeled after Oregon's 1997 law, these laws allow terminally ill individuals to legally obtain and use prescriptions for lethal doses of medications as long as strict guidelines are followed. Close monitoring by Oregon's Health Department has not found any evidence of abuse of, nor widespread use by, very sick patients (Oregon Health Authority, 2017). Additional state legislatures are likely to approve aid-in-dying laws in future years. Social workers are not authorized to directly assist clients to hasten their deaths, even in states with aid-in-dying legislation, and should understand that doing so could have serious legal implications.

Payment Reforms to Promote Palliative Care

Although the palliative care team provides a coordinated approach to medical, psychosocial, and spiritual care, the U.S. health care system primarily reimburses medical services provided by physicians, nurse practitioners, and physician assistants. Nonmedical team services—including the psychosocial support provided by social workers and spiritual care provided by chaplains—must be absorbed by the hospital, or supported financially by foundation grants and by corporate and individual philanthropy. This model does not sustain a team approach that integrates psychosocial care. Currently, payment for interdisciplinary care under Medicare is available only to hospice patients, and not for palliative care provided in hospitals or at home.

Stakeholders are advocating for numerous APMs to support interdisciplinary palliative care. These APMs are vital to fully integrating psychosocial care provided by social workers into the team model and sustaining these services over time. New payment policies to transform reimbursement for palliative care are anticipated over the next few years. This is especially important for seriously ill individuals who are not yet eligible for, or who decline, hospice care.

Palliative Care Training

The shortage of palliative care professionals in all disciplines has been documented (IOM, 2008). As the number of Medicare beneficiaries is expected to double over the next 20 years, more health care professionals will be needed to meet the full range of medical, psychosocial, and spiritual needs of patients with serious illness. The federal Palliative Care and Hospice Education and Training Act (PCHETA) has been introduced in multiple congressional sessions to expand the palliative care workforce, including social workers (PCHETA, 2017). Among its key provisions, PCHETA would support palliative care training for social work students, palliative care fellowships for social work faculty, and incentive awards for social work students to pursue careers in palliative care through teaching or practice. This bill will likely gather increasing support as the need for palliative care services increases.

RESEARCH

Many studies have been conducted on a wide range of topics in palliative care. Research has demonstrated the benefits of palliative care, including improved quality of life, reduced patient and caregiver burden, and lower health care costs. Symptoms that accompany life-limiting illness, including pain and depression, are lower among patients receiving palliative care (Laguna, Goldstein, Allen, Braun, & Enguidanos, 2012). Higher quality of care and patient outcomes (Kamal, Gradison, Maguire, Taylor, & Abernethy, 2014; Smith, Bernacki, & Block, 2015), greater patient and family satisfaction, and better bereavement outcomes are found among those receiving palliative care (Meier, 2011; Roza, Lee, Meier, & Goldstein, 2015; Smith et al., 2015). In addition to decreasing distressing symptoms, palliative care delivered simultaneously with usual medical treatment may prolong life (Temel et al., 2010). The benefits of advance care planning have also been demonstrated (Hannon et al., 2012; Hudson et al., 2008).

Palliative care decreases costs. Inpatient palliative care consult teams reduce hospital costs due to shorter duration of stay, less time in intensive care, and improved use of hospital resources, and report a higher likelihood of discharge to hospice care in an appropriate setting (May, Normand, & Morrison, 2014; Morrison et al., 2008; Smith, Brick, O'Hara, & Normand, 2014). Home-based palliative care may decrease hospital length of stay (Chen et al., 2015) and ICU-based palliative care may decrease time spent in the ICU (Khandelwal et al., 2015).

There is much to be learned about how to best deliver palliative care in community-based settings, nursing homes, assisted living facilities, outpatient settings, and home care. Models that integrate health care and social services need to be developed and evaluated to determine whether they reduce hospitalizations and health care costs while improving quality of life for patients and families. Research is needed on delivering better palliative care to members of diverse racial and ethnic groups, persons from the lesbian, gay, bisexual, and transgender (LGBT) community, homeless persons, incarcerated persons, cognitively impaired individuals, refugees, and many cultural groups and special populations. Research is also needed to understand how to address religious and spiritual aspects of patient care (Alcorn et al., 2010). Increasingly, health care services are delivered by for-profit hospitals and hospice agencies. Evaluating how this affects the quality of care is important.

Evidence supports the effectiveness of advance care planning and advance directives, but more research is needed to understand the most effective models for this. Family meetings are associated with positive outcomes, including less time in the ICU, earlier withdrawal of technology, and timely referral to palliative care and hospice (Curtis et al., 2001), but research is needed to determine whether the family meeting is associated with higher patient and family satisfaction, improved bereavement, or results in any negative outcomes, and if so, how to minimize these. Evidence-based approaches are necessary to understand how the setting, length, and number and composition of participants affect the outcomes of family meetings. Despite the demonstrated value of palliative care in increasing quality of life and decreasing costs, funding for palliative care research is limited. Less than 1% of the National Institutes of Health (NIH) budget is allocated to palliative care (Hughes & Smith, 2014). Additional barriers to palliative care research are lack of institutional capacity to conduct research and difficulties and ethical concerns in conducting research on very seriously ill patients.

More widespread inclusion of social workers on palliative teams and eligibility for reimbursement by Medicare and other insurers would be promoted if there was evidence demonstrating the benefit of social work on the palliative care team. This includes the contribution of social workers to improving quality of life, increasing patient and family satisfaction with palliative care services, and reducing health care costs. There is little education on palliative care in MSW programs (Berkman & Stein, 2017; Sumser, Remke, Leimena, Altilio, & Otis-Green, 2015). Although very few, there are some excellent models in MSW programs and post-MSW fellowship and certificate programs. Evaluating models of educating social workers in both generalist and specialty-level palliative care is needed.

CONCLUSION

Palliative care is a relatively new and growing social work specialty. It is a deeply rewarding practice area because it involves developing and using advanced clinical skills, is stimulating and challenging, involves interdisciplinary collaboration, and, most importantly, offers the opportunity for making a very meaningful contribution to patients and family members as they experience one of the most important transitions in their lives. As the U.S. population ages and more effective treatments are developed to extend the lives of seriously ill individuals, and as palliative care gains wider acceptance and is introduced earlier in the course of illness, the need for palliative social work will increase. There is also a great need for social workers in a wide range of health care and social service settings to have generalist-level competence in palliative care. This will enable them to provide basic palliative care to patients and family members who are experiencing serious or life-limiting illness. Opportunities for education and training of palliative social workers at both the specialist and generalist levels are needed to have an adequate number of social workers with palliative expertise to meet the ever-growing needs of patients and their family members.

Chapter Discussion Questions

1. What are some important ethical issues that arise in palliative care?

2. What policies need to be revised in order to provide better palliative care in the United States?

3. What are some of the important ways that the cultural values of the patient and the social worker affect palliative social work practice?

4. What research evidence would be helpful to: (a) improve clinical palliative social work practice and (b) change policies related to palliative social work practice?

CASE EXAMPLE AND DISCUSSION QUESTIONS

Case Example 9.2

Presenting Problem: Mrs. Y is rushed to the hospital after complaining of chest pain and collapsing in the bathroom. She is sent to the emergency room (ER) in a major medical center. Her husband and children accompany her.

Social History: Mrs. Y is a 48-year-old, first-generation Chinese immigrant. She is a hostess in a busy restaurant in Chinatown. Mr. and Mrs. Y speak almost no English. Their children explain medical information to them. Their 15-year-old daughter is the most fluent in English.

Medical History: Mrs. Y is diagnosed with end-stage congestive heart failure with a prognosis of weeks to months. She must stop working and alter her diet and lifestyle. The cardiologist, ER nurse, physician's assistant, and family stand around Mrs. Y's bed in an open cubicle. It is now 10:00 p.m. on a Friday night and the hospital interpreter has left. The ER is crowded and noisy, so the staff decides against using the language line. The cardiologist asks the daughter to translate. She reviews the treatment options for Mrs. Y, including medication and open-heart surgery. She asks the daughter to stress that time is short and her mother should get her affairs in order. The daughter translates for her parents and siblings. The staff notes her calm and mature demeanor.

Questions for Discussion

1. Is it appropriate to appoint the 15-year-old daughter as the family spokesperson?

2. Is disclosing the diagnosis and prognosis a professional imperative? What if the family adheres to cultural taboos that prohibit disclosure as bad luck? How can we find out the patient's preferences for information disclosure?

3. How could this event affect the family dynamics in the future?

4. What are the pros and cons of using an untrained family member as an interpreter?

REFERENCES

Alcorn, S. R., Balboni, M. J., Prigerson, H. G., Reynolds, A., Phelps, A. C., Wright, A. A., . . . Balboni, T. A. (2010). "If God wanted me yesterday, I wouldn't be here today": Religious and spiritual themes in patients' experiences of advanced cancer. *Journal of Palliative Medicine, 13*(5), 581–588. doi:10.1089/jpm.2009.0343

Altilio, T., & Colón, Y. (2007). Cultural perspectives in pain management: Implications for social worker and other psychosocial professionals. *Pain Practitioner, 17*(2), 25–29.

Altilio, T., & Otis-Green, S. (2005). "Res Ipsa Loquitur". . . it speaks for itself . . . social work—values, pain, and palliative care. *Journal of Social Work in End-of-Life and Palliative Care, 1*(4), 3–6. doi:10.1300/J457v01n04_02

Altilio, T., Otis-Green, S., & Dahlin, C. M. (2008). Applying the National Quality Forum Preferred Practices for Palliative and Hospice Care: A social work perspective. *Journal of Social Work in End-of-Life and Palliative Care, 4*(1), 3–16. doi:10.1080/15524250802071999

Amella, E. J. (2003). Geriatrics and palliative care: Collaboration for quality of life until death. *Journal of Hospice & Palliative Nursing, 5*(1), 40–48. doi:10.1097/00129191-200301000-00018

American Academy of Hospice and Palliative Medicine. (2008). Statement on access to palliative care and hospice. Retrieved from http://aahpm.org/positions/access

Astrow, A. B., Wexler, A., Texeira, K., He, M. K., & Sulmasy, D. P. (2007). Is failure to meet spiritual needs associated with cancer patients' perceptions of quality of care and their satisfaction with care? *Journal of Clinical Oncology, 25*(36), 5753–5757. doi:10.1200/jco.2007.12.4362

Bakitas, M., Kryworuchko, J., Matlock, D. D., & Volandes, A. E. (2011). Palliative medicine and decision science: The critical need for a shared agenda to foster informed patient choice in serious illness. *Journal of Palliative Medicine, 14*(10), 1109–1116. doi:10.1089/jpm.2011.0032

Barclay, J. S., Blackhall, L. J., & Tulsky, J. A. (2007). Communication strategies and cultural issues in the delivery of bad news. *Journal of Palliative Medicine, 10*(4), 958–977. doi:10.1089/jpm.2007.9929

Barry, M. J., & Edgman-Levitan, S. (2012). Shared decision making—The pinnacle of patient-centered care. *New England Journal of Medicine, 366*(9), 780–781. doi:10.1056/NEJMp1109283

Beauchamp, T. L., & Childress, J. F. (2012). *Principles of biomedical ethics* (7th ed.). New York, NY: Oxford University Press.

Berkman, C., & Stein, G. L. (2017). Palliative and end-of-life care in the masters of social work curriculum. *Palliative and Supportive Care,* 1–9. doi:10.1017/S147895151700013X

Berkman, C. S., & Ko, E. (2009). Preferences for disclosure of information about serious illness among older Korean American immigrants in New York City. *Journal of Palliative Medicine, 12*(4), 351–357. doi:10.1089/jpm.2008.0236

Berkman, C. S., & Ko, E. (2010). What and when Korean American older adults want to know about serious illness. *Journal of Psychosocial Oncology, 28*(3), 244–259. doi:10.1080/07347331003689029

Berlinger, N., Jennings, B., & Wolf, S. M. (2013). *The Hastings Center guidelines for decisions on life-sustaining treatment and care near end-of-life* (2nd ed.). New York, NY: Oxford University Press.

Billings, J. A. (2011). The end-of-life family meeting in intensive care part II: Family-centered decision making. *Journal of Palliative Medicine, 14*(9), 1051–1057. doi:10.1089/jpm.2011.0038-b

Bishop, L., Flick, T., & Wildman, V. (2015). *Best practices for using telehealth in palliative care.* Alexandria, VA. Retrieved from https://www.nhpco.org/sites/default/files/public/palliativecare/PALLIATIVECARE_Telehealth.pdf

Blacker, S., & Christ, G. (2011). Defining social work's role and leadership contributions in palliative care. In T. Altilio & S. Otis-Green (Eds.), *Oxford textbook of palliative social work* (pp. 21–30). New York, NY: Oxford University Press.

Block, R. G. (2015). Interventions for adolescents living with cancer. In G. Christ, C. Messner, & L. Behar (Eds.), *Handbook of oncology social work* (1st ed., pp. 457–463). New York, NY: Oxford University Press.

Brangman, S., & Periyakoil, V. S. (2014). *Doorway thoughts: Cross-cultural health care for older adults.* New York, NY: American Geriatrics Society.

Breitbart, W., Poppito, S., Rosenfeld, B., Vickers, A. J., Li, Y., Abbey, J., . . . Cassileth, B. R. (2012). Pilot randomized controlled trial of individual meaning-centered psychotherapy for patients with advanced cancer. *Journal of Clinical Oncology, 30*(12), 1304–1309. doi:10.1200/jco.2011.36.2517

Center to Advance Palliative Care. (2017). About palliative care. Retrieved from https://www.capc.org/about/palliative-care/

Centers for Medicare and Medicaid Services. (2015). 80 Federal Register 70956. Retrieved from https://www.federalregister.gov/documents/2015/07/15/2015-16875/medicare-program-revisions-to-payment-policies-under-the-physician-fee-schedule-and-other-revisions

Centers for Medicare and Medicaid Services. (2017). Medicare Care Choices Model. Retrieved from https://innovation.cms.gov/initiatives/Medicare-Care-Choices/

Chen, C. Y., Thorsteinsdottir, B., Cha, S. S., Hanson, G. J., Peterson, S. M., Rahman, P. A., . . . Takahashi, P. Y. (2015). Health care outcomes and advance care planning in older adults who receive home-based palliative care: A pilot cohort study. *Journal of Palliative Medicine, 18*(1), 38–44. doi:10.1089/jpm.2014.0150

Chochinov, H. M. (2012). *Dignity therapy: Final words for final days.* New York, NY: Oxford University Press.

Cincotta, N. (2004). The end of life at the beginning of life: Working with dying children and their families. In J. Berzoff & P. R. Silverman (Eds.), *Living with dying* (pp. 318–347). New York, NY: Columbia University Press.

Clark, E. J. (2011). Self-care as best practice in palliative care. In T. Altilio & S. Otis-Green (Eds.), *Oxford textbook of palliative social work* (pp. 771–777). New York, NY: Oxford University Press.

Committee on Improving the Quality of Cancer Care: Addressing the Challenges of an Aging Population, Board on Health Care Services, and Institute of Medicine. (2013). *Delivering high-quality cancer care: Charting a new course for a system in crisis.* Washington, DC: National Academies Press.

Curtis, J. R., Patrick, D. L., Shannon, S. E., Treece, P. D., Engelberg, R. A., & Rubenfeld, G. D. (2001). The family conference as a focus to improve communication about end-of-life care in the intensive care unit: Opportunities for improvement. *Critical Care Medicine, 29*(2), N26–N33. doi:10.1164/rccm.2501004

Daaleman, T. P., Williams, C. S., Hamilton, V. L., & Zimmerman, S. (2008). Spiritual care at the end of life in long-term care. *Medical Care, 46*(1), 85–91. doi:10.1097/MLR.0b013e3181468b5d

Del Rio, N. (2004). A framework for multicultural end-of-life care: Enhancing social work practice. In J. Berzoff & P. R. Silverman (Eds.), *Living with dying* (pp. 439–461). New York, NY: Columbia University Press.

Delgado-Guay, M. O. (2014). Spirituality and religiosity in supportive and palliative care. *Current Opinion in Supportive and Palliative Care, 8*(3), 308–313. doi:10.1097/spc.0000000000000079

Delgado-Guay, M. O., Chisholm, G., Williams, J., Frisbee-Hume, S., Ferguson, A. O., & Bruera, E. (2016). Frequency, intensity, and correlates of spiritual pain in advanced cancer patients assessed in a supportive/palliative care clinic. *Palliative and Supportive Care, 14*(4), 341–348. doi:10.1017/s147895151500108x

Delgado-Guay, M. O., Parsons, H. A., Hui, D., De la Cruz, M. G., Thorney, S., & Bruera, E. (2013). Spirituality, religiosity, and spiritual pain among caregivers of patients with advanced cancer. *The American Journal of Hospice and Palliative Care, 30*(5), 455–461. doi:10.1177/1049909112458030

Fadiman, A. (2012). *The spirit catches you and you fall down: A Hmong Child, her American doctors, and the collision of two cultures* (2nd ed.). New York, NY: Farrar, Straus, and Giroux.

Farrell, T. W., Widera, E., Rosenberg, L., Rubin, C. D., Naik, A. D., Braun, U., . . . Shega, J. (2016). AGS position statement: Making medical treatment decisions for unbefriended older adults. *Journal of the American Geriatrics Society.* doi:10.1111/jgs.14586

Frankl, V. E. (2006). *Man's search for meaning.* New York, NY: Simon & Schuster.

Glajchen, M., & Gerbino, S. (2016). Communication in palliative social work. In E. Wittenberg-Lyles, B. R. Ferrell, J. Goldsmith, T. Smith, S. L. Ragan, M. Glajchen, & G. F. Handzo (Eds.), *Oxford textbook of palliative care communication.* Oxford, NY: Oxford University Press.

Hall, S., Petkova, H., Tsouros, A. D., Constantini, M., & Higginson, I. J. (2011). *Palliative care for older people: Better practices.* Copenhagen, Denmark: World Health Organization.

Hannon, B., O'Reilly, V., Bennett, K., Breen, K., & Lawlor, P. G. (2012). Meeting the family: Measuring effectiveness of family meetings in a specialist inpatient palliative care unit. *Palliative and Supportive Care, 10*(1), 43–49. doi:10.1017/s1478951511000575

Hernandez, P., Gangsei, D., & Engstrom, D. (2007). Vicarious resilience: A new concept in work with those who survive trauma. *Family Process, 46*(2), 229–241. doi:10.1111/j.1545-5300.2007.00206.x

Hickey, K. (2007). Minors' rights in medical decision making. *JONAS Healthc Law Ethics Regul, 9*(3), 100–104; quiz 105–106. doi:10.1097/01.NHL.0000287968.36429.a9

Hickman, S., Sabatino, C., Moss, A., & Nester, J. (2008). The POLST (Physician Orders for Life-Sustaining Treatment) paradigm to improve end-of-life care: Potential state legal barriers to implementation. *Journal of Law Medical Ethics, 36*(1), 119–140. doi:10.1111/j.1748-720X.2008.00242.x

Hudson, P., Quinn, K., O'Hanlon, B., & Aranda, S. (2008). Family meetings in palliative care: Multidisciplinary clinical practice guidelines. *BMC Palliative Care, 7*(1), 1–12. doi:10.1186/1472-684x-7-12

Hughes, M. T., & Smith, T. J. (2014). The growth of palliative care in the United States. *Annual Review of Public Health, 35,* 459–475. doi:10.1146/annurev-publhealth-032013-182406

Institute of Medicine. (2008). *Retooling for an aging America: Building the health care workforce.* Washington, DC: National Academies Press.

Institute of Medicine. (2014). *Dying in America: Improving quality and honoring individual preferences near the end of life.* Washington, DC: National Academies Press.

Jennings, B., Ryndes, T., D'Onofrio, C., & Baily, M. A. (2003). Access to hospice care: Expanding boundaries, overcoming barriers. *The Hastings Center Report, Special Supplement* (March–April). Retrieved from http://www.thehastingscenter.org/wp-content/uploads/access_hospice_care.pdf

Jones, B. L. (2005). Pediatric palliative and end-of-life care: The role of social work in pediatric oncology. *Journal of Social Work in End-of-Life and Palliative Care, 1*(4), 35–61. doi:10.1300/J457v01n04_04

Joubert, L., Hocking, A., & Hampson, R. (2013). Social work in oncology: Managing vicarious trauma—the positive impact of professional supervision. *Social Work in Health Care, 52*(2–3), 296–310. doi:10.1080/00981389.2012.737902

Kamal, A. H., Gradison, M., Maguire, J. M., Taylor, D., & Abernethy, A. P. (2014). Quality measures for palliative care in patients with cancer: A systematic review. *Journal of Oncology Practice, 10*(4), 281–287. doi:10.1200/jop.2013.001212

Kapo, J., Morrison, L. J., & Liao, S. (2007). Palliative care for the older adult. *Journal of Palliative Medicine, 10*(1), 185–209. doi:10.1089/jpm.2006.9989

Khandelwal, N., Kross, E. K., Engelberg, R. A., Coe, N. B., Long, A. C., & Curtis, J. R. (2015). Estimating the effect of palliative care interventions and advance care planning on ICU utilization: A systematic review. *Critical Care Medicine, 43*(5), 1102–1111. doi:10.1097/ ccm.0000000000000852

Kite, S. (2006). Palliative care for older people. *Age and Ageing, 35*(5), 459–460. doi:10.1093/ ageing/afl069

Kleinman, A. (1988). *The illness narratives: Suffering, healing, and the human condition*. New York, NY: Basic Books.

Kroenke, K., & Spitzer, R. L. (2002). The PHQ-9: A new depression diagnostic and severity measure. *Psychiatric Annals, 32*(9), 1–7.

Laguna, J., Goldstein, R., Allen, J., Braun, W., & Enguidanos, S. (2012). Inpatient palliative care and patient pain: Pre- and post-outcomes. *Journal of Pain and Symptom Management, 43*(6), 1051–1059. doi:10.1016/j.jpainsymman.2011.06.023

Lasch, K. E. (2002). Culture and pain. *Pain: Clinical Updates, 10*(5).

Lipsky, L. V. D., & Burk, C. (2009). *Trauma stewardship: An everyday guide to caring for self while caring for others*. San Francisco, CA: Berrett-Koehler Publishers.

Lynn, J. (2005). Living long in fragile health: The new demographics shape end of life care. *The Hastings Center Report, Spec No*, S14–S18.

Mathieu, F. (2012). *The compassion fatigue workbook*. New York, NY: Taylor & Francis Group.

May, P., Normand, C., & Morrison, R. S. (2014). Economic impact of hospital inpatient palliative care consultation: Review of current evidence and directions for future research. *Journal of Palliative Medicine, 17*(9), 1054–1063. doi:10.1089/jpm.2013.0594

McCabe, M. S., & Coyle, N. (2014). Ethical and legal issues in palliative care. *Seminars in Oncology Nursing, 30*(4), 287–295. doi:10.1016/j.soncn.2014.08.011

Meier, D. E. (2011). Increased access to palliative care and hospice services: Opportunities to improve value in health care. *The Milbank Quarterly, 89*(3), 343–380. doi:10.1111/j.1468-0009.2011.00632.x

Moadel, A., Morgan, C., Fatone, A., Grennan, J., Carter, J., Laruffa, G., . . . Dutcher, J. (1999). Seeking meaning and hope: Self-reported spiritual and existential needs among an ethnically-diverse cancer patient population. *Psychooncology, 8*(5), 378–385. doi:10.1002/ (SICI)1099-1611(199909/10)8:5<378::AID-PON406>3.0.CO;2-A

Morrison, R. S., Penrod, J. D., Cassel, J. B., Caust-Ellenbogen, M., Litke, A., Spragens, L., & Meier, D. E. (2008). Cost savings associated with US hospital palliative care consultation programs. *Archives of Internal Medicine, 168*(16), 1783–1790. doi:10.1001/ archinte.168.16.1783

Mudigonda, P., & Mudigonda, T. (2010). Palliative cancer care ethics: Principles and challenges in the Indian setting. *Indian Journal of Palliative Care, 16*(3), 107–110. doi:10.4103/0973-1075.73639

Mystakidou, K., Parpa, E., Tsilila, E., Katsouda, E., & Vlahos, L. (2004). Cancer information disclosure in different cultural contexts. *Support Care Cancer, 12*(3), 147–154. doi:10.1007/s00520-003-0552-7

N.Y. Public Health Law. (2010). §2994-d.1.

National Association of Social Workers. (2004). NASW standards for palliative & end-of-life care. Retrieved from https://www.socialworkers.org/LinkClick. aspx?fileticket=xBMd58VwEhk%3D&portalid=0

National Association of Social Workers. (2015). *Advanced Certified Hospice and Palliative Social Worker* (ACHP-SW). Washington, DC: Author.

National Hospice and Palliative Care Organization. (2016). Facts and figures: Hospice care in America. Retrieved from https://www.nhpco.org/sites/default/files/public/ Statistics_Research/2016_Facts_Figures.pdf

National Hospice and Palliative Care Organization. (2017). Hospice Care. Retrieved from https://www.nhpco.org/about/hospice-care

National Learning Consortium. (2013). Shared decision making. Retrieved from https:// www.healthit.gov/sites/default/files/nlc_shared_decision_making_fact_sheet.pdf

National Quality Forum. (2006). *A national framework and preferred practices for palliative and hospice care quality.* Washington, DC: Author.

Neenan, M. (2009). *Developing resilience: A cognitive-behavioural approach.* New York, NY: Routledge.

Nelson-Becker, H., Nakashima, M., & Canda, E. R. (2006). Spiritual assessment in aging. *Journal of Gerontological Social Work, 48*(3–4), 331–347. doi:10.1300/J083v48n03_04

Oregon Health Authority. (2017). Public health division. Oregon Death with Dignity Act: Data summary 2016. Retrieved from https://public.health.oregon.gov/ProviderPartnerResources/ EvaluationResearch/DeathwithDignityAct/Pages/ar-index.aspx

Orloff, S. F. (2015). Pediatric hospice and palliative care: The invaluable role of social work. In G. Christ, C. Messner, & L. Behar (Eds.), *Handbook of oncology social work* (1st ed., pp. 75–86). New York, NY: Oxford University Press.

Otis-Green, S., Sherman, R., Perez, M., & Baird, R. P. (2002). An integrated psychosocial-spiritual model for cancer pain management. *Cancer Practice, 10* (Suppl 1), S58–S65.

Palliative Care and Hospice Education and Training Act. (2017). H.R. 1676//S. 693, Congress.

Patient Choice and Quality Care Act. (2017). S.1334. Sponsor: Sen. Warner, Mark R. [D-VA]. Retrieved from https://www.congress.gov/bill/115th-congress/senate-bill/1334

Puchalski, C., Ferrell, B., Virani, R., Otis-Green, S., Baird, P., Bull, J., . . . Sulmasy, D. (2009). Improving the quality of spiritual care as a dimension of palliative care: The report of the Consensus Conference. *Journal of Palliative Medicine, 12*(10), 885–904. doi:10.1089/jpm.2009.0142

Redfoot, D., Feinberg, L., & Houser, A. (2013). The aging of the baby boom and the growing care gap: A look at future declines in the availability of family caregivers. Retrieved from http://www.aarp.org/home-family/caregiving/info-08-2013/the-aging-of -the-baby-boom-and-the-growing-care-gap-AARP-ppi-ltc.html

Reese, D. J., Raymer, M., Orloff, S. F., Gerbino, S., Valade, R., Dawson, S., . . . Huber, R. (2006). The Social Work Assessment Tool (SWAT). *Journal of Social Work in End-of-Life and Palliative Care, 2*(2), 65–95. doi:10.1300/J457v02n02_05

Remke, S. S. (2015). Pediatric palliative care. In G. Christ, C. Messner, & L. Behar (Eds.), *Handbook of oncology social work* (1st ed., pp. 499–504). New York, NY: Oxford University Press.

Roza, K. A., Lee, E. J., Meier, D. E., & Goldstein, N. E. (2015). A survey of bereaved family members to assess quality of care on a palliative care unit. *Journal of Palliative Medicine, 18*(4), 358–365. doi:10.1089/jpm.2014.0172

Scott, K., Thiel, M. M., & Dahlin, C. M. (2008). The essential elements of spirituality in end-of-life care. *Chaplaincy Today, 24*(2), 15–21. doi:10.1093/geront/gnv037

Simon, C. E., Pryce, J. G., Roff, L. L., & Klemmack, D. (2005). Secondary traumatic stress and oncology social work: Protecting compassion from fatigue and compromising the worker's worldview. *Journal of Psychosocial Oncology, 23*(4), 1–14.

Smith, G., Bernacki, R., & Block, S. D. (2015). The role of palliative care in population management and accountable care organizations. *Journal of Palliative Medicine, 18*(6), 486–494. doi:10.1089/jpm.2014.0231

Smith, S., Brick, A., O'Hara, S., & Normand, C. (2014). Evidence on the cost and cost-effectiveness of palliative care: A literature review. *Palliative Medicine, 28*(2), 130–150. doi:10.1177/0269216313493466

Sormanti, M. (2015). Understanding bereavement: How theory, research, and practice inform what we do. In G. Christ, C. Messner, & L. Behar (Eds.), *Handbook of Oncology Social Work* (1st ed., pp. 543–551). New York, NY: Oxford University Press.

Span, P. (2017, January 16). Physician aid in dying gains acceptance in the U.S. *New York Times*.

Stark, D. (2011). Teamwork in palliative care: An integrative approach. In T. Altilio & S. Otis-Green (Eds.), *Oxford textbook of palliative social work* (pp. 415–424). New York, NY: Oxford University Press.

Stein, G. L., & Bonuck, K. A. (2001). Attitudes on end-of-life care and advance care planning in the lesbian and gay community. *Journal of Palliative Medicine, 4*(2), 173–190. doi:10.1089/109662101750290218

Stein, G. L., Cagle, J. G., & Christ, G. H. (2016). Social work involvement in advance care planning: Findings from a large survey of social workers in hospice and palliative care settings. *Journal of Palliative Medicine, 20*(3), 253–259. doi:10.1089/jpm.2016.0352

Stroebe, M., & Schut, H. (1999). The dual process model of coping with bereavement: Rationale and description. *Death Studies, 23*(3), 197–224. doi:10.1080/074811899201046

Sulmasy, D. P. (2002). A biopsychosocial-spiritual model for the care of patients at the end of life. *Gerontologist, 42* (Spec No 3), 24–33. doi:10.1093/geront/42.suppl_3.24

Sumser, B., Remke, S., Leimena, M., Altilio, T., & Otis-Green, S. (2015). The serendipitous survey: A look at primary and specialist palliative social work practice, preparation, and competence. *Journal of Palliative Medicine, 18*(10), 881–883. doi:10.1089/jpm.2015.0022

Taylor, H. (2015). Legal and ethical issues in end-of-life care: Implications for primary health care. *Primary Health Care, 25*(5), 34–41.

Temel, J. S., Greer, J. A., Muzikansky, A., Gallagher, E. R., Admane, S., Jackson, V. A., . . . Lynch, T. J. (2010). Early palliative care for patients with metastatic non–small-cell lung cancer. *New England Journal of Medicine, 363*(8), 733–742. doi:10.1056/NEJMoa1000678

The Regence Foundation. (2011). Living well at the end of life: A national conversation. Retrieved from http://syndication.nationaljournal.com/communications/NationalJournalRegenceToplines.pdf

University of Minnesota Center for Bioethics. (2005). End of life care: An ethical overview. Retrieved from http://www.ahc.umn.edu/img/assets/26104/End_of_Life.pdf

Vacco v. Quill. (1997). 521 U.S. 793.

Washington v. Glucksberg. (1997). 521 U.S. 702.

Wiener, L., & Sansom-Daly, U. M. (2015). Interventions for children under age 15 living with cancer. In G. Christ, C. Messner, & L. Behar (Eds.), *Handbook of oncology social work* (1st ed., pp. 447–455). New York, NY: Oxford University Press.

Winkelman, W. D., Lauderdale, K., Balboni, M. J., Phelps, A. C., Peteet, J. R., Block, S. D., . . . Balboni, T. A. (2011). The relationship of spiritual concerns to the quality of life of advanced cancer patients: Preliminary findings. *Journal of Palliative Medicine, 14*(9), 1022–1028. doi:10.1089/jpm.2010.0536

Worden, J. W. (2008). *Grief counseling and grief therapy: A handbook for the mental health practitioner* (4th ed.). New York, NY: Springer Publishing.

World Health Organization. (2017). WHO definition of palliative care. Retrieved from http://www.who.int/cancer/palliative/definition/en/

10

Correctional Health Care and Psychosocial Care

Tina Maschi, Keith Morgen, Carolyn Brouard, and Jaclyn Smith

The numbers of justice-involved juveniles and adults who end up in prison are staggering, especially in the United States, the country with the largest incarcerated population. The Institute for Criminal Justice Policy estimates that there are 11 million people incarcerated worldwide (Walmsley, 2016). Over half are held in custody in the following eight countries: America (2.2 million), China (1.65 million), Russia (640,000), Brazil (607,000), India (418,000), Thailand 311,000), Mexico (255,000), and Iran (225,000). Among the justice-involved population of all ages, there are high rates of comorbid health, substance abuse, mental health problems, and health disparities, especially among racial and ethnic minorities.

Across the globe, the health and behavioral health status of people in prison is generally worse compared to their community counterparts. Physical or mental health conditions may include: developmental and learning disabilities, attention deficit disorders, anxiety disorders, arthritis, cancer, heart or lung disease, or cognitive impairment or dementia. In general, health and behavioral health conditions are found at much higher rates in the prison population than in the general population. Upward of 96% of incarcerated juveniles and adults report histories of trauma and associated posttraumatic stress symptoms or disorders (Maschi, Morgen, Zgoba, Courtney, & Ristow, 2011). Additionally, across U.S. prisons and abroad, upward of 40% to 70% have substance use problems. Rates of communicable diseases, such as tuberculosis, are up to 84 times higher in prisons than in the general population and the cause is largely attributed to poor nutrition and overcrowded prison conditions. Suicide risk is also high in prisons. Incarcerated adults are seven times more likely to commit suicide than community-dwelling people. Incarcerated youth have the highest suicide risk and are18 times more likely to commit suicide than youth in the general population (World Health Organization [WHO], 2014). Tobacco is another significant health risk among the incarcerated. Global statistics show an average smoking rate of 28% among incarcerated (WHO, 2014).

There are high numbers of vulnerable populations in U.S. prisons and abroad to the extent that the United Nations Office on Drugs and Crimes (UNODC) has created a special needs handbook (UNODC, 2009). The UNODC recognizes the incarcerated populations with special needs to include youth, women, persons with disabilities and serious physical and mental illnesses, ethnic minorities and indigenous peoples, foreign-born (immigrants), lesbian, gay, bisexual, and transgender (LGBT) people, older people, and persons with terminal illnesses and on death row.

Social workers are trained with a specialized skill to work with individuals, families, and systems, and the profession is integral to helping address the complex health, social, and legal needs of the correctional population. For example, the United Nations' Nelson Mandela Rule (rules 74 and 78) noted that the professional specialists required in a correctional setting to optimize the health and well-being of incarcerated people and staff include social workers as well as interprofessional partners, such as psychiatrists, psychologists, and teachers (Penal Reform International [PRI], 2016). Given the intersection of public health and criminal justice, there is a global imperative to prepare social workers to fulfill this role in correctional health care, as well as advocate for improved health care conditions in the criminal justice system (CJS). Even as policies shift to reduce the number of incarcerated people or improve conditions, there is also a need for social workers to develop and refine community diversion and reentry treatment programs that integrate health and social care services, including assessment and treatment, psychoeducation, case management, program development and evaluation, and advocacy.

Correctional health and behavioral health care are concerns for the social work profession as well as the general public. In reality, prisons are part of the community and only separated from the community by barbwire fences. Additionally, incarcerated juveniles, adults, and older adults eventually will return to their communities after they have served their sentences. Therefore, preserving the health of our community members even when incarcerated should be of great interest to the larger community. Moreover, there is a cost saving to have all community members in good health. Maintaining health while incarcerated improves the overall total population health, reduces health and justice disparities, reduces overall health care costs and recidivism, improves public safety, and reduces the overall size of prison populations and the associated financial burden (American Civil Liberties Union [ACLU], 2012).

This chapter is designed to provide social workers with an introduction to correctional health and psychosocial care with a focus on prison health care. It provides an overview of the role of health and justice disparities as a mass incarceration driver and an overview of core themes of social work practice in a correctional setting. In addition, it presents examples of human rights instruments and laws that address health and criminal justice issues so that social workers can judge the extent to which correctional settings in which they work or may work are consistent with these standards. Also included is a review of relevant research and evidence-based practices (EBPs) for the justice population that can help guide the social work response. The chapter concludes with case studies and discussion questions to assist social workers to better understand practice, policy, and research issues significant for the future correctional health care delivery system.

THE CONTINUUM OF CARE AND JUSTICE

Although this chapter focuses largely on correctional health and behavioral health care in prisons, it is important to understand the CJS and the legal pathways to prison. It is also important to understand how the CJS intersects with health care services in the community and/or when they are embedded in a host justice setting. As shown in Figure 10.1, the continuum of care and justice model shows the trajectory of health care and justice points of contact in which social workers may be involved. As for the CJS, the first encounter a youth or adult who is alleged to have committed a crime is the police. If arrested, the individual may be placed in detention or jail before

appearing before the courts. If sentenced in the courts, the judge may give a dispo-
sition for release, probation, placement in an alternative to incarceration program,
or placement in secure care juvenile or adult correctional setting, such as federal or
state prison. After serving his or her sentence, the individual is released on parole or
under the supervision of community corrections. However, in some cases, the person
completes his or her maximum sentence and is released to the community with no
parole-reporting requirement.

As for health care services, the continuum of care across the life course (from birth to
death) includes community-based hospital services, such as use of the emergency room,
inpatient services (e.g., surgery, injuries, or illnesses that require medically supervised
recovery time), or outpatient clinical services. Additional services include primary care,
outpatient and inpatient specialized care, home-based health services (e.g., for persons
with disabilities), assisted living, long-term care, and hospice/end-of-life care.

Figure 10.1 also represents the health and criminal justice pathways of health and justice
disparities (Maschi, 2017). Discrimination based on race, class, gender, sexual orientation,
mental health, and immigration status is overrepresented in the CJS; however, at the
same time, discrimination leads to less access to health care services in the community.
Therefore, in any discussion of the CJS, it is important to discuss health and justice disparities, especially as they relate to race, class, and geographic location. Although racism
is a global social issue, in particular, racial inequalities in the U.S. general population are
widely known and have been well documented. Minority populations have less access to
care, receive poorer quality of care, and experience worse health outcomes than Whites
(Adler & Newman, 2002; Adler & Rehkopf, 2008; Groman & Ginsburg, 2004; Smedley,
Stith, & Nelson, 2003). As for criminal justice involvement, the Sentencing Project (2013)

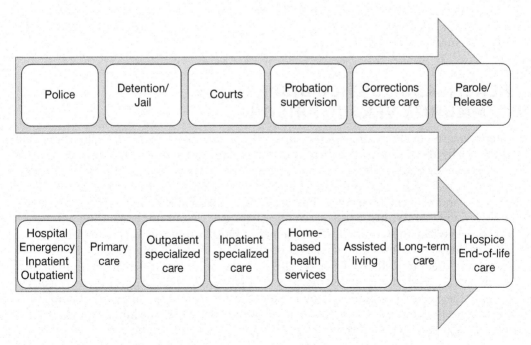

Figure 10.1 Tracking of the pathways of justice and health disparities along the continuum of the health and justice systems.

reported that for Black males in their 30s, 1 in every 10 is in prison or jail on any given day. Black men have a lifetime likelihood of imprisonment of 1 in 3, compared to 1 in 17 for White men. Black men are incarcerated at a rate 6.7 times the rate of White men (Guerino, Harrison, & Sabol, 2011).

The intersection between the criminal justice and health systems reveals disproportionate health and justice disparities based on race, class, and geographic location. Justice-involved individuals more often experience higher rates of chronic, acute, and behavioral health problems compared to the general population. People from low-income communities, especially racial and ethnic minority low-income communities, are more likely to be arrested and also be medically underserved. If behavioral health conditions go undetected and untreated, such as mental health and substance use issues, it also increases the likelihood of arrest and imprisonment. For people in custody in a jail or prison, the common occurrence of overcrowding increases the risk of the spread of communicable diseases, including HIV/AIDS, and lack of access to quality health services. Upon community reentry, formerly incarcerated people experience barriers to health and mental health services often due to stigma of incarceration and providers' reluctance to serve them and/or lack of health insurance (Baillargeon, Binswanger, Penn, Williams, & Murray, 2009; Maschi, Morrissey, & Leigey, 2013).

As for age group similarities, a large percentage of both the young and the old in prison commonly experienced life course cumulative disadvantage. These social determinants of health and criminal justice involvement include homelessness; poverty and financial problems; low educational attainment; lack of family support and family problems; lack of access to care; and trauma, violence, abuse, and other stressful life events (e.g., being a victim and/or witness to violence and living in a poverty-stricken neighborhood) prior to incarceration (Sampson & Lauritsen, 1997; WHO, 2014). As for participatory or political well-being, voting rights may be denied, especially for formerly incarcerated persons with felony convictions (ACLU, 2010). Obtaining access to needed social welfare benefits, including housing and health care, including for veterans, may be difficult (ACLU, 2010, 2012; Mesurier, 2011).

HEALTH AND JUSTICE DISPARITIES: COMMUNITY VERSUS PRISON

There is a growing body of evidence supporting racial disparities in the CJS from racial profiling by the police to the disproportionate confinement of racial/ethnic groups (e.g., Alexander, 2010). However, there is also a body of evidence that racial disparities in regard to health show mixed results in prison settings. For example, Binswanger, Krueger, and Steiner (2009) noted that while minorities experience more criminal justice involvement than Whites, "critical scientific gaps exist in our understanding of the relationship between the CJS and the persistence of racial/ethnic health inequalities" (p. 1). Some evidence suggests that incarceration may have a stabilizing effect on health, and may therefore diminish or reverse the direction of racial disparities in health in prison. Mumola's (2007) study compared mortality rates of incarcerated people in state prisons to those of the general population, showing that the incarcerated sample had overall lower death rates than the non-incarcerated. While White and Hispanic inmate mortality was slightly higher than the mortality rates of their counterparts in the general population, the opposite was found among incarcerated Blacks who had lower mortality compared to non-incarcerated Blacks. In state prisons, Black and Hispanic prison mortality rates were comparable, while the mortality rates of Whites were 67% higher in comparison to their community counterparts. It is important to note the methodological limitations of Mumola's study, which has been criticized for ignoring important factors in mortality, such as age and race differences, between the sample and reference populations (Patterson, 2010).

However, other studies have supported Mumola's findings. For example, in a nationally representative sample, Rosen, Hammond, Wohl, and Golin (2012) found that incarcerated Blacks had less morbidity when compared to incarcerated Whites. Racial differences in the use of health care were in the opposite direction of those observed in non-incarcerated populations. That is, Black inmates were more likely to access prison services than their White counterparts. Using combined national and state correctional data and age-specific death rates for the U.S. population, Patterson (2010) found a similar pattern of higher mortality among Whites and lower mortality among Blacks in the incarcerated population compared to the non-incarcerated.

There is a dearth of research that addresses racial health disparities among the older incarcerated population. A recent study by Merten, Bishop, and Williams (2012) of incarcerated males, aged 45 to 80, found that Blacks reported less illness than their White counterparts. The suggested moderators for this finding were that Blacks compared to Whites had a greater valuation of life, less loneliness, and lower levels of depressed mood. Spirituality and religion also may impact health among the incarcerated. For example, Allen et al. (2013) examined positive and negative religious coping among older inmates in Alabama. They found that incarcerated people who reported greater levels of positive religious coping reported significantly lower levels of depression. In addition to emotional and spiritual health, other resources that influence better health in prison may include access to various types of services beyond institutionalized health care including recreation, education, and social support. For example, Browning, Miller, and Spruance (2001) found that incarcerated people who consistently received visits from relatives had better parole outcomes, whereas those with no visitors had higher rates of parole violation and recidivism. Similarly, in a study by Maschi, Leibowitz, Rees, and Pappacena (2016), using a sample of 625 incarcerated males aged 50 and older, it was found that incarcerated older Black men appeared to be more resilient than older White men based on a number of emotional and social factors. Black men reported higher levels of emotional health, coping with stress, service usage, social supports, and overall health compared to their White counterparts (Maschi et al., 2016). Overall, these findings suggest that access to internal and external coping resources, including improved access to care in prison or the community, may assist with improving health equity among diverse racial/ethnic groups. It also suggests that social workers and other professionals in the community need to improve prevention efforts to improve health and well-being among diverse justice-involved individuals.

Despite the growing evidence for a reduction in racial health disparities among the incarcerated, there has been little empirical exploration of the association with health among the incarcerated and a follow-up discourse as to why this phenomenon may exist. Suggested explanations for the health improvements experienced by Black inmates include more immediate access to institutionalized health care, more routine nutrition, a reduction of behavioral and lifestyle risk factors, and a more structured environment that may be more conducive to disease self-management (Harzke et al., 2010; Massoglia, 2006; Patterson, 2010). Massoglia (2008), however, found that incarceration may have some mediating effects on Black/White health disparities, but nonetheless, in the long term, incarceration has a more negative impact on Black males' physical health and thereby reestablishes preexisting racial disparities in health. Disproportionate rates of

Table 10.1 Possible Pathways and Social Work/Psychology Activities

	Police	Detention/Jail	Courts	Probation	Corrections	Parole
Possible pathways	Arrest Diversion Release	Diversion Bail release Dismissal	Sentenced Dismissal	Completed Violation of probation		Parole supervision No parole
Health, mental health, and/or substance abuse interventions care	Intake Assessment Crisis intervention Treatment Research and evaluation Advocacy	Intake Institutional Inpatient Outpatient services Discharge plans Research and evaluation Advocacy	Intake Assessment Crisis intervention Treatment Referrals Research and evaluation Advocacy	Intake Community-based inpatient/ outpatient services and treatment Research and evaluation Advocacy	Intake Institutional inpatient/ outpatient services and treatment Research and evaluation Advocacy	Intake Community-based inpatient/ outpatient services and treatment Research and evaluation Advocacy

imprisonment and longer sentencing patterns are a major contributing factor in producing health problems in later life among Blacks, including exposure to infectious diseases such as hepatitis and tuberculosis. However, in a different study, Massoglia (2006) reported that during interviews with male inmates in Minnesota, Black inmates' mental health was much less negatively affected by their incarceration experience than that of White inmates.

Lastly, with the deinstitutionalization movement of the 1960s, the largest mental health treatment provider in the United States became the CJS (Houser & Belenko, 2015). Even today, jails and prisons have significantly greater proportions of persons with mental illness, substance use, and co-occurring disorders (Substance Abuse and Mental Health Services Administration [SAMHSA], 2017). For instance, current research shows almost half a million inmates have mental health issues in our country's jails and prisons (Kretschmar, Butcher, Kanary, & Devens, 2015). Furthermore, Maschi, Kwak, Ko, and Morrissey (2012) discussed prior research stating that approximately 65% of prisoners have a documented mental health disorder (e.g., PTSD, anxiety, depression, impulse control disorder). Specifically, 70% of younger prisoners (ages 17–22) have a mental health disorder (Goncalves, Endrass, Rossegger, & Dirkzwager, 2016). As problematic and epidemic the problem of untreated/undertreated mental health and addiction issues may be in the prison systems nationwide, a recent report from the Vera Institute stated that jails are even more problematic and basically serve as a de facto psychiatric holding facility for persons with mental illness (Kretschmar et al., 2015; Steadman, Osher, Robbins, Case, & Samuels, 2009). With the high rates of mental health concerns, substance abuse issues, and co-occurring disorders among inmates, few jails or prisons provide sufficient services that address these problems (Hunt, Peters, & Kremling, 2015).

PRACTICE

Social workers, often in collaboration with psychologists and medical professionals (physicians and nurses), serve a role in integrating health and justice whether it be working with justice-involved individuals, families, or communities in community settings or legal settings. For example, a social worker employed in the hospital in an emergency room or hospice facility may work with incarcerated and/or formerly incarcerated patients. A social worker employed in a prison may also work in a regional medical unit inside of a prison or provide discharge planning services for soon-to-be-released prisoners who have chronic or serious and/or terminal illnesses. Table 10.1 shows the types of activities in which a social worker may be engaged across health, mental health, and/or justice settings, such as conducting intake assessments, crisis intervention, inpatient or outpatient health, mental health, or substance abuse treatment (e.g., counseling and/or psychoeducation), case management, discharge planning, research and evaluation (including program development), and/or advocacy. As for correctional settings, such as prisons, the trajectory of health and mental health services is most often embedded in the prison system from hospitals and primary care to end-of-life hospice care. Social workers who work in community corrections often provide direct services or treatment, such as counseling and/or case management services linking formerly incarcerated individuals to community health, mental health, and substance abuse service providers, such as public health homes. Regardless of the employment settings of social workers, it is inevitable that some of their clients will have criminal justice histories. Therefore, in order to best serve their clients, social workers must be prepared to address not only health, mental health, and social issues, but legal, including criminal justice, issues as well (Maschi, Shi, Forseth, Laureano, & Viola, 2017).

The Nature of Prisons: Punishment Versus Rehabilitation and the Role of Psychosocial Care in Correctional Settings

Unlike prisons, jails were not designed for longer term placement of juveniles and adults sentenced to long-term placement. The underlying criminal justice philosophy applied to prisons was to punish, deter, incapacitate criminal offenders, especially violent offenders, from committing future crimes (Maschi, Bradley, & Ward, 2009). This philosophy was codified in law, and prisons were built as concrete reminders that punishment was the dominant paradigm compared to rehabilitation with the exception of juveniles in the juvenile justice system. People sentenced to prison for crimes lose their freedom and their social connection to society and are expected to use the prison experience to reflect upon and then change their criminogenic thinking and behavior. As well documented in the case of the U.S. prison system, using a punitive approach has overshadowed concerns for the quality of life, personal safety, and well-being of incarcerated people, especially vulnerable populations of youth and the elderly (e.g., ACLU, 2012). For example, most prisoners live in four-by-four foot prison cells often without windows. In congregate settings, prisoners share public mess halls and courtyards where violence may erupt (Kinsella, 2004). Prolonged solitary confinement is commonly used as an intervention strategy that has long-term physical and mental health consequences for those placed in it (Haney, 2001). Evidence suggests that when people are sentenced to prison, they lose not only their freedom but also, all too often, lose their health and quality of life (Haney, 2001). Hence, promoting quality of life by providing quality health and mental health care for people of all ages has been a struggle for an ill-prepared correctional workforce. Social workers can play an important role in providing assessment, interventions, and advocacy that promote rehabilitation as opposed to punishment approaches to criminal justice matters.

Prison is also a culture of violence. Prison is often characterized as a frightening and traumatizing environment since aggression, violence, and bullying are integrated into its fabric. Persons who are young or old and/or have physical and/or mental disabilities are at an increased vulnerability to victimization by other prisoners or staff (Maschi, Sutfin, & O'Connell, 2012). Vulnerable groups are often targets of other inmates or staff including harassment or bullying, such as being made fun of often in an attempt to provoke them to respond in self-defense (Maschi, Viola, & Koskinen, 2015). If that self-defense response is violent, it may result in a disciplinary action. Vulnerable populations, such as youth, women, LGBT people, and the elderly, experience sexual victimization by other prisoners because they are less able to defend themselves (e.g., Maschi et al., 2015). Professional staff, such as social workers, psychologists, and medical staff, often may be involved in system reform or advocacy on behalf of vulnerable clients.

Case Example 10.1

Jorge is a 56-year-old male from Puerto Rico and the youngest of nine children. He has a history of trauma and criminal offending that has included the unexpected death of his father at age 5, childhood sexual victimization, poverty, prostitution, drug dealing, substance abuse (heroin addiction), and recidivism (incarcerated two times). At age 17, he reported committing armed robbery to support his heroin addiction and was sentenced to 20 years in prison. During his prison term, he continued to use drugs. He violated parole within 15 months of release after being charged with sexual offense of a minor and possession of

(continued)

controlled dangerous substances, and as a result, is now serving his second and current 45-year sentence. In prison, he has spent eight of the past 15 years in solitary confinement. He perceives prison as "an overcrowded monster" designed to hold, degrade, and punish people. He views the staff as disinterested and disengaged and is despondent over the limited access to counseling and education rehabilitative services. Jorge was diagnosed with cancer 6 months ago while in prison and is projected to receive parole in 14 years when he is in his late 70s. He has not had any contact with family in over 5 years and reports feeling depressed.

As noted in Case Example 10.1, Jorge is an older incarcerated Latino man with a host of needs that a social worker can assist with. He was diagnosed with a serious illness, has a history of trauma and adverse life experiences, substance use, and repeat offending. He is also dealing with the psychological and emotional stress of prison exacerbated by being placed in prolonged solitary confinement and has had no family contact for over 5 years. Depending on how progressed his cancer is, Jorge may also be a candidate for compassionate release based on his declining health status. In an ideal prison setting, a social worker assigned to Jorge would work with an interdisciplinary team that would consist of, at minimum, a doctor, nurse, psychiatrist, and psychologist, to address the health and mental health care needs. Based on Jorge's health status, the team would make a decision if Jorge would be transferred from a general prison population setting to a special hospital unit that addresses the needs of incarcerated people with serious health conditions.

Given that Jorge has had negative experiences with the health providers in prison, the social worker would provide weekly counseling sessions with Jorge if he is interested. He would also be referred for psychoeducational programming that might include: stress, chronic disease, diet and exercise management programs and peer support groups. The social worker also might educate the other professionals about the mitigating factors and the psychosocial experiences that have influenced Jorge's attitudes and behaviors, including trauma, adversity, and discrimination. The social worker also would more than likely monitor Jorge's health status and assist him with completing necessary documentation for consideration for compassionate release and support or even advocate for his release. The social worker also may engage the family (including facilitating family visits), and set up a discharge plan if Jorge were to be released due to his failing health to a skilled nursing home. Given that Jorge has a sexual offense history, the social worker would use a community partner agency that accepts clients with a criminal offense history.

INVOLUNTARY MEDICATION ISSUES

An important practice issue that social workers, psychologists, and other allied professionals may be confronted with is the use of involuntary psychotropic medication in prison (see Table 10.2). Although many states do permit nonemergency involuntary psychotropic medication of those in prisons and jails, the involuntary hospitalization of inmates is a much more difficult procedure. Many of the states indicated that involuntary admission, though technically possible, is nearly impossible due to legal procedures and a lack of inpatient beds. Consequently, if prisons and jails are becoming de facto mental health facilities, resources must be invested to provide mental health/addiction services on prison grounds. The CJS's mental health treatment for those requiring longer term care for moderate/severe disorders is symptomatic of the larger nationwide inpatient, long-term bed shortage.

Table 10.2 Involuntary Nonemergency Medication and Hospitalization Laws for State Prisons and Jails

State	Nonemergency Involuntary Inpatient or Outpatient Admission of Inmate Permitted in Jails/Prisons?	Nonemergency Involuntary Medication Administration in Jails/Prisons?
AL	YES	NO
AK	Unclear	YES
AZ	YES	YES
AR	Unclear	YES
CA	Unclear	YES
CO	Unclear	YES
CT	Unclear	YES
DE	Unclear	YES
DC	YES	YES
FL	Unclear	YES
GA	YES	YES
HI	Unclear	YES
ID	YES	YES
IL	Unclear	YES
IN	Unclear	YES
IA	YES	YES
KS	YES	YES
KY	Unclear	YES
LA	YES	YES
ME	YES	YES
MD	YES	NO
MA	YES	NO
MI	Unclear	YES
MN	NO	NO
MS	YES	YES
MO	Unclear	YES

(continued)

Table 10.2 Involuntary Nonemergency Medication and Hospitalization Laws for State Prisons and Jails (*continued*)

State	Nonemergency Involuntary Inpatient or Outpatient Admission of Inmate Permitted in Jails/Prisons?	Nonemergency Involuntary Medication Administration in Jails/Prisons?
MN	Unclear	YES
NE	YES	YES
NV	Unclear	YES
NH	Unclear	Unclear
NJ	YES	YES
NM	Unclear	YES
NY	YES	Unclear
NC	YES	YES
ND	YES	YES
OH	Unclear	YES
OK	NO	YES
OR	Unclear	YES
PA	YES	NO
RI	Unclear	YES
SC	YES	NO
SD	Unclear	YES
TN	Unclear	YES
TX	Unclear	YES
UT	Unclear	YES
VT	Unclear	YES
VA	Unclear	NO
WA	Unclear	YES
WV	YES	YES
WI	YES	YES
WY	YES	YES

Source: Table produced from data in a Treatment Advocacy Center report by Torrey, Zdanowicz, Kennard, Lamb, Eslinger, Biasotti, and Fuller. (2014). *The treatment of persons with mental illness in prisons and jails: A state survey.* Retrieved from http://www.treatmentadvocacycenter.org/storage/documents/treatment-behind-bars/treatment-behind-bars.pdf

To prepare social workers for field education and practice, their access to appropriate specialized training needs to be strengthened. First, graduate programs in social work, psychology, and allied professions need to increase and enhance their forensic-track offerings. For example, the American Psychiatric Association [APA] (2004) advocates for increased practicum and internship training in jails and prisons. These experiences would serve as the foundation for the next generation of professionals, including social workers, psychologists, and other health professionals to receive training vital to this population. This training should also address the relevant mental health and addiction needs of this population, as well as provide increased emphasis on older adult care. Second, there is a need within this training—and beyond—to refocus efforts on how to incorporate psychotherapeutic theories and interventions within the CJS.

Galietta, Fineran, Fava, and Rosenfeld (2010) noted the lack of randomized controlled trials (RCTs) in the adult forensic population. Thus, perhaps a return to basic clinical and diagnostic theoretical ideas—without too much effort to create manualized/specialized services for prisoners—may be the clinical training and practice waves of the future. For example, many have argued for a return to the basic principles when utilizing cognitive behavioral therapy with a forensic population (e.g., Bayliss, Miller, & Henderson, 2010; DeMatteo, 2010; Ivanoff & Schmidt, 2010). SAMHSA (2015) reviewed basic clinical treatment and diagnostic matters for working in the CJS system. This document was not a manual on how to conduct treatment in the CJS, but rather how to simply reconsider clinical and diagnostic matters relevant to this population. A close read of many parts of this document finds basic, foundational addiction and mental health theory. Finally, Morgen (2015) reviewed how to incorporate basic existential therapy principles in work with an offender. Again, this was not a reconceptualization of existential theory; rather, it was an application of existential theory in another clinical setting. Perhaps the field has been trying too hard to create RCTs and empirically based treatments (EBTs) for the forensic setting. A back-to-basics approach may better serve this population.

POLICY

International and national policies that can inform social workers', psychologists', and allied professionals' approach to correctional health and mental health in the United States include: the Universal Declaration of Human Rights (UDHR; United Nations [UN], 1948); the UN Standard Minimum Rules for the Treatment of Prisoners also newly referred to as the Nelson Mandela Rules (PRI, 2016); the International Covenant on Civil and Political Rights (ICCPR; UN, 1966a); the International Covenant on Economic, Social, and Cultural Rights (ICESC; UN, 1966b); the Convention Against Torture and Other Cruel, Inhuman or Degrading Treatment or Punishment; the Body of Principles for the Protection of All Persons Under Any Form of Detention or Imprisonment; the Basic Principles for the Treatment of Prisoners; and the United Nations Standard Minimum Rules for the Administration of Juvenile Justice (or the "Beijing Rules"). All of these human rights documents (also commonly referred to as instruments) are designed to protect and promote prisoner rights, including health/mental health and health care in prison. These documents universally affirm the tenet that prisoners retain fundamental human rights. These instruments also are binding on governments to the extent that the norms set out in them expand the broader standards contained in other human rights treaties (Human Rights Watch [HRW], 2015). We highlight in the following select segments of the UDHR and the Nelson Mandela Rules, which are most relevant to social work practice in health and mental health care in prison.

Universal Declaration of Human Rights and Core Covenants

The UDHR was ratified in 1948 as a response to the atrocities of World War II (UN, 1948). The UDHR preamble underscores the norm of "respect for the inherent dignity and equal and inalienable rights" of all human beings, which in this case clearly includes prisoners (UN, 1948). Of the 30 UDHR articles, five are of particular relevance to prisoners of all ages. Article 25 states that "Everyone has the right to a standard of living adequate for the health and well-being of himself" (UN, 1948, p. 5). These guarantees are relevant before, during, and after prison term, and include housing, medical and mental health, and social services, as well as the right to security in case of unemployment, sickness, disability, or old age (UN, 1948). Article 3 states "everyone has the right to life, liberty, and the security of person" (UN, 1948, p. 3) and Article 5 states "no one shall be subjected to torture or to cruel, inhuman, or degrading treatment or punishment" (UN, 1948, p. 3). These articles provide a broad blueprint for designing and implementing international policies and legal standards that protect vulnerable populations, especially from victimization and inadequate health care, while in prison. Article 22 emphasizes that "everyone has the right to social security" (UN, 1948, p. 5). Social security is consistent with the concept of human agency and right of every person to have the optimal opportunity to achieve cultural, economic, and social well-being in his or her country, including people in prison (UN, 1948).

Two UN covenants, the ICCPR (UN, 1966a) and the ICESC (UN, 1966b), further explicate the right to services, including for prisoners' rights. Article 10 in the ICCPR specifies prison rehabilitation as a key component. It states that "the penitentiary system shall comprise treatment of prisoners and the essential aim shall be their reformation and social rehabilitation" (UN, 1966a, p. 3). Article 12 of the ICESC recognizes "the right of everyone to the enjoyment of the highest attainable standard of physical and mental health" (UN, 1966b, p. 4). This includes continual improvement of environmental conditions; the prevention, treatment, and control of the spread of diseases; and adequate medical services (UN, 1966b). Adopting international policies based on these provisions would assist in promoting well-being among prisoners across their life span, especially in older adulthood when they are most vulnerable to age-related health decline.

The 2015 Nelson Mandela Rules

The 2015 Nelson Mandela Rules are a revised version of the original 1955 Standard Minimum Rules for the Treatment of Prisoners (or Standard Minimum Rules [SMRs]). In 2015, the United Nations General Assembly unanimously adopted the Mandela Rules, which laid out the minimum standards for good prison management (PRI, 2016). There are five basic principles found in the rules that can guide social work practice consistent with the profession's ethical mandates when practicing in correctional health care: (a) incarcerated people must be treated with respect for their inherent dignity and value as human beings; (b) they must be treated according to their needs, without discrimination; (c) torture or other ill-treatment is prohibited; (d) the purpose of prison is to protect society and reduce reoffending; and (e) the safety of prisoners, staff, service providers, and visitors is a central concern at all times.

The Mandela Rules also clarify the roles of prison health staff, including social workers. Prison health staff should be independent from prison authorities and security staff and be contracted by health care providers (as opposed to corrections). Prison health staff also have the sole duty to provide compassionate care for their patients and should never be involved in security concerns or punishment of prisoners. The clarification of role and responsibilities can help guide social workers in resolving ethical dilemmas, such as the institution's denial of treatment to a prisoner that may result in dual loyalty conflicts between serving the patient or the institution.

The Mandela Rules also have provisions for access to physical and mental health care (Rules 24–29, 31). According to the Rules, it is the responsibility of the state when individuals are deprived of their liberty (incarcerated) that health care be provided at the same level of care as in the community. Additionally, in order to ensure continuity of care between prison and the community, prison health care should be organized in close cooperation with community health services.

The role of health care professionals (Rules 25, 30–34) in prison must be separate from that of the prison administration. The same ethical and professional standards apply to prison health care staff as those outside prison. Their role in prison is to evaluate, promote, and treat the physical and mental health of their patients in prison. This includes treatment and care for infectious diseases, substance dependencies, mental health, and dental care. Health care staff must not be involved in prison management issues, such as disciplinary measures, and their clinical decisions must not be overruled or ignored by nonmedical prison staff. Prison health care staff have a duty to report any signs of torture or other inhumane treatment.

These principles and rules can help social workers when dealing with ethical dilemmas, such as dual loyalty conflicts. This may include reporting abuse and/or providing clinical services and advocacy when torture and cruel, inhumane, and unusual punishment occurs; the physical or sexual assault of a prisoner by a correctional officer; or institutional neglect in the case of prolonged solitary confinement and subsequent physical and mental deterioration of the incarcerated individual (PRI, 2016).

Select U.S. Laws and Policies

Although there has been movement toward the provision of constitutional right to health care with the Patient Protection and Affordable Care Act (ACA) in the United States, there is a well-recognized human right to adequate health care in prison. The U.S. Supreme Court has legal provisions that state that the deliberate indifference to a prisoner's serious illness constitutes cruel and unusual punishment in violation of the Eighth Amendment (e.g., *Estelle v. Gamble*, 1976). The Court stated in its opinion that the "denial of medical care may result in pain and suffering which no one suggests would serve any penological purpose" (429 US 97). Health justice demands that the dignity and worth of each person be accounted for in the allocation of scarce resources (Maschi, Viola, & Sun, 2013). Human rights philosophy argues that all individuals should be treated with dignity and respect. This includes individuals with physical and mental health issues, and criminal offense histories (Wronka, 2008). This clearly is not the case when individuals are denied health care and/or are dying in prison without appropriate care.

Another useful law in improving the prison system for individuals with health and mental health issues is the Americans with Disabilities Act (ADA). In 1998, the U.S. Supreme Court held in *Pennsylvania Dept. of Corrections v. Yeskey*, 524 U.S. 206 (1998) that the ADA applies to persons in prisons and jails. Prison wardens in the United States stated that compliance with the ADA inadvertently improved their services for other vulnerable populations, such as frail elders (National Institute of Corrections [NIC], 2010). ADA-compliant standards in prisons have included environmental modifications, such as handrails in inmate cells, showers, hallways, and communal settings (NIC, 2010). Some prisons have created specialized mental health or chronic health management or geriatric services to best ensure comprehensive services for older prisoners.

At the state and local levels, parole reform has become increasingly an issue of public concern, especially with juveniles convicted with life sentences who reach old age in prison. Two legal provisions that address health and justice are clemency and compassionate and geriatric release policies (Office of Inspector General, U.S. Department of Justice, 2015). Clemency generally refers to an act of mercy in which a public official, such as a governor or president, has the power to reduce the harshness of punishment or sentencing of prisoners (Shear, 2016). Clemency is a policy issue that has gained increased attention during the Obama administration and often affected legal protections of older adults in prison (Shear, 2016). For example, a *New York Times* article documents Obama's "merciful" record at the federal level in which he granted 78 pardons and 153 commutations to incarcerated people who largely received long-term sentences for drug convictions during the 1980s tough-on-crime era.

Compassionate and geriatric release laws also have gained increased attention by scholars, policy makers, and the general public. For example, Maschi et al. (2016) conducted a study of compassionate and geriatric release laws in the United States. In a search of the LexisNexis legal database using the keyword search terms compassionate release, medical parole, geriatric prison release, elderly (or seriously ill) and prison, 47 federal and state laws were identified using inductive and deductive analysis strategies. Of the possible 52 federal and state corrections systems (50 states, Washington, DC, and Federal Corrections), 47 have laws allowing incarcerated people, or their families, to petition for early release based on advanced age or health. Six major categories of these laws were identified: (a) physical/mental health, (b) age, (c) pathway to release decision, (d) post release support, (e) nature of the crime (personal and criminal justice history), and (f) stage of review. The federal government has also called for the reform of compassionate and geriatric release laws given that many incarcerated people have not been released based on their current provisions (Office of Inspector General, U.S. Department of Justice, 2015).

This article used a human rights approach to assess the laws, policies, and practices to the extent that provisions of existing compassionate and geriatric release laws meet basis human rights principles (Maschi et al., 2016). The principles of the human rights framework are: dignity and worth of the person, the five domains of human rights (i.e., political, civil, social, economic, and cultural), participation, nondiscrimination, and transparency and accountability (UN, 1948). The Compassionate and Geriatric Release Checklist (CGR-C; Maschi, 2016) was created for social workers and allied professionals, policy makers, advocates, and other key stakeholders to use as an assessment tool to develop or amend existing compassionate or geriatric release laws. This tool can also be used by social workers to prepare expert testimony for local, state, or federal hearings, or as an educational or professional training exercise. Applying a human rights framework, the checklist consists of seven assessment categories for compassionate and geriatric release laws: dignity and respect of the person; promotion of political, civil, economic, social, and cultural rights; nondiscrimination; participation; transparency; accountability; and special populations served. For a copy of this checklist, please email your request to: tmaschi59@gmail.com.

In the CGR checklist, assessment category 1 consists of items that address the principle of dignity and respect of the person. It includes such items as the humane treatment of vulnerable populations in prison. Assessment category 2 addresses the promotion of political, civil, economic, social, and cultural rights. It includes such items as the use of legal language such as cruel or inhumane if release from prison and access to benefits post release is denied. Assessment category 3 refers to nondiscrimination. It includes items such as how a law does not discriminate based on age, criminal justice history, or other background factors. Assessment category 4, participation, includes such items as the involvement of the incarcerated individual and family members, victims and/or their family members, and professionals. Assessment category 5, transparency, includes items such as parole or judicial decisions that are based on sound evidence, including reliable risk assessment. Assessment category 5 refers to accountability and includes items such as that the law specifies time limits for each stage of the review. Assessment category 6 addresses special populations issues, and includes the UN's special needs categories (UNODC, 2009) such as older persons, persons with disabilities, and terminal illnesses, persons with serious and/or long-term prison sentences.

A human rights–based analysis using this checklist suggests that most of the provisions of each U.S. compassionate and geriatric release often fall short of meeting the basic human rights principles that speak to the dignity and worth of the incarcerated person, family, and victim rights and supports, and accountability and transparency on the part of the judicial and correctional systems to grant release.

Additionally, the majority of the U.S. compassionate and geriatric release laws fell short of nondiscrimination provisions. This is especially true when assessing the level of risk of incarcerated people with histories of sex or violent offenses. Based on available research, this type of provision is overly restrictive. For example, in a study investigating whether risk factors for recidivism remained stable across age groups ($N = 1,303$), the findings showed that rates decreased in older age groups (ages 55 and older; Fazel, Sjostedt, Langstrom, & Grann, 2006). Given these findings about older age and the reduced risk for recidivism, it is important to underscore that incarcerated individuals with violent offense histories (despite their failing health status) or elderly in U.S. federal and state prisons are often nevertheless excluded from compassionate or geriatric release provisions (HRW, 2012).

RESEARCH

For the last 40 years or so, the criminal justice field has been moving slowly but inexorably toward the use of scientific evidence to develop programs and interventions designed to prevent and reduce crime and victimization and promote health and well-being. There are now many resources that can provide funders and program managers with detailed information on EBPs in almost all areas of criminal justice. Many questions and challenges remain regarding the implementation of these EBPs, and researchers and scholars are now turning their attention to these issues. Policy makers need to advocate for programs and initiatives that are supported by solid empirical evidence. With diminishing resources available for funding criminal justice issues, understanding how to identify and implement EBPs will be critical for decision makers in all areas of the justice system.

In the 1970s, Robert Martinson issued his now infamous synthesis of research in corrections (Martinson, 1974), followed by a book by Lipton, Martinson, and Wilks (1975). Both of these sources seemed to lead to the conclusion that "nothing works" in rehabilitating offenders. In the 1980s, numerous reviews were conducted to rebut Martinson, along with research into the effectiveness of alternative ways of preventing crime (Welsh & Farrington, 2007). This included a series of publications by the Canadian psychologist Paul Gendreau and his colleagues with titles such as "Effective Correctional Treatment: Bibliotherapy for Cynics" (1979) and "Treatment in Corrections: Martinson was Wrong" (1981).

There is no standard definition of what constitutes EBP. The Office of Justice Programs (OJP, 2017) "considers programs and practices to be evidence-based when their effectiveness has been positively demonstrated by causal evidence, generally obtained through one or more outcome evaluations," where "causal evidence depends on the use of scientific methods to rule out, to the extent possible, alternative explanations for the documented change." The National Center for Injury Prevention and Control's (2017) Continuum of Evidence Effectiveness illustrates distinctions between evidence-based and promising programs and practices (see more at: www.ncjp.org/saas/ebps#sthash. VjdV5ABi.dpuf).

The federal government developed resources for community service providers to access model criminal justice programs. For example, the Office of Juvenile Justice and Delinquency Prevention (OJJDP) established the Model Programs Guide (MPG) in 2000. The MPG was originally developed as a tool to support the Title V Community Prevention Grants Program, and was expanded in 2005 to include substance abuse, mental health, and education programs. The MPG contains over 200 juvenile justice programs in the areas of prevention, immediate sanctions, intermediate sanctions, residential, and reentry. Programs are rated as "exemplary," "effective," or "promising" based on the conceptual framework of the program; the program fidelity; the evaluation design; and the empirical evidence demonstrating the prevention or reduction of problem behavior, the reduction of risk factors related to problem behavior, or the enhancement of protective factors related to problem behavior. Ratings were established by a peer review panel, and are now based on the same rating instrument used by CrimeSolutions.gov.

These eight evidence-based guidelines include: (1) Assess actuarial risk/needs; (2) Enhance intrinsic motivation; (3) Target interventions: a. Risk principle: Prioritize supervision and treatment resources for higher risk offenders, b. Need principle: Target interventions to criminogenic needs. Responsivity principle: Be responsive to temperament, learning style, motivation, culture, and gender when assigning programs. Dosage: Structure 40% to 70% of high-risk offenders' time for 3 to 9 months. Treatment: Integrate treatment into the full sentence/sanction requirements; (4) Skill train with directed practice (use cognitive behavioral treatment methods); (5) Increase positive reinforcement; (6) Engage ongoing support in natural communities; (7) Measure relevant processes/practices; and (8) Provide measurement feedback (OJJDP, 2000).

The What Works in Reentry Clearinghouse (whatworks.csgjusticecenter.org) is a BJA-funded initiative established by the Council of State Governments in 2012 and designed to provide information on evidence-based reentry interventions. The site contains information about 56 initiatives in six focus areas (brand name programs, employment, family-based programs, housing, mental health, and substance abuse). Interventions are rated on a five-point scale: strong or modest evidence of a beneficial effect; no statistically significant findings; and strong or modest evidence of a harmful effect. The ratings were made by experts using standardized coding instruments.

Even from this brief summary of available resources, we can see that different organizations and agencies take different approaches to identifying EBPs. Users should review the information provided on the websites carefully to determine what criteria and procedures are used to identify EBPs. In particular, users should be aware of the number of studies that support a particular program or practice, and whether these studies used RCTs or quasi-experimental designs. The Blueprints for Healthy Youth Development website provides a list of 500 youth programs rated on at least one of six federal or private organization EBP websites, including CrimeSolutions.gov and the OJJDP MPG (see www.blueprintsprograms.com/resources.php).

In recent years, knowledge about how best to implement programs and practices has been increasing rapidly. One of the leading organizations in this "implementation science" movement has been the National Implementation Research Network (NIRN,

2017). The NIRN website (nirn.fpg.unc.edu) provides a wealth of information on implementation. Those interested can begin with a comprehensive report produced by NIRN that summarizes what is known about implementation research (Fixsen, Naoom, Blase, Friedman, & Wallace, 2005).

CONCLUSION

This chapter provided a brief overview of correctional health care with a focus on social work and psychosocial care with allied professionals. In both the United States and abroad, health and justice disparities persist in that the CJS has become the de facto health and mental health care system. Social workers and allied professionals who work in the system can most effectively work in correctional settings when they are competent in generalist and specialized care that integrates research, practice, policy, and advocacy skills. The adoption of empirically supported practices and EBPs may serve to improve health and well-being and reduce the cycle of recidivism for the most vulnerable of individuals and groups in our society. Social workers in collaboration with psychologists and other allied professionals can make a significant difference in improving care when working in a team-based fashion within and across systems of care.

CHAPTER DISCUSSION QUESTIONS

1. Please review the United Nations Standard Minimum Rules for the Treatment of Prisoners and/or Nelson Mandela Rules. Please discuss the ways in which social workers in correctional settings can practice a compassionate and rehabilitation approach as compared to the punishment approach.

2. Discuss reasons why legislation, such as compassionate release laws, is warranted. That is, what are the pros and cons of releasing incarcerated persons with serious or terminal illnesses early from prison?

3. Discuss the ways in which social workers can play a role at the micro, mezzo, and macro levels in facilitating the promotion of the social determinants of health and justice.

4. Using the case vignettes, conduct an assessment of the health, mental health, substance use, and legal issues described. Discuss some of the assessment and intervention strategies that might be recommended.

5. Using an online evidence-based practice database noted in this chapter, find an intervention of interest. Briefly summarize the intervention, including the problem it addresses, the population it targets, a description of the intervention, and available empirical evidence supporting its effectiveness. Share your findings with a small and large group that includes a follow-up discussion.

6. As a professional or graduate student in social work or clinical/counseling psychology, review the National Association of Social Workers (NASW) or APA Code of Ethics. How does a forensic social worker or clinical/counseling psychologist ethically manage their caseload considering the current status of limited adequate mental health/addiction care within the prison system?

CASE EXAMPLE AND DISCUSSION QUESTIONS

Case Example 10.2

Mary is a 64-year-old, Caucasian, Catholic woman who is incarcerated in a maximum security facility for women. She identifies herself as a lesbian. As a child, she experienced the divorce of her parents, abandonment by her mother, and sexual, physical, and verbal abuse by her father, whom she described as having serious mental health issues. At age 25, Mary married a man 10 years younger, had two children, and divorced. This is her first criminal conviction, and she is serving a 10-year prison sentence (85% minimum) for conspiracy and the attempted murder of her abusive husband, which she describes as self-defense. Mary describes this sentence as unfair and unjust based on mitigating circumstances. She has a medical history of hypertension, vision impairment, and osteoporosis that makes it difficult for her to walk or use a top bunk bed. At age 64, Mary's extensive dental problems have resulted in a premature need for dentures. She describes her current prison experience as "degrading, especially the way correctional officers treat inmates." Although she reports feelings of depression and despair, Mary reports that she copes with her prison experience by "finding meaning" in it through spirituality. Despite her ill health, Mary is resistant to using prison health care services. Her projected parole date is in 2 years, when she will be 66 years old. Because of the distance, Mary has not had any in-person visits with her family members since her incarceration but corresponds monthly by mail with her two adult children and four grandchildren and every 3 months by phone. She says that she misses her family immensely.

Questions for Discussion

1. As a social worker for this case, write a case presentation that you would give to an interdisciplinary team meeting that consists of a doctor, nurse, psychologist, and psychiatrist.

2. What are one or two treatment goals that you would work with her while in prison?

3. How might you involve Mary's family while in prison or preparing for her release?

REFERENCES

Adler, N. E., & Newman, K. (2002). Socioeconomic disparities in health: Pathways and policies. *Health Affairs (Millwood), 21*, 60–76.

Adler, N. E., & Rehkopf, D. H. (2008). U.S. disparities in health: Descriptions, causes, and mechanisms. *Annual Review of Public Health, 29*, 235–252. doi:10.1146/annurev .publhealth.29.020907.090852

Alexander, M. (2010). *The new Jim Crow: Mass incarceration in the age of colorblindness*. New York, NY: The New Press.

Allen, R. S., Harris, G. M., Crowther, M. R., Oliver, J. S., Cavanaugh, R., & Phillips, L. L. (2013). Does religiousness and spirituality moderate the relations between physical and mental health among aging prisoners? *International Journal Geriatric Psychiatry, 28*, 710–717. doi:10.1002/gps.3874

American Civil Liberties Union. (2010). Voting with a criminal offense history. Retrieved from http://www.aclu.org/racial-justice-voting-rights/voting-criminal-record-executive-summary

American Civil Liberties Union. (2012). At America's expense: The mass incarceration of the elderly. Retrieved from https://www.aclu.org/criminal-law-reform/report-americas-expense-mass-incarceration-elderly

American Psychiatric Association. (2004). *Diagnostic and statistical manual of mental disorders* (4th ed., text revision). Washington, DC: Author.

Baillargeon, J., Binswanger, I. A., Penn, J. V., Williams, B. A., & Murray, O. J. (2009). Psychiatric disorders and repeat incarcerations: the revolving prison door. *American Journal of Psychiatry, 166*, 103–109. doi:10.1176/appi.ajp.2008.08030416

Bayliss, C. M., Miller, A. K., & Henderson, C. E. (2010). Psychopathy development and implications for early intervention. *Journal of Cognitive Psychotherapy, 24*(2), 71–80.

Binswanger, I. A., Krueger, P. M., & Steiner, J. F. (2009). Prevalence of chronic medical conditions among jail and prison inmates in the USA compared with the general population. *Journal of Epidemiological Community Health, 63*(11), 912–919. doi:10.1136/jech.2009.090662

Browning, S. L., Miller, R. R., & Spruance, L. M. (2001). Criminal incarceration dividing the ties that bind: Black men and their families. *Journal of African American Men, 6*(1), 87–102.

DeMatteo, D. (2010). A proposed prevention intervention for nondrug-dependent drug court clients. *Journal of Cognitive Psychotherapy, 24*(2), 104–115.

Estelle v. Gamble. (1976). 429 U.S. 97.

Fazel, S., Sjostedt, G., Langstrom, N., & Grann, M. (2006). Risk factors for criminal recidivism in older sexual offenders. *Sexual Abuse: A Journal of Research and Treatment, 18*(2), 159–167. doi:10.1177/107906320601800204

Fixsen, D. L., Naoom, S. F., Blase, K. A., Friedman, R. M., & Wallace, F. (2005). *Implementation research: A synthesis of the literature* (FMHI #231). Tampa, FL: University of South Florida, Louis de la Parte Florida Mental Health Institute, The National Implementation Research Network.

Galietta, M., Fineran, V., Fava, J., & Rosenfeld, B. (2010). Antisocial and psychopathic individuals. In D. McKay, J. S. Abramowitz, S. Taylor, D. McKay, J. S. Abramowitz, & S. Taylor (Eds.), *Cognitive-behavioral therapy for refractory cases: Turning failure into success* (pp. 385–405). Washington, DC: American Psychological Association.

Gendreau, P. (1981). Treatment in corrections: Martinson was wrong. *Canadian Psychology, 22*, 332–338.

Gendreau, P., & Ross, R. R. (1979). Effective correctional treatment: Bibliotherapy for cynics. *Crime and Delinquency, 25*, 463–489.

Goncalves, L. C., Endrass, J., Rossegger, A., & Dirkzwager, A. J. E. (2016). A longitudinal study of mental health symptoms in young prisoners: Exploring the influence of personal factors and the correctional climate. *BMC Psychiatry, 16*, 1–11. doi:10.1186/s12888-016-0803-z

Groman, R., & Ginsburg, J. (2004). Racial and ethnic disparities in health care: A position paper of the American College of Physicians. *Annals of Internal Medicine, 141*(3), 226–232.

Guerino, P., Harrison, P., & Sabol, W. (2011). *Prisoners in 2010.* U.S. Department of Justice, Bureau of Justice Statistics. Retrieved from http://bjs.ojp.usdoj.gov/content/pub/pdf/p10.pdf

Haney, C. (2001). The psychological impact of incarceration. Retrieved from http://aspe
.hhs.gov/hsp/prison2home02/Haney.htm

Harzke, A. J., Baillargeon, J. G., Pruitt, S. L., Pulvino, J. S., Paar, D. P., & Kelley, M. F. (2010).
Prevalence of chronic medical conditions among inmates in the Texas prison system.
Journal of Urban Health, 3, 486–503. doi:10.1007/s11524-010-9448-2

Houser, K., & Belenko, S. (2015). Disciplinary responses to misconduct among female
prison inmates with mental illness, substance use disorders, and co-occurring disorders. *Psychiatric Rehabilitation Journal, 38*, 24–34. doi:10.1037/prj0000110

Human Rights Watch. (2012). Old behind bars: The aging prison population in
the United States. Retrieved from http://www.hrw.org/reports/2012/01/27/
old-behind-bars

Human Rights Watch. (2015). *World report.* New York, NY: Seven Stories Press.

Hunt, E., Peters, R. H., & Kremling, J. (2015). Behavioral health treatment history among
persons in the justice system: Findings from the arrestee drug abuse monitoring II
program. *Psychiatric Rehabilitation Journal, 38*, 7–15. doi:10.1037/prj0000132

Ivanoff, A., & Schmidt, H. I. (2010). Functional assessment in forensic settings: A valuable
tool for preventing and treating egregious behavior. *Journal of Cognitive Psychotherapy,
24*(2), 81–91.

Kinsella, C. (2004). *Correctional health care costs.* Lexington, KY: The Council of State
Governments. Retrieved from http://www.csg.org/knowledgecenter/docs/
TA0401CorrHealth.pdf

Kretschmar, J. M., Butcher, F., Kanary, P. J., & Devens, R. (2015). Responding to the mental
health and substance abuse needs of youth in the juvenile justice system: Ohio's
behavioral health/juvenile justice initiative. *American Journal of Orthopsychiatry, 85*,
515–521. doi:10.1037/ort0000139

Lipton, D., Martinson, R., & Wilks, J. (1975). *The effectiveness of correctional treatment: A
survey of treatment evaluation studies.* New York, NY: Praeger.

Martinson, R. (Spring 1974). What works?—Questions and answers about prison reform.
The Public Interest, 22–54.

Maschi, T. (2017). *Continuum pathway for health and justice.* Illustration developed by
Maschi. New York, NY.

Maschi, T., Bradley, C., & Ward, K. (Eds.). (2009). *Forensic social work: Psychosocial and legal
issues in diverse practice settings.* New York, NY: Springer Publishing.

Maschi, T., Kwak, J., Ko, E., & Morrissey, M. B. (2012). Forget me not: Dementia in prison.
Gerontologist, 52(4), 441–451. doi:10.1093/geront/gnr131

Maschi, T., Leibowitz, G., Rees, J., & Pappacena, L. (2016). Analysis of United States compassionate and geriatric release laws: Applying a human rights approach to global
prisoner health. *Journal of Human Rights and Social Work, 1*, 165–174.

Maschi, T., Morgen, K., Zgoba, K., Courtney, D., & Ristow, J. (2011). Age, cumulative trauma
and stressful life events, and post-traumatic stress symptoms among older adults
in prison: do subjective impressions matter? *Gerontologist, 51*, 675–686. doi:10.1093/
geront/gnr074

Maschi, T., Morrissey, M.B., & Leigey, M. (2013). The case for human agency, well-being,
and community reintegration for people aging in prison: A statewide case analysis.
Journal of Correctional Health Care, 19(3), 194–201. doi:10.1177/1078345813486445

Maschi, T., Shi., Q., Forseth, K., Laureano, P., & Viola, D (2017). Exploring the association between race and health among older adults in prison. *Social Work in Public Health, 32*(3), 143–153. doi:10.1080/19371918.2016.1160342

Maschi, T., Sutfin, S., & O'Connell, B. (2012). Aging, mental health, and the criminal justice system: A content analysis of the literature. *Journal of Forensic Social Work, 2,* 162–185.

Maschi, T., Viola, D., & Koskinen, L. (2015). Trauma, stress, and coping among older adults in prison: Towards a human rights and intergenerational family justice action agenda. *Traumatology, 21*(3), 188–200. doi:10.1037/trm0000021

Maschi, T., Viola, D., & Sun, F. (2013). The high cost of the international aging prisoner crisis: Well-being as the common denominator for action. *The Gerontologist, 53*(4), 543–554. doi:10.1093/geront/gns125

Massoglia, M. (2006). Race and the impact of incarceration on midlife mental health: Where whiteness is not a privilege. Retrieved from http://citation.allacademic.com/meta/p126233_index.html

Massoglia, M. (2008). Incarceration, health, and racial disparities in health. *Law & Society Review, 42*(2), 275–306. doi:10.1111/j.1540-5893.2008.00342.x

Merten, M. J., Bishop, A. J., & Williams, A. L. (2012). Prisoner health and valuation of life, loneliness, and depressed mood. *American Journal of Health Behavior, 36*(2), 275–288. doi:10.5993/AJHB.36.2.12

Mesurier, R. (2011). *Supporting older people in prison: Ideas for practice.* UK: Age UK. Retrieved from http://www.ageuk.org.uk/documents/en-gb/for-professionals/government-and-society/older%20prisoners%20guide_pro.pdf?dtrk=true

Morgen, K. (2015, March). Older adult substance use disorder: National trends at facility and client levels. Paper presented at the Eastern Psychological Association Conference, Philadelphia, PA.

Mumola, C. J. (2007). *Medical causes of death in state prisons, 2001–2004* (NCJ 216340). Washington, DC: Bureau of Justice Statistics, U.S. Department of Justice.

National Center for Injury Prevention and Control. (2017). Continuum of Evidence Effectiveness. Retrieved from http://www.ncjp.org/saas/ebps#sthash.VjdV5ABi.dpuf

National Implementation Research Network. (2017). Retrieved from http://nirn.fpg.unc.edu/

National Institute of Corrections. (2010). Effectively managing aging and geriatric offenders. Retrieved from http://nicic.gov/Library/024363

Office of Justice Programs. (2017). What is an evidence-based program. Retrieved from https://www.ojpdiagnosticcenter.org/services/ebp

Office of Juvenile Justice and Delinquency Prevention. (2000). Model Programs Guide (MPG). Retrieved from https://www.ojjdp.gov/mpg/

Office of Inspector General, U.S. Department of Justice. (2015). The impact of an aging inmate population on the Federal Bureau of Prisons. Washington, DC: Author.

Patterson, E. J. (2010). Incarcerating death: Mortality in U.S. state correctional facilities, 1985–1998. *Demography, 47*(3), 587–607.

Penal Reform International. (2016). *The revised United Nations standard minimum rules for the treatment of prisoners (Nelson Mandela rules): Short guide.* London: Author.

Pennsylvania Dept. of Corrections v. Yeskey, 524 U.S. 206 (1998).

Rosen, D. L., Hammond, W. P., Wohl, D. A., & Golin, C. E. (2012). Disease prevalence and use of health care among a national sample of black and white male state prisoners. *Journal of Health Care for the Poor and Underserved, 23*(1), 254–272. doi:10.1353/hpu.2012.0033

Sampson, R. J., & Lauristen, J. H. (1997). A life-course theory of cumulative disadvantage and the stability of delinquency. In T. Thornberry (Ed.), *Advances in criminological theory and delinquency* (Vol. 7, pp. 1–29). New Brunswick, NJ: Transaction Publishers.

Sentencing Project. (2013). Racial disparity. The Sentencing Project web site. Retrieved from http://www.sentencingproject.org/template/page.cfm?id=122.

Shear, M. (2016). Obama's 78 Pardons and 153 Commutations Extend Record of Mercy. Retrieved from http://www.nytimes.com/2016/12/19/us/politics/obama -commutations-pardons-clemency.html?_r=0

Smedley, B., Stith, A., & Nelson, A. (2003). *Unequal treatment: Confronting racial and ethnic disparities in health care*. Washington, DC: National Academies Press.

Steadman, H. J., Osher, F. C., Robbins, P. C., Case, B., & Samuels, S. (2009). Prevalence of serious mental illness among jail inmates. *Psychiatric Services, 60*(6), 761–765. doi:10.1176/ps.2009.60.6.761

Substance Abuse and Mental Health Services Administration. (2015). *Screening and assessment of co-occurring disorders in the justice system*. HHS Publication No. (SMA)-15-4930. Rockville, MD: Author.

Substance Abuse and Mental Health Services Administration. (2017). SAMHSA's National Registry of Evidence-Based Programs and Practices. Retrieved from https://www .samhsa.gov/nrepp

United Nations. (1948). The Universal Declaration of Human Right. Retrieved from http://www.un.org/en/documents/udhr/

United Nations. (1966a). International Covenant on Economic, Social, and Cultural Rights. Retrieved from http://www.ohchr.org/EN/ProfessionalInterest/Pages/CESCR.aspx

United Nations. (1966b). International Covenant on Political and Civil Rights. Retrieved from http://www.ohchr.org/EN/ProfessionalInterest/Pages/CCPR.aspx

United Nations Office on Drugs and Crime. (2009). *Handbook on prisoners with special needs*. Retrieved from http://www.unodc.org/pdf/criminal_justice/Handbook_on_ Prisoners_with_Special_Needs.pdf

Walmsley, R. (2016). *World Female Imprisonment List* (3rd ed.). Institute for Criminal Policy Research. Retrieved from http://www.prisonstudies.org/sites/default/files/ resources/downloads/world_female_imprisonment_list_third_edition_0.pdf

Welsh, B. C., & Farrington, D. P. (2007). Save Children from a Life of Crime. *Criminology & Public Policy, 6,* 871–879.

World Health Organization. (2014). *Prisons and Health*. Retrieved from http://www .euro.who.int/__data/assets/pdf_file/0005/249188/Prisons-and-Health.pdf?ua=1

Wronka, J. (2008). *Human rights and social justice: Social action and service for the helping and health professions*. Thousand Oaks, CA: Sage Publication.

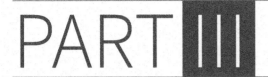

PART III

Working With Special Populations

11

Child and Family Health

Abigail M. Ross, Madeline K. Wachman, and Michelle Falcon

Poor health in childhood impedes healthy development across the life span. While the United States is the wealthiest country in the world, indicators for the health and well-being of U.S. children are far below those of other developed countries (World Health Organization [WHO], 2015), are characterized by widespread disparities by race, geographic location, and socio-economic status (Seith & Isaksen, 2011), and may be worsening on selected measures. From 2011 to 2013, the U.S. infant mortality rate was 6%, yet the rate for Black or African American infants was 11.3%. Results of a recent survey indicated that, of parents with a child between the ages of 10 months and 5 years, less than 1% received a standardized screening for developmental or behavioral problems; however, 26.2%, of the screened sample was determined to be at moderate or high risk (National Health Interview Survey, 2014). Between 2012 and 2014, increases in diagnoses of asthma, attention deficit hyperactivity disorder, food and skin allergies, and serious emotional or behavioral difficulties increased, with disproportionate increases in those living below the federal poverty line. In 2014, only 71.6% of children received their combined seven-vaccine series, yet the percentage dropped to 65.7% in families that fell below the poverty line (Centers for Disease Control and Prevention [CDC], 2015).

There is widespread agreement in the scientific community that the effects of social determinants of health, and poverty in particular, are particularly powerful for children. For children, health and access to care are contingent primarily upon structures in their social context, including and especially the family system (McNeil, 2010). Given the emphasis on person-in-environment underscored in social work training and the breadth of settings in which social workers practice, social workers are well positioned to play a vital role in promoting and ensuring the health and well-being of children—and their families—through micro, mezzo, and policy-oriented prevention and intervention. While there are many definitions of child and family in existence, this chapter focuses on current practice, policy, and research specific to minor children and their families in the United States with the goal of identifying critical considerations for social workers practicing across the continuum of health and health care.

BACKGROUND

Komro, Flay, Biglan, and The Promise Neighborhoods Research Consortium (2011) have proposed a framework for understanding how the social determinants of health affect the healthy development of children. Similar to the person-in-environment model (Bronfenbrenner, 2009), this framework consists of distal influences (e.g., neighborhood and family poverty, access to health care, social capital/marginalization), proximal environments (e.g., family, school, and peers), and biological mediators (e.g., stress reactivity and neurological development) in relation to outcomes of physical and psychological health, academic performance, and social and emotional competence (Biglan, 2014). Nurturing environments that promote healthy development of children and youth have three main characteristics, in that they: (a) minimize the incidence of biologically and psychologically toxic events, including adverse childhood experiences (ACEs); (b) actively teach and encourage pro-social behavior while minimizing opportunities for problem behavior; and (c) encourage personal agency (Biglan, Flay, Embry, & Sandler, 2012).

Families and caregivers are perhaps the most important proximal influence on the healthy development of children and youth (Biglan, 2014) and assume a central role in nurturing, promoting, and maintaining the health and well-being of their children. Families and caregivers are a main priority of Healthy People 2020 (HP2020); most HP2020 multidisciplinary public health interventions designed for children and youth are organized around or incorporate the following goals: (a) fostering knowledgeable and nurturing families, parents, and caregivers; (b) creating safe and supportive environments in homes, schools, and communities; and (c) increasing access to high-quality health care (U.S. Department of Health and Human Services, 2011). The following section describes selected approaches to pediatric health and health care delivery that operate from the assumption that the family plays a critical role in ensuring optimal health of children and youth.

PRACTICE

Family-Centered Care

Within the larger health care arena, family-centered care (FCC), described as a collaborative partnership approach to health care decision making between providers and families, has long been considered the standard of pediatric health care practice across hospitals, clinics, and other health care settings (Kuo et al., 2012). As a philosophy of care and care delivery, FCC is widely recognized across disciplines, health care systems, federal and state legislative bodies, and the Institute of Medicine (IOM) as essential to efforts designed to achieve optimal patient health, health care quality, and patient satisfaction (American Academy of Pediatrics [AAP], Committee on Hospital Care, 2003; IOM, 2001; Stange et al., 2010). While agreement on specific FCC tasks, actions, and practices has not yet been reached (Bamm & Rosenbaum, 2008; Jolley & Shields, 2009), there is general consensus across key stakeholder groups that core principles characterizing FCC include:

- Open, unbiased, and timely information sharing
- A respectful working relationship in which diversity, culture, language, and care preferences are honored
- Shared decision making that draws on needs, strengths, and values of all involved
- Flexibility and negotiation of desired health outcomes
- A collaborative approach to decision making and care provision, wherein the family is considered a critical partner in achieving desired outcomes (Kuo et al., 2012)

FCC is particularly appropriate when providing care to children, as parents and caregivers are heavily involved in the care of their children, are often in the position of making decisions on their behalf, and typically function as conduits to acquisition of care. Similar to patient-centered care, FCC prioritizes the patient–provider interaction, but is unique

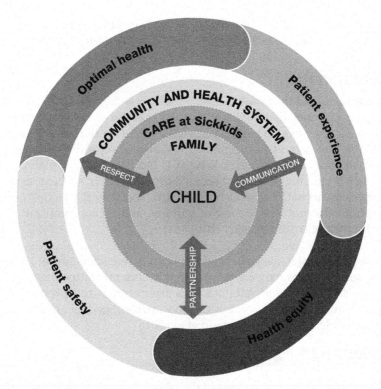

Figure 11.1 Model of child and family-centered care.
Source: Adapted from the Child Family Centered Care Model, Patient Family Resources developed by The Hospital for Sick Children (SickKids). http://www.sickkids.ca/patient-family-resources/child -family-centred-care/59043-54345%20stat%20CFCCmodel4.pdf © 2014. Adapted and reprinted with permission from The Hospital for Sick Children (SickKids).

in that it also incorporates the needs of all family members (Shields, Pratt, & Hunter, 2006). Specifically, the AAP considers FCC to be an integral component of the pediatric patient-centered medical home (AAP, 2016; AAP, Committee on Hospital Care, 2003), and the Maternal and Child Health Bureau (MCHB) regards FCC as a core objective for care of children with special health care needs (Figure 11.1; MCHB, n.d.).

The Family Health Paradigm

Within the social work discipline specifically, the family health approach to social work practice with children and families (Pardeck & Yuen, 1999) is especially helpful to consider. Grounded in family developmental and systems theories, the family health paradigm conceptualizes family health as "a state of holistic well-being of the family system that is manifested by the development of, and continuous interaction among, the physical, mental, emotional, social, economic, cultural, and spiritual dimensions of the family which results in the holistic well-being of the family and its members" (p. 1). When employing a family health approach, the family is viewed as a dynamic system that functions to maintain health, has the capacity to support individual members, influences health decisions, and attaches meaning to both health and illness. A family health approach draws specifically on the capacity of the family as an agent of facilitation and/or change (Yuen, 2005).

Care Coordination

Inherent in both FCC and the family health paradigm is the concept of care coordination (CC), a series of activities that facilitate both negotiation of services across disciplines within specific settings (e.g., hospitals) as well as creation of new relationships across and among different providers, organizations, and community collaterals spanning both medical and nonmedical arenas. While CC has been studied extensively in other disciplines, such as nursing (McClanahan & Weismuller, 2015), a recent review identified three primary elements of CC as related to pediatric social work practice: (a) assessment, (b) identification and problem solving of barriers, and (c) communication (Monterio, Arnold, Locke, Steinhorn, & Shanske, 2016).

Conducted from a strengths perspective, the biopsychosocial assessment includes objective data pertaining to the patient and the family (e.g., demographics, family structure, current relationships, employment and educational status, medical and mental health diagnoses, cultural and religious background, risk and protective factors), as well as assessments of family dynamics, values, perceptions, overall functioning, and approaches to problem solving (Monterio et al., 2016).

Case Example 11.1

Milagros is a 15-year-old Latina adolescent (U.S.-born) who was brought to the emergency room (ER) by her mother for physical symptoms including inability to tolerate food, frequent urination, and extreme thirst. After a standard emergency evaluation, the medical team determined that Milagros's symptoms were consistent with a diagnosis of diabetic ketoacidosis, resulting from inadequate levels of insulin produced by the body. Milagros was subsequently admitted to a medical inpatient unit at the same hospital for stabilization and management. The inpatient medical team was concerned that Milagros was not complying with the recommended treatment plan, as the family has not been attending their follow-up appointments since receiving the diagnosis approximately 6 months ago.

Milagros lives with her mother and two younger brothers in Section 8 housing. Her parents are not married. Her mother was born in Mexico and her English is limited; she holds multiple part-time jobs in the local area. Her father is not actively involved in her or her family's life. While Milagros has historically been a good student, her academic performance has steadily declined since receiving the diagnosis of type 2 diabetes 6 months ago. Milagros reports that she does not experience difficulty managing insulin injections and the requisite dietary changes accompanying the recent diagnosis are "fine." She notes that a meaningful romantic relationship ended shortly after receiving the diagnosis, and that she has been finding it more difficult to function in school and has stopped hanging out with her friends. She also told the emergency medical team that "the world feels overwhelming" and disclosed that she has taken to cutting to alleviate some of her anxiety, although she denies intent to kill herself. She has asked the team not to share this information with her mother because she "does not want to be a disappointment." Her mother reports that she thinks her daughter takes the insulin as needed and that she has not been able to accompany her daughter to follow-up appointments due to conflicts with her work schedule. She mentions that she experiences physiological symptoms of stomach pain and difficulty sleeping, but that these do not impair her ability to work.

Employing a family health and FCC approach, the biopsychosocial assessment includes perspectives of the individual as well as the family system, assessments of family communication patterns, cohesion, power dynamics, and constructions of reality. A thorough biopsychosocial assessment promotes the social worker's ability to engage a family, facilitate connections to appropriate resources, and communicate with other providers. When conducting a biopsychosocial assessment, the social worker interviews both the child and the caregiver separately to obtain relevant data including demographics and information related to family structure, current relationships, employment and educational status, medical diagnoses, mental health issues and symptom presentation, and environmental risk and protective factors. Upon completion of the biopsychosocial assessment, the social worker creates a case formulation that links predisposing, precipitating, and perpetuating factors influencing the child's and family's presenting problem or circumstance. Recognizing the potential for communication patterns to function as perpetuating factors—both within the family system and between the family and collaterals—maximizes the potential for delivery of higher quality care. In the case of Milagros, suboptimal communication patterns within the family, and between the family and the interprofessional team, perpetuated the lack of family engagement, thereby interfering with Milagros's health and well-being.

In health care settings, social workers frequently assume the role of identifying existing and potential barriers that may interfere with a family's capacity to access health care or execute a care plan, potentially putting child safety at risk. Barriers that require problem solving may include literacy and language issues that prevent clear communication of recommendations, cultural differences in perception of health and illness, housing instability, food insecurity, transportation, or parental challenges with mental health, substance use or other problems (Monterio et al., 2016). For example, because of experiences with other family members who died as a result of untreated diabetes symptoms, Milagros's mother believed that diabetes was not treatable, and thus did not prioritize attendance of follow-up appointments because both she and her daughter did not want to "receive bad news." Consistent with both FCC and family health approaches, addressing barriers through CC includes facilitation of linkages to formal and informal resources, enhancing family self-efficacy through empowerment-oriented interventions, and engaging in advocacy to promote social justice and acquire appropriate services. In this case, the social worker worked with Milagros and her mother to develop a different perception of all possible health trajectories associated with diabetes and manage anxiety around medical appointments. After completing a comprehensive suicide assessment and determining that Milagros was not at acute risk, the social worker facilitated referrals to outpatient mental health resources for both Milagros and her mother that were located within their community.

The third major theme characterizing CC in pediatric social work practice is communication—with the family, the interprofessional team, and other collaterals such as schools and additional community-based supports. Understanding and using the family's preferred modes of communication, their fluency in and preferred modes of technology (e.g., telephone, text message, email), as well as factors that may interfere with their abilities to communicate (e.g., number of minutes allocated to a cellular telephone, prepaid data plans) will enhance their capacity to engage in recommended plans of care (Monterio et al., 2016). In addition, social workers frequently serve as translators between the family and interprofessional teams, as families may not necessarily understand diagnoses as explained by medical professionals, treatment recommendations, or the health care system in general. For example, Milagros's mother did not understand that insulin was required to be taken daily, was not able to absorb the information relevant to her daughter's diagnosis of diabetes at the time of receiving the diagnosis for a number of reasons, and experienced the health care system as intimidating. To ensure that Milagros and her mother were able to acquire appropriate care, the social worker's referrals were characterized by closed-loop communication among providers, warm hand-offs, and check-ins with the family after discharge from the inpatient unit (Monterio et al., 2016).

Trauma-Informed Care and Practice

The prevalence of trauma in childhood has been well documented and is described in detail in the research segment of this chapter. While not unique to social work practice with children and families, trauma-informed care and practice (TICP), often referred to as "trauma-informed care" or "trauma-informed practice," is a strengths-based approach to working with clients that both recognizes and acknowledges trauma and its prevalence as well as maintains awareness and sensitivity to its dynamics in all aspects of service delivery (Bateman & Henderson, 2013). Distinct from trauma-specific or trauma-centered interventions that are explicitly designed to address trauma and its sequelae, trauma-informed approaches seek to engage people who have experienced trauma, recognize the presence of trauma symptoms, and acknowledge the role that trauma has contributed to their current challenges (Courtois 2001; Martsolf & Draucker, 2005; Wright, Woo, Muller, Fernandes, & Kraftcheck, 2003). Generally, TICP is organized around principles of safety, trustworthiness and transparency, peer support, collaboration and mutuality, empowerment, voice and choice, and cultural, historical, and gender issues (Substance Abuse and Mental Health Services Administration [SAMHSA], 2014).

While research shows that the provider–patient relationship is a central component of providing trauma-informed care for children and youth (e.g., Brown, King, & Wissow, 2017), TICP emphasizes the importance of organizational-level investment (Bloom & Farragher, 2010). SAMHSA recognizes organizations or systems that are trauma-informed as those that "realize the widespread impact of trauma and understands potential paths for recovery; recognize the signs and symptoms of trauma in clients, families, staff, and others involved with the system and respond by fully integrating knowledge about trauma into policies, procedures, and practices; and seeks to actively resist re-traumatization" (SAMHSA, 2014, p. 9). Many systems (e.g., child welfare, education) have adopted trauma-informed approaches (see Ko et al., 2008).

Special Considerations

While an extensive review of human development, milestones, and appropriate interventions is beyond the scope of this chapter, adolescence in particular is a developmental stage associated with the onset of a number of health and mental health problems, most of which are largely preventable (Mulye et al., 2009). Developmentally, the biological changes of puberty and the need to negotiate key developmental tasks (e.g., differentiation) combined with normative experimentation place adolescents at increased sensitivity and susceptibility to environmental influences in their social context. While the health trajectories of adolescents are often mediated by their health behaviors (McNeely & Blanchard, 2009), adolescents who reside in neighborhoods characterized by concentrated poverty are at risk of a variety of negative outcomes, including substance use, risky sexual behaviors, and poor mental and physical health outcomes (Leventhal & Brooks-Gunn, 2004). In addition to chronic or comorbid medical illness (Qin, Webb, Kapur, & Sorensen, 2013) as illustrated in the case of Milagros, these factors place individuals at increased risk of suicide, which is now the second leading cause of death for youth ages 15 to 19 (AAP, 2016).

When working with adolescents and their families, social workers must consider the legal ability of minors to consent to their own sensitive health care decisions (e.g., mental health services, sexual and reproductive health care), as well as applications of confidentiality as determined by the Health Insurance Portability and Accountability Act of 1996 (HIPAA). The age of consent varies significantly across states. In many states, consent laws apply to minors 12 years of age or older. Twenty-one states and the District of Columbia explicitly allow minors to consent for contraceptive services; 25 states allow minors to consent under specific circumstances (e.g., those who are married, pregnant, or already are parents themselves), and four states offer no explicit policy (Guttmacher Institute, 2017). While beyond the scope of this child, social workers must be mindful of their role as mandated reporters when screening for risk for and incidence of child maltreatment.

While lesbian, gay, bisexual, trans, and queer (LGBTQ) health is covered extensively in Chapter 15, youth who identify as part of the LGTBQ community experience a unique set of health care challenges. For example, parents/caregivers of LGBTQ youth who do not support their child's sexual identity/gender expression may make medical decisions that do not align with the wishes of their child, or may not permit the child to engage in services or community groups. Additional barriers faced by transgender youth and their families include a lack of availability of gender-affirming health care and limited health insurance coverage for it (Gridley et al., 2016).

POLICY

Federal funding for children's health covers a range of health and developmental issues—from pregnancy to young adulthood—such as access to insurance, child welfare, infant mortality prevention, screening, and services to children with special health care needs. The federal government plays a substantial role in providing incentives to states to invest in and promote primary and preventive health and social services for children and families, such as the Federal Medical Assistance Program (FMAP) and the Enhanced Federal Matched Assistance Program (eFMAP) through Medicaid and the Children's Health Insurance Program (CHIP). Administered at the state level, Medicaid and CHIP are two means-based public insurance programs that are critical to ensuring the health and well-being of children and families. Jointly funded by matched federal and state dollars, Medicaid and CHIP serve as the foundation for low-income children and pregnant women, covering over one third of children and 39.5% of children with special health care needs specifically (Dworetzky & Ablavsky, 2016). While states also provide funding for services, there is wide variability in state-level programming, funding contribution levels, and policy implementation.

Medicaid and CHIP: Similarities and Differences in Coverage, Eligibility, and Services

Medicaid is required for children ages 0 to 19 with family income up to 138% of the federal poverty level (FPL), although some states have increased the income eligibility maximum. As of January 2017, through Medicaid, 49 states cover children and 34 states cover pregnant women with incomes at or above 200% FPL (Brooks, Wagnerman, Artiga, Cornachione, & Ubri, 2017). Federally matched funds are guaranteed to match the full amount of state expenditures. Of particular relevance for children and families, Medicaid's Early and Periodic Screening, Diagnosis, and Treatment (EPSDT) program is designed to provide preventive and medically necessary diagnostic and treatment services for children with chronic health problems and special health care needs, including health promotion, dental, developmental, and medical services. Case management, care coordination, and establishing linkages between primary health care providers and other services (e.g., schools and other community-based services) are critical components of EPSDT.

CHIP is available to children with family income that exceeds the Medicaid income cap, but not enough to afford private health coverage. While CHIP benefits vary by state, all states provide comprehensive coverage (e.g., immunizations and well-baby/well-child care) at no cost. Under CHIP, states receive enhanced matching funds up to 300% FPL. States that have elected to raise the Medicaid eligibility income cap receive the federally matched Medicaid match rate. There is no federal mandate for EPSDT services under CHIP.

The reach of CHIP and Medicaid has increased with the enactment of the Patient Protection and Affordable Care Act (ACA, 2010; P.L.111-148). Together, Medicaid and CHIP have decreased the uninsured rate for children by more than half, from 14% to 5% as of June 2016 (Zammitti, Cohen, & Martinez, 2016). In 2016, several states took up options to expand access to coverage for children and pregnant women. Since the enactment of the ACA and the expansion of Medicaid in some states, Medicaid and CHIP enrollment has increased by a net of 17 million people (Medicaid, 2017). There is strong evidence that children with health insurance are more likely to attend school, graduate from high school, and live healthier lives than children who are uninsured (Cohodes, Grossman, Kleiner, & Lovenheim, 2014).

Importantly, the 2015 Medicaid expansion currently provides increased coverage to low-income adults, many of whom are working parents. This coverage includes behavioral and substance abuse services. Such services are essential to child and family well-being, given the well-documented link between child and family health. Continuing to invest in the health and well-being of children and families will likely result in improved adult health outcomes—and thereby reductions in costs and overall demands on the health care system—over the life cycle (see Table 11.1).

Table 11.1 Overview of Federal Policies Impacting Children and Family Health

Federal Law/Program	Overview
Children's Health Insurance Program (CHIP, Title XXI of the Social Security Act)	Federal–state partnership that provides health coverage to families who earn too much to qualify for Medicaid, but not enough to afford private insurance.[a]
Medicaid (Title XIX of the Social Security Act)	Means-tested entitlement program that provides health coverage to low-income families. Funded jointly by states and federal government.[b]
Early and Periodic Screening, Diagnosis and Treatment (EPSDT)	Medicaid's preventive child health program for children and adolescents under 21 years old. Provides screening services, including comprehensive physical exams, immunizations, vision, dental, and hearing services, as well as linkages to services to provide treatment.[c]

(continued)

Table 11.1 Overview of Federal Policies Impacting Children and Family Health (*continued*)

Federal Law/Program	Overview
Maternal & Child Health Block Grant (MCHBG, Title V of the Social Security Act)	Provides federal funds to state public health agencies to provide services and promote health of pregnant women, mothers, and children. Grant funds are allocated to states based on a matching formula between states and the federal government.[d]
Substance Abuse and Mental Health Services Administration (SAMHSA) Community Mental Health Services Block Grants	Provides financial assistance to states and territories to enable them to carry out the state's plan for providing comprehensive community mental health services to adults and children.[e]
Maternal, Infant, and Early Childhood Home Visiting (MIECHV) Program	Established as part of the Affordable Care Act focused on evidence-based home visiting services to provide services and referrals for expectant and new parents and their children.[f]
Earned Income Tax Credit (EITC) and the Child Tax Credit	Refundable income credits for working people with low to moderate income in order to reduce the tax burden.[g]
Supplemental Nutrition Assistance Program (SNAP)	SNAP offers nutrition assistance with the goal of alleviating food insecurity for families and children.[h]
Special Supplemental Nutrition Program for Women, Infants, and Children (WIC)	WIC provides federal grants to states for supplemental foods, health and nutrition education, and referrals for women and children.[i]

[a]Children's Health Insurance Program. Medicaid website. Retrieved from www.medicaid.gov/chip/chip-program-information.html

[b]Medicaid. Medicaid website. Retrieved from www.cms.hhs.gov/home/medicaid.asp

[c]Early and Periodic Screening, Diagnostic, and Treatment. Medicaid website. Retrieved from http://www.cms.hhs.gov/MedicaidEarlyPeriodicScrn/

[d]Maternal and Child Health Bureau. Health Resources & Services Administration website. Retrieved from mchb.hrsa.gov/

[e]Community Mental Health Services Block Grant. Substance Abuse and Mental Health Services Administration website. Retrieved from mentalhealth.samhsa.gov/cmhs/

[f]Maternal, Infant, and Early Childhood Home Visiting Program (MIECHV Program). Retrieved from mchb.hrsa.gov/maternal-child-health-initiatives/home-visiting-overview

[g]Earned Income Tax Credit. Internal Revenue Service website. Retrieved from www.irs.gov/credits-deductions/individuals/earned-income-tax-credit

[h]Supplemental Nutrition Assistance Program. United States Department of Agriculture Food & Nutrition Service website. Retrieved from www.fns.usda.gov/snap/supplemental-nutrition-assistance-program-snap

[i]Women, Infants, and Children (WIC) Program. United States Department of Agriculture Food & Nutrition Service website. Retrieved from www.fns.usda.gov/wic/women-infants-and-children-wic

The Maternal, Infant, and Early Childhood Home Visiting Program

A significant proportion of the federal funding on children and youth health has been targeted toward families with very young children (i.e., birth to 5 years). The federally funded Maternal, Infant, and Early Childhood Home Visiting (MIECHV) program serves families and young children through allocation of funding to states for provision of evidence-based home visiting programs (MIECHV Program, 2016). In order to receive funds, state grantees must demonstrate the capacity for effective implementation, which includes referring and monitoring coordination across agencies and systems. The focus on identification, screening, referral, and collaboration, aims to bolster linkages between systems and ensures children and families do not fall through the cracks (Stark, Gebhard, & DiLauro, 2014). Development of early childhood systems of care that include home visiting programming is an essential goal of the program.

Social Determinants of Health

While policies developed to address adverse health impacts of the social determinants of health are reviewed in Chapter 3, it is important to note that the effects of these policies—positive or negative—may disproportionately affect child health. While an extensive review of U.S. social policy is beyond the scope of this chapter, we highlight the Earned Income Tax Credit (EITC) program for consideration. The EITC provides tax refunds to families and is the largest federal income support program in the country (Center on Budget and Policy Priorities, 2011). By increasing the family's income, low-wage families may be more likely to utilize health care and engage in healthy behaviors (e.g., purchase healthier food). Research into family EITC use showed lower rates of low birth weight children, fewer preterm births, and increased prenatal care among these families (Hoynes, Miller, & Simon, 2015; Strully, Rehkopf, & Xuan, 2010).

State Innovation: A Case Example

Most federally or jointly funded programs, including Medicaid, CHIP, and MIECHV, require state-level oversight and administration. As efforts to either expand existing programs and/or allocate funding for specific initiatives is at the discretion of states, some states have become incubators for innovative policy and programming. In response to the Rosie D class action lawsuit, which was filed on behalf of Medicaid-enrolled children and youth with serious emotional disturbance (SED), Massachusetts developed the Children's Behavioral Health Initiative (CBHI), a statewide interagency initiative that provides a continuum of home- and community-based behavioral health services with the goal of strengthening and establishing a comprehensive community-driven system of care. In Massachusetts, the state Medicaid program (MassHealth) provides coverage for all services along the continuum of home- and community-based behavioral health services. In addition to improvements in mental health screening during pediatric primary care visits in Massachusetts (Romano-Clarke et al., 2014), there is also evidence that CBHI has had a broader positive effect on child and family health. From 2009 to 2012, there was a 32% reduction in youth psychiatric inpatient admissions and a 30% reduction in length of stay during inpatient admissions, leading to a 40% reduction in inpatient services expenditures (Massachusetts Attorney General, 2013; Stroul, Pires, Boyce, Krivelyova, & Walrath, 2014). In addition, the advent of mobile crisis intervention teams led to a decline in the use of ER visits for youth receiving CBHI services; about half of crisis encounters (56%) occurred in a community location rather than in an ED (Massachusetts Attorney General, 2013; Stroul et al., 2014).

RESEARCH

Findings from the ACE study (Felitti et al., 1998) provide a foundation for understanding how effective social work prevention and intervention efforts with children and their families can improve health outcomes in adulthood. Conceptually, the ACE study represented a significant departure from traditional biomedical models that do not necessarily account for the social environment or individual experiences. Conducted over 10 years, the ACE study was the first large-scale epidemiological study to examine associations between ACEs and health conditions in adulthood. ACE study participants were self-selected subscribers of a large health maintenance organization (HMO) who presented for medical evaluation at a health clinic. Sixty-eight percent of participants ($N = 17,421$) agreed to participate and completed a questionnaire about 10 discrete categories of ACEs occurring prior to age 18. Specific categories included: emotional abuse; physical abuse; sexual abuse; neglect; familial substance abuse; familial mental health problems; familial incarceration; witnessing domestic violence; parental divorce/separation; and loss of a parent by death or abandonment. Based on the number of categories (as opposed to frequency of occurrences), an ACE score was created on a scale of 0 to 10 (Felitti et al., 1998).

In general, results showed that ACEs are widespread, that they are interrelated, that they are associated with numerous health risk behaviors and health problems in adulthood, and that the more ACE categories one experienced, the higher the likelihood of adverse health outcomes in adulthood (Dong, Anda, et al., 2004; Felitti et al., 1998). Specifically, one in four respondents reported that they experienced at least two categories of ACEs, and one in 16 experienced at least four. Sixty-six percent of female respondents reported experiences in ACE categories of abuse, family discord, or witnessing violence (Felitti et al., 1998). Retrospective reports of ACEs were associated with chronic obstructive pulmonary disease (COPD; Anda et al., 2007), cancer (Brown et al., 2010), liver disease (Dong, Dube, Felitti, Giles, & Anda, 2003), and heart disease (Dong, Giles, et al., 2004; Dube, Anda, Felitti, Edwards, & Croft, 2002). Greater likelihood of a number of health risk behaviors, including smoking, sexual risk behaviors, obesity, and substance abuse, was also positively associated with ACE score (Anda et al., 2007; Dong et al., 2003; Dube et al., 2002; Edwards, Anda, Gu, Dube, & Felitti, 2007; Felitti et al., 1998). Higher ACE scores were associated with severe and persistent mental health problems (Chapman et al., 2004; Dube et al., 2001). For example, the likelihood of depression climbed 460% for participants reporting ACE scores greater than four. Childhood and adolescent suicide attempts increased 51-fold, or 5,100% and 30-fold, or 3,000%, for individuals reporting an ACE score of 7 or more.

It is important to note that of the 17,421 participants, approximately 77% were White, 72% had attended college, and 62% were over 50 years of age. In addition, experiences such as abject poverty, community violence, historical/intergenerational trauma, forced relocations, racism, stigma, and religious or linguistic persecution were not included in ACE measurement.

Currently, about one quarter of children in the United States are living in poverty and five children die due to firearm-related deaths each day. Moreover, racial and ethnic disparities in health are ubiquitous. For example, when compared to their White counterparts, African American children have significantly higher rates of deaths from asthma, hospitalizations, and ER visits; lower likelihood of kidney transplantation; the largest percentages and numbers of new HIV and AIDS diagnoses across age groups and via perinatal transmission; and later autism diagnoses (Flores, 2010). The pervasive nature of these racial disparities indicates that structural and systemic changes that promote health equity are much needed.

There is evidence to suggest that both environmental risks as well as the quality of interpersonal relationships may function as mechanisms through which ACEs lead to health risk behaviors and poor health outcomes in adulthood (for a review, see Larkin, Felitti, & Anda, 2014). With regard to mechanisms for preventing ACEs and mitigating their effects when they do occur, trauma-informed universal, targeted, and indicated interventions that emphasize protective factors have the potential to reduce ACEs as well as assist children and their families in developing adaptive coping responses that foster physiological and psychological health.

CONCLUSION

Despite the fact that the effects of the built and social environment, poverty, and ACEs on long-term health trajectories are well documented (e.g., CDC, 2010; Dube, Felitti, Dong, Giles, & Anda, 2003; Felitti et al., 1998), only 8% of federal expenditures are allocated to children, even though children account for 24% of the U.S. population ("First Focus," 2014; U.S. Census Bureau, 2013). Key elements of policy and practice that have the potential to optimize child and family health and require more investment are (a) coordination of service delivery within and across systems, (b) continuity of services and supports that span the breadth of developmental milestones, and (c) multilevel preventive interventions designed to address social determinants of health.

In practice, social workers are well equipped to work at the intersection of many systems and in a variety of settings where services are provided to children and families. Social workers have the potential to play an integral role in transforming the health care delivery system to a more trauma-informed service system that is able to provide appropriate ACE responses. As noted in this chapter, when children transition across developmental stages, the locations in which they receive health and health care also change. While it is critical to continue to invest in early childhood systems of care, research shows that health and social services for children and families are less coordinated, limited in scope, and underfunded once they enter formal school systems, and that these programs increasingly target children and adolescents as individuals, as opposed to family systems (Pardeck & Yuen, 2001). While increases in autonomy are developmentally appropriate milestones throughout childhood and adolescence, families and family health remain critical indicators of child well-being. As such, services must continue to incorporate a family-centered and inclusive approach.

With respect to policy and programming, the financing of health care and social services, combined with the lack of incentives to coordinate across systems, requires more attention. Alternative service delivery models (e.g., patient-centered medical homes, accountable care organizations), and investigations of alternative payment and reimbursement mechanisms may provide an opportunity to reduce silos across practice settings through improved communication, coordination, and ultimately, provision of care. Financing of CC initiatives that prioritize developmental transitions across systems, as well as alternative delivery and payment efforts that incentivize integration across systems, are critical for improving population health for children and families.

Many of these decisions are determined through policy development, yet research shows a marked disconnect between the strong presence social workers have at the clinical practice level and the paucity of involvement at the policy level (Bachman et al., 2017). As such, social workers must direct substantial efforts toward advocacy interventions that ensure that these issues are addressed at the policy level (Avalere Health, 2017; Sharfstein, 2017).

CHAPTER DISCUSSION QUESTIONS

1. This chapter described FCC, family health, and care coordination in a pediatric health care setting. How might these practices be applied in other settings (e.g., schools, clinics, shelters, etc.) that affect child and family health and well-being?

2. What health policies and programs covered in this chapter are relevant to your social work practice with children and families?

3. There are a number of programs and policies that are designed for very young children (e.g., birth to 5 years) and their families. Discuss why you believe this age group has received such a high level of federal funding (compared to other age groups) and the benefits and challenges that may come from these policies.

4. Research on the health of children and families has revealed the association between ACEs on negative health outcomes in adulthood. What systems-level interventions might be able to alter these trajectories?

5. This chapter has discussed a number of challenges to child and family health. In what arenas might social work be underutilized, and how might the profession address this challenge?

CASE EXAMPLE AND DISCUSSION QUESTIONS

Case Example 11.2

Sandra is a 4-year-old White child who presents to a local primary care clinic as a result of a child protective investigation. The 51A was filed by the local daycare after Sandra repeatedly presented with dirty clothes and her mother, Leah, appeared disheveled and disoriented at pickup on numerous occasions. The child protective worker arranged the visit for Sandra and her mother. Per mother's report, the child protective worker "told me if we came to this appointment, then they would get out of my life." Sandra's mother has a history of depression and substance abuse and the family has experienced periods of housing instability; they recently secured Section 8 housing after spending 7 months in a shelter. Leah is concerned that Sandra will "lose her slot" at the daycare center if a child protective case is opened, which would interfere with mom's ability to attend work at the local factory. Notably, Sandra is behind on her vaccinations, as Leah is convinced that vaccinations caused her nephew's autism. Leah does not appear to see the utility of the primary care clinic visit, and states that she would "just like to get this part [her meeting with you] over with." Sandra has a younger brother who is 21 months old.

Questions for Discussion

1. As the social worker in the primary care clinic, how would you use FCC and the family health paradigm with Sandra and Leah?

2. What components of CC might be required for Sandra and her family? How would you implement them?

3. Which social determinants of health might be affecting Sandra and her family? How might you use trauma-informed approaches to develop interventions that address these?

REFERENCES

Affordable Care Act. (2010). See Public Law 111-148 below.

American Academy of Pediatrics. (2016). Suicide and suicide attempts in adolescence. *Pediatrics, 138*(1), e1–e11. doi:10.1542/peds.2016-1420

American Academy of Pediatrics, Committee on Hospital Care. (2003). Family-centered care and the pediatrician's role. *Pediatrics, 112*, 691–697. doi:10.1542/peds.112.3.691

Anda, R. F., Brown, D. W., Felitti, V. J., Bremmer, J. D., Dube, S. R., & Giles, W. H. (2007). Adverse childhood experiences and prescribed psychotropic medication in adults. *American Journal of Preventative Medicine, 32*(5), 389–394. doi:10.1016/j.amepre.2007.01.005

Avalere Health. (May 18, 2017). The impact of medicaid capped funding on children. Prepared for the Children's Hospital Association. Retrieved from http://go.avalere.com/acton/attachment/12909/f-0483/1/-/-/-/-/Avalere%20-%20Childrens%20Hospital%20Association%20Report%20on%20Medicaid%20Capped%20Funding%20embargo.pdf

Bachman, S., Wachman, M., Manning, L., Cohen, A. M., Seifert, R. W., Jones, D. K., . . . Riley, P. (2017). Social work's role in Medicaid reform: A qualitative study. *American Journal of Public Health, 107*(S3), S250–S255. doi:10.2105/AJPH.2017.304002

Bamm, E. L., & Rosenbaum, P. (August 2008). Family-centered theory: Origins, development, barriers, and supports to implementation in rehabilitation medicine. *Archives of Physical Medicine and Rehabilitation. 89*(8), 1618–1624. doi:10.1016/j.apmr.2007.12.034

Bateman, J., & Henderson, C. (2013). Trauma-informed care and practice: Towards a cultural shift in policy reform across mental health and human services in Australia—a national strategic direction. Retrieved from http://www.mhcc.org.au/media/44467/nticp_strategic_direction_journal_article__vf4_-_jan_2014_.pdf

Biglan, A. (February 2014). A comprehensive framework for nurturing the well-being of children and adolescents. Report submitted to the U.S. Department of Health and Human Services; contract #HHSP23320095648WC. Retrieved from https://gucchdta-center.georgetown.edu/resources/WP1%20%20Comprehensive%20Framework%20508%20v5.pdf

Biglan, A., Flay, B. R., Embry, D. D., & Sandler, I. (2012). Nurturing environments and the next generation of prevention research and practice. *American Psychologist, 67*, 257–271.

Bloom, S. L., & Farragher, B. (2010). *Destroying sanctuary: The crisis in human service delivery systems.* New York, NY: Oxford University Press.

Bronfenbrenner, U. (2009). *The ecology of human development.* Cambridge, MA: Harvard University Press.

Brooks, T., Wagnerman, K., Artiga, S., Cornachione, E., & Ubri, P. (January 12, 2017). Kaiser Family Foundation. Retrieved from http://kff.org/medicaid/report/medicaid-and-chip-eligibility-enrollment-renewal-and-cost-sharing-policies-as-of-january-2017-findings-from-a-50-state-survey/

Brown, D. W., Anda, R. F., Felitti, V. J., Edwards, V. J., Malarcher, A. M., Croft, J. B., & Giles, W. H. (2010). Adverse childhood experiences are associated with the risk of lung cancer: A prospective cohort study. *BMC Public Health, 10*(20). Retrieved from http://www.biomedcentral.com/1471-2458/10/20

Brown, J. D., King, M. A., & Wissow, L. S. (2017). The central role of relationships to trauma-informed integrated care for children and youth. *Academic Pediatrics, 17*, S94–S101. doi:10.1016/j.acap.2017.01.013

Center on Budget and Policy Priorities. (2011). Policy basics: The earned income tax credit. Washington, DC: Center on Budget and Policy Priorities. Retrieved from http://www.cbpp.org/cms/index.cfm?fa=view&id=2505

Centers for Disease Control and Prevention. (2010). Adverse childhood experiences reported by adults—five states. *Morbidity & Mortality Weekly Report, 59*(49), 1609.

Centers for Disease Control and Prevention. (2015). Health, United States, 2015—Child and adolescent health. Retrieved from www.cdc.gov/nchs/hus/child.htm

Chapman, D. P., Whitfield, C. L., Felitti, V. J., Dube, S. R., Edwards, V. J., & Anda, R. F. (2004). Adverse childhood experiences and the risk of depressive disorders in adulthood. *Journal of Affective Disorders, 82*(2), 217–225. doi:10.1016/j.jad.2003.12.013

Cohodes, S., Grossman, D., Kleiner, S., & Lovenheim, M. (2014). The effect of child health insurance access on schooling: Evidence from public insurance expansions. (No. w20178). National Bureau of Economic Research. Retrieved from http://www.nber.org/papers/w20178

Courtois, C. (2001). Healing the incest wound: A treatment update with attention to recovered-memory issues. *American Journal of Psychotherapy, 51*, 464–496.

Dong, M., Anda, R. F., Felitti, V. J., Dube, S. R., Williamson, D. F., Thompson, T. J., . . . Giles, W. H. (2004). The interrelatedness of multiple forms of childhood abuse, neglect, and household dysfunction. *Child Abuse & Neglect, 28*, 771–784. doi:10.1016/j.chiabu.2004.01.008

Dong, M., Dube, S. R., Felitti, V. J., Giles, W. H., & Anda, R. F. (2003). Adverse childhood experiences and self-reported liver disease: New insights into the causal pathway. *Archives of Internal Medicine, 163*, 1949–1956. doi:10.1001/archinte.163.16.1949

Dong, M., Giles, W. H., Felitti, V. J., Dube, S. R., Williams, J. E., Chapman, D. P., & Anda, R. F. (2004). Insights into causal pathways for ischemic heart disease: Adverse childhood experiences study. *Circulation, 110*(13), 1761–1766. doi:10.1161/01.CIR.0000143074.54995.7F

Dube, S. R., Anda, R. F., Felitti, V. J., Chapman, D. P., Williamson, D. F., & Giles, W. H. (2001). Childhood abuse, household dysfunction, and the risk of attempted suicide throughout the life span: Findings from the adverse childhood experiences study. *Journal of the American Medical Association, 286*(24), 3089–3096. doi:10.1001/jama.286.24.3089

Dube, S. R., Anda, R. F., Felitti, V. J., Edwards, V. J., & Croft, J. B. (2002). Adverse childhood experiences and personal alcohol abuse as an adult. *Addictive Behaviors, 27*, 713–725. doi:10.1016/S0306-4603(01)00204-0

Dube, S. R., Felitti, V. J., Dong, M., Giles, W. H., & Anda R. F. (2003). The impact of adverse childhood experiences on health problems: Evidence from four birth cohorts dating back to 1900. *Preventive Medicine, 37*(3), 268–277. doi:10.1016/S0091-7435(03)00123-3

Dworetzky, B. A., & Ablavsky, E. (2016). Medicaid and CHIP: What's the difference? Retrieved from the Center for Advancing Health Policy & Practice website, http://cahpp.org/resources/medicaid-chip-difference/

Edwards, V. J., Anda, R. F., Gu, D., Dube, S. R., & Felitti, V. J. (2007). Adverse childhood experiences and smoking persistence in adults with smoking-related symptoms and illness. *Permanente Journal, 11*, 5–7. doi:10.7812/TPP/06-110

Felitti, V. J., Anda, R. F., Nordenberg, D., Williamson, D. F., Spitz, A. M., Edwards, V., & Marks, J. S. (1998). Relationship of childhood abuse and household dysfunction to many of the leading causes of death in adults: The adverse childhood experiences (ACE) study. *American Journal of Preventive Medicine, 14*(4), 245–258. doi:10.1016/S0749-3797(98)00017-8

First Focus Children's Budget. (2014). Retrieved from http://firstfocus.net/resources/report/childrens-budget-2014/

Flores, G. (2010). Technical report: Racial and ethnic disparities in the health and health care of children. *Pediatrics, 125*(4), e979–e1020. doi:10.1542/peds.2010-0188

Gridley, S. J., Crouch, J. M., Evans, Y., Eng, W., Antoon, E., Lyapustina, M., . . . Breland, D. J. (2016). Youth and caregiver perspectives on barriers to gender-affirming health care for transgender youth. *Journal of Adolescent Health, 59*(3), 254–261. doi:10.1016/j. jadohealth.2016.03.017

Guttmacher Institute. (2017, December 1). Minors' access to contraceptive services. Retrieved from www.guttmacher.org/state-policy/explore/minors-access-contraceptive-services

Hoynes, H. W., Miller, D. L., & Simon, D. (2015). Income, the earned income tax credit, and infant health. *American Economic Journal: Economic Policy, 71*, 172–211.

Institute of Medicine. (2001). *Crossing the Quality Chasm: A New Health System for the 21st Century.* Washington, DC: National Academies Press. Retrieved from https://www. ncbi.nlm.nih.gov/books/NBK222274/

Jolley, J., & Shields, L. (2009).The evolution of family-centered care. *Journal of Pediatric Nursing, 24*(2), 164–170. doi:10.1016/j.pedn.2008.03.010

Ko, S., Ford, J., Kassam-Adams, N., Berkowitz, S., Wilson, C., Wong, M., . . . Layne, C. (2008). Creating trauma-informed systems: Child welfare, education, first responders, health care, and juvenile justice. *Professional Psychology: Research and Practice, 39*(4), 396–404. doi:10.1037/0735-7028.39.4.396

Komro, K. A., Flay, B. R., Biglan, A., & The Promise Neighborhoods Research Consortium. (2011). Creating nurturing environments: A science-based framework for promoting child health and development within high-poverty neighborhoods. *Clinical Child and Family Psychology Review, 14*, 111–134. doi:10.1007/s10567-011-0095-2

Kuo, D., Houtrow, A., Arango, P., Kuhlthau, K., Simmons, J., & Neff, J. (2012). Family-centered care: Current applications and future directions in pediatric health care. *Maternal and Child Health Journal, 16*, 297–305.

Larkin, H., Felitti, V., & Anda, R. (2014). Social work and adverse childhood experiences research: Implications for practice and health policy. *Social Work in Public Health, 29*(1), 1–16. doi:10.1080/19371918.2011.619433

Leventhal, T., & Brooks-Gunn, J. (July 2004). A randomized study of neighborhood effects on low-income children's educational options. *Developmental Psychology, 40*(4), 488–507. doi:10.1037/0012-1649.40.4.488

Martsolf, D., & Draucker, C. (2005). Psychotherapy approaches for adult survivors of childhood sexual abuse: An integrative review of outcomes research. *Issues in Mental Health Nursing, 26*, 801–825. doi:10.1080/01612840500184012

Massachusetts Attorney General. (2013). Report on implementation of Rosie D. Settlement agreement submitted to United States District Court. Springfield, MA: District of Massachusetts.

Maternal and Child Health Bureau. (n.d.). Retrieved from the Health Resources & Services Administration website: http://mchb.hrsa.gov/

Maternal, Infant, and Early Childhood Home Visiting Program. (July, 2016 Update). Retrieved from https://mchb.hrsa.gov/maternal-child-health-initiatives/home-visiting-overview

McClanahan, R., & Weissmuller, P.C. (2015). School nurses and care coordination for children with complex needs: An integrative review. *Journal of School Nursing, 31*(1), 34–43. doi:10.1177/1059840514550484

McNeely, C., & Blanchard, J. (2009). The teen years explained: A guide to healthy adolescent development. Baltimore, MD: Johns Hopkins Bloomberg School of Public Health, Center for Adolescent Health. Retrieved from http://www.jhsph.edu/adolescenthealth

McNeil, T. (2010). Family as a social determinant of health: Implications for governments and institutions to promote the health and well-being of families. *Health care Quarterly, 14S*, 60–67. doi:10.12927/hcq.2010.21984

Medicaid. (April 2017). Medicaid and CHIP enrollment data highlights. Retrieved from https://www.medicaid.gov/medicaid/program-information/medicaid-and-chip -enrollment-data/report-highlights/index.html

Monterio, C., Arnold, J., Locke, S., Steinhorn, L., & Shanske, S. (2016). Social workers as care coordinators: Leaders in ensuring effective, compassionate care. *Social Work in Health Care, 55*(3), 191–213. doi:10.1080/00981389.2015.1093579

Mulye, T.P., Park, M.J., Nelson, C.D., Adams, S.H., Irwin, C.E., Jr., & Brindis, C. (2009). Trends in adolescent and young adult health in the United States. *Journal of Adolescent Health, 45*(1), 8–24. Retrieved from http://download.journals.elsevierhealth.com/ pdfs/journals/1054-139X/PIIS1054139X09001244.pdf

National Health Interview Survey. (2014). National survey of children's health, results comparison 2007–2011/12: Results comparison 2007–2011/12 NSCH national chart-book profile for nationwide. Child and adolescent health measurement initiative, Data resource center for child and adolescent health. Retrieved from www.childhealthdata.org

Pardeck, J. T., & Yuen, F. K. O. (Eds.). (1999). *Family health: A holistic approach to social work practice*. Westport, CT: Auburn House.

Pardeck, J.T., & Yuen, F.Y. (2001). Family health. *Journal of Health & Social Policy, 13*(3), 59–67.

Public Law 111-148: 124 Stat. 119: The Patient Protection and Affordable Care Act (ACA). (March 23, 2010; H.R. 3590). Washington, DC: U.S. Government Publishing Office. Retrieved from https://www.gpo.gov/

Qin, P., Webb, R., Kapur, N., & Sorensen, H.T. (2013). Hospitalization for physical illness and risk of subsequent suicide: A population study. *Journal of Internal Medicine, 273*, 48–58. doi:10.1111/j.1365-2796.2012.02572.x

Romano-Clarke, G., Tang, M.H., Xerras, D.C., Egan, H.S., Pasinski, R.C., Kamin, H.S., Murphy, J.M. (2014). Have rates of behavioral health assessment and treatment increased for Massachusetts children since the Rosie D. decision? A report from two primary care practices. *Clinical Pediatrics, 53*(3), 243–249. doi:10.1177/0009922813507993

Seith, D., & Isaksen, E. (2011). Who are America's poor children? Examining health disparities among children in the United States. In *Report Prepared by the National Center for Children in Poverty*. New York, NY: Columbia University Academic Commons. doi: 10.7916/D8WW7RNB

Sharfstein, J. (May 17, 2017). JAMA Forum: After 50 years, a leap backward for children? *Journal of the American Medication Association (JAMA)*. Retrieved from https://newsat-jama.jama.com/2017/05/17/jama-forum-after-50-years-a-leap-backward-for-children/

Shields, L., Pratt, J., & Hunter, J. (2006). Family-centred care: A review of qualitative studies. *Journal of Clinical Nursing, 15*(10), 1317–1323. doi:10.1111/j.1365-2702.2006.01433.x

Stange, K. C., Nutting, P. A., Miller, W. L., Jaen, C. R., Crabtree, B. F., Flocke, S. A., & Gill, J.M. (2010). Defining and measuring the patient-centered medical home. *Journal of General Internal Medicine, 25*(6), 601–612. doi:10.1007/s11606-010-1291-3

Stark, D.R., Gebhard, B., & DiLauro, E. (2014). The maternal, infant, and early child home visiting program: Smart investments build strong systems for young children. Washington, DC: Zero to Three, Policy Center. Retrieved from http://www.zerotothree .org/policy/homevisiting/docs/ztt-homevisiting_final.pdf

Stroul, B., Pires, S., Boyce, S., Krivelyova, A., & Walrath, C. (2014). *Return on investment in systems of care for children with behavioral health challenges*. Washington, DC: Georgetown

University Center for Child and Human Development, National Technical Assistance Center for Children's Mental Health.

Strully, K.W., Rehkopf, D.H., & Xuan, Z. (2010). Effects of prenatal poverty on infant health: State earned income tax credits and birth weight. *American Sociological Review, 754*, 534–562. doi:10.1177/0003122410374086

Substance Abuse and Mental Health Services Administration. (2014). SAMHSA's concept of trauma and guidance for a trauma-informed approach. Rockville, MD. Retrieved from http://www.traumainformedcareproject.org/resources/SAMHSA%20TIC.pdf

U.S. Census Bureau. (2013). Children characteristics: 2012 American Community Survey 1-year estimates. Retrieved from https://factfinder.census.gov/bkmk/table/1.0/en/ACS/13_1YR/DP02

U.S. Department of Health and Human Services. (2011). Healthy People 2020. Retrieved from https://www.healthypeople.gov/2020/topics-objectives/topic/maternal-infant-and-child-health

World Health Organization. (2015). World Health Statistics 2015. Retrieved from http://apps.who.int/iris/bitstream/10665/170250/1/9789240694439_eng.pdf

Wright, D., Woo, W., Muller, R., Fernandes, C., & Kraftcheck, E. (2003). An investigation of trauma-centered inpatient treatment for adult survivors of abuse. *Child Abuse and Neglect, 27*, 393–411. doi:10.1016/S0145-2134(03)00026-7

Yuen, F. K. O. (2005). *Social work practice with children and families: A family health approach.* Binghamton, NY. Haworth Social Work Press.

Zammitti, E.P., Cohen, R.A., & Martinez, M.E. (November 2016). Health insurance coverage: Early release of estimates from the national health interview survey, January–June 2016. National Center for Health Statistics. Retrieved from http://www.cdc.gov/nchs/data/nhis/earlyrelease/insur201611.pdf

Health Care and Work With Older Adults and Their Caregivers

Manoj Pardasani and Priscilla D. Allen

The population of older adults in the United States has grown exponentially over the past few decades. Individuals ages 65 and over numbered 47.8 million in 2015, an increase of 30% since 2005 (Administration on Aging, 2016). This number is projected to more than double to over 98 million by 2060 (U.S. Census, 2017). Currently, one in seven individuals living in the United States is 65 years old or older. By 2040, one in five will be in that age category (U.S. Census, 2017).

Although social policies and practice models have tried to address the needs of this growing population, they have not kept pace with this radical transformation in our society. Since 1900, the percentage of Americans age 65 and older has more than tripled from 4.1% in 1900 to 14.5% in 2014, and adults age 60 and over have increased 32.5% from 48.9 million to 64.8 million (Administration on Aging, 2016). Not only has the number been steadily increasing, but so has the life expectancy of this cohort. Individuals reaching age 65 have an average life expectancy of an additional 19.3 years (Administration on Aging, 2016). In 2015, there were 27.6 million individuals ages 65 to 74, 13.9 million individuals ages 75 to 84, and 6.3 million individuals age 85 and older (Administration on Aging, 2016). The physical, mental, and functional health of all these individuals varies greatly. Thus, older adults requiring health care and other support services now need to be viewed on a continuum-of-care model rather than as a homogeneous group.

The older adult population is also growing increasingly diverse with respect to ethnicity and diversity. Non-White older adults have increased from 6.5 million in 2004 to 10 million in 2014 and are projected to increase to 21.1 million in 2030 (Federal Interagency Forum on Aging-Related Statistics, 2016), representing 28% of all older adults in the United States. Between 2014 and 2030, the White older adult population is projected to increase by 46%, while the non-White cohort will increase by 110% (Federal Interagency Forum on Aging-Related Statistics, 2016).

Even as this population grows in number, not all older adults need or use the same degree and frequency of services and entitlements. However, those individuals who are most vulnerable or lack adequate resources are most in need. For instance, older women outnumber older men—there are approximately five older women to every four older men in the country (Population Reference Bureau, 2015). About 29% (13.3 million) of individuals age 65 and older live alone (9.2 million women and 4.1 million men). This number does not include older adults who reside in long-term care facilities like nursing homes (Administration on Aging, 2016). Almost half of all older women (46%) live alone (Administration on Aging, 2016). Despite a plethora of income support and other entitlement programs, over 4.5 million older adults (10%) lived below the poverty level in 2014 (Population Reference Bureau, 2015). In 2014, approximately four out of five older adults (84%) reported Social Security as their major source of income. Social Security constituted 90% or more of the income received by one third of all older adults in the same year (Population Reference Bureau, 2015).

As people live longer, the need for caregiving increases as well. About 34.2 million Americans provide unpaid care to an adult age 50 or older (National Alliance for Caregiving & AARP, 2015). Also, about 15.7 million adult family caregivers care for someone who has Alzheimer's disease (AD) or other dementia (Alzheimer's Association, 2015). The overwhelming majority of caregivers (75%) are female, and female caregivers spend more time providing care than males do (21.9 vs. 17.4 hours per week; National Alliance for Caregiving & AARP, 2015). There are at least 3 million self-identified lesbian, gay, bisexual, and transgender (LGBT) persons aged 55+ in the United States, a number expected to double in the next two decades (Espinoza, 2014). Nearly one in 10 caregivers (9%) self-identify as LGBT (National Alliance for Caregiving & AARP, 2015). Supports and services are critically needed for both the caregivers and the care recipients.

The purpose of this chapter is to look at the unique challenges of meeting the comprehensive health care needs of this population. This chapter examines the implications for social policy and gerontological practice and highlights the current models of entitlements and support services for older adults while identifying unmet needs and gaps. A summary of health status of older adults in the United States is presented in Table 12.1.

Table 12.1 Health Status of Older Adults in the United States

- Between 2012 and 2014, most older adults had at least one chronic health condition and many had multiple conditions. The most frequently occurring chronic conditions among older adults were arthritis (49%), heart disease (30%), cancer (24%), diabetes (21%), and hypertension (71%).
- Among older adults ages 65 to 74, the share of men who were obese increased from 24% to 36% from 1988–1994 to 2009–2012, and the proportion of women ages 65 to 74 who were obese increased from 27% to 44%. In 2015, about 30% of adults age 60 and older reported height/weight combinations that placed them among the obese.
- In 2014, about 12% of older adults reported participating in leisure-time aerobic and muscle-strengthening activities that met the 2008 federal physical activity guidelines. The percentage of older adults meeting the guidelines decreased with age, ranging from 15% among people ages 65 to 74 to 5% among people age 85 and over.
- In 2015, only 8% reported that they smoked and 7% reported excessive alcohol consumption.
- In 2015, less than 3% reported that they had experienced psychological distress.
- In 2014, 6.8 million people age 65 and over stayed in a hospital overnight at least one night in a 1-year period. Among this group of older adults, 11% stayed overnight one time, 3% stayed overnight twice, and 2% stayed overnight three or more times.
- In 2014, older adults averaged more office visits with doctors than younger adults. Among people age 75 and over, 20% had 10 or more visits to a doctor or other health care professional in a 1-year period compared with 13% among people ages 45 to 64.

(continued)

Table 12.1 Health Status of Older Adults in the United States (*continued*)

- In 2014, some type of disability (i.e., difficulty in hearing, vision, cognition, ambulation, self-care, or independent living) was reported by 36% of people age 65 and over.
- In 2013, 30% of community-resident Medicare beneficiaries age 65 and over reported difficulty in performing one or more activities of daily living (ADLs) and an additional 12% reported difficulty with one or more instrumental ADLs. By contrast, 95% of institutionalized Medicare beneficiaries age 65 and over had difficulties with one or more ADLs, and 81% of them had difficulty with three or more ADLs.

Source: Adapted from Administration on Aging. (2016). *A profile of older Americans*. Washington, DC: Administration for Community Living, U.S. Department of Health and Human Services.

PRACTICE

Given the projected growth in the older adult population, according to the National Association of Social Workers (NASW), health care with older adults is considered the fastest-growing area for social workers (NASW, 2017a). The increasing health care needs of older adults pose unique challenges in a rapidly changing health system in which social workers are the key agents called upon to facilitate and navigate complex cases, often after a health crisis occurs and with diminished resources. Social workers can be essential partners in advancing care and services for our society (McInnis-Dittrich, 2014). Despite the evolving role of social workers, they have unique skills to enhance the quality of life for elders and to activate person-centered care. This chapter provides a discussion of practice, research, and policy issues, including the implications of preventive care to minimize risks and to implement improved planning.

NASW projects that some 70,000 new social workers will be needed by 2030 to meet the needs of an aging population (Pace, 2014). However, gerontological social workers account for only 5% of all practitioners as we enter the second decade of the 21st century (NASW, 2017a). Social work is especially important as many agencies continue to hire undertrained personnel and other professionals to do the work of certified and licensed social workers, potentially increasing the vulnerability of elders (Bern-Klug, 2008). This is due partly to a lower supply of social workers interested in working with older adults, as well as the stagnating budgets of many organizations serving this population. The lack of trained social workers could also be due to a lack of understanding about the range of skills using contextual and specialized knowledge that social workers bring to the field. Some may say that a person's own internalized fear of aging leads them to work with younger, more vital-perceived clients (Allen, Cherry, & Palmore, 2009). Yet, in fact, work with older adults may be some of the most rewarding in the field as it considers the older adults' life ecology, their family system, socio-environmental and cultural contexts, policy and research relevance, and informed practice within a comprehensive perspective. Working with older adults requires a savvy and persistent professional who can manage care coordination and advocacy in times of need that may be acute, chronic, or intermittent in nature, working in typical health care settings, providing nutritional assistance, health literacy, and health promotion programs. Many older adults continue to work in later life or may have primary caregiver responsibilities for minor children. Social workers provide services such as support groups, education, career counseling, job referral services, and professional training classes. They also work with an aging adult's family members to develop long-term health care plans and connect them with vital services and assistance.

Culturally Competent Practice With Older Adults

Cultural competence is acquired when social workers recognize both the humility as well as the power required to respect and appreciate the unique characteristics and experiences of clients. Cultural competence is never fixed, but is an ongoing process for practitioners driven by an earnest curiosity in people's unique perspective while recognizing that the belief system for the worker is almost always different from the client, and it is the client's perspective that counts. Skills include working to understand diversity and tradition and the unique ways individuals, families, groups, and communities experience lifelong patterns of being, shaped by such forces as oppression for some people and privilege for some others.

NASW provides a detailed array of practice standards in their 2003 publication *Standards and Indicators for Cultural Competence in Social Work Practice*. These standards promote the implementation of cultural and linguistic competence at three intersecting levels: the individual, institutional, and societal (NASW, 2015). Cultural competence requires social workers to "examine their own cultural backgrounds and identities while seeking out the necessary knowledge, skills, and values that can enhance the delivery of services to people with varying cultural experiences associated with their race, ethnicity, gender, class, sexual orientation, religion, age, or disability or other cultural factors" (NASW, 2015, p. 65). In health care, cultural competence requires social workers to be responsive to the health beliefs and practices of diverse populations and integrate that knowledge into their outreach and intervention efforts. Being a culturally competent social worker requires the "use of an intersectionality approach to practice, examining forms of oppression, discrimination, and domination through diversity components of race and ethnicity, immigration and refugee status, religion and spirituality, sexual orientation and gender identity and expression, social class, and abilities" (NASW, 2015, p. 10).

Perhaps the most pressing reality is that older people face ageism that needs to be addressed in practice on a daily basis in a society where youth is revered. It is key that social workers understand the unique intersectionality and cumulative disadvantages of age factors such as race, ethnicity, class, sexual orientation, sex, gender identity, religion, and political affiliation.

As ethical practitioners, social workers strive to uphold the rights of an older person and to encourage self-determination, which may be even more imperative given that so many in health care and in families often attempt to diminish the older adult's ability to make informed decisions. Under the NASW Code of Ethics (2017b) social workers need to respect each individual and ensure that the individual's autonomy and self-determination is ensured. Thus, culturally competent social workers engage, educate, empower, intervene, connect, and advocate for the rights of all older adults while taking into consideration the cultural lens through which they (including our older adult consumers and their families) view the world and make decisions.

As mentioned earlier, the older adult population in the United States is increasingly diverse in terms of age, race/ethnicity, education levels, income status, health status, and living situations. A monolithic system of services and programs cannot meet the plethora of needs of this booming cohort. Older adults may be at different stages in the aging life span with respect to their need for health care and supportive services, access to resources, knowledge of services and programs, and motivation to seek assistance. Most experts believe that service models should be designed and offered incrementally along an aging continuum of care. In other words, as older adults age,

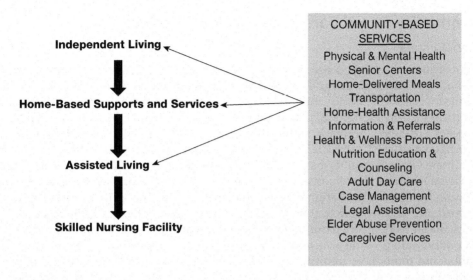

Figure 12.1 The aging continuum-of-care model.

their need for services, programs, and other supports grows concurrently with their age. An individual in their 60s may still be working, is usually ambulatory, relatively healthy, and in need of limited health care services. However, as this individual ages, the number of chronic health conditions may increase, frailty may set in, the person may become less ambulatory and more homebound, and the need for comprehensive health care increases. Thus, if services and programs could be "scaled up" in step with growing needs across the continuum, older adults could be taken care of comprehensively and effectively.

As seen in Figure 12.1, the aging continuum of care extends from older adults living independently in their own homes surrounded by their traditional social supports to requiring home-based assistance in order to continue to live in their familiar surroundings. Some older adults can live out the rest of their lives in their own homes while others may become frail and have significant needs for assistance and monitoring. These older adults may need to move into assisted living facilities where they have their own living space, and health care and other services are provided onsite to promote health and well-being. For other older adults who develop significant chronic health issues, disabilities, or cognitive impairment (such as dementia), skilled nursing facilities can provide comprehensive care in a safe and nurturing environment. As the older adult moves from one context to another, the service model can be scaled up to ensure quality of life. Along this continuum of care, it is important to remember that it is not just the older adult who is the target of intervention, but the family as well.

Because institutional care (long-term care facilities) is increasingly very expensive and seen as a service of last resort, greater emphasis is placed on community-based programs and services to promote "aging-in-place." The goal of the integrated network of community-based services is to preserve an older adult's independence as long as possible and delay institutionalization, thereby upholding his or her dignity and self-determination. In the next section, there is a discussion of some critical practice issues related to community-based care, as well as institutional care (skilled nursing facilities).

Community-Based Care (Independent) Models

Senior Centers

Senior centers have long been a cornerstone of community-based services for independent older adults and are an integral component of the aging continuum of care. They play a significant role in the health and well-being of older adults by providing opportunities for nutrition, recreation, socialization, volunteer development, information and referral, advocacy, education, outreach, and health promotion (Krout, 1998; Leest, 1995; National Council on Aging [NCOA], 2015). Senior centers function as community focal points that coordinate vital community-based social and nutrition supports that help older Americans remain independent in their communities (NCOA, 2015; Torres-Gil, Spencer-Suarez, & Rudinica, 2014). The National Institute of Senior Centers (2012) reports that there are currently 11,000 publicly funded senior centers serving older adults in the United States. Social workers are required to conduct outreach to engage community-dwelling older adults and provide a vast array of services that increase knowledge of health prevention and promotion, influence behavioral changes to improve mental and physical health, and increase socialization. It is essential to understand the design and effect of evidence-based interventions that could benefit seniors, in addition to using comprehensive care coordination to meet the diverse needs of their consumers. Social workers can also use senior centers to organize older adults on issues that affect their lives and coordinate social action and political advocacy to bring about a change. Senior centers can serve as clearing houses for information that is vital to the lives of older adults and their families. Thus, it is imperative for social workers in senior centers to be well versed in group dynamics, practice with families, benefits and entitlements, and the network of service providers in a community.

Home-Based Case Management

A primary contributor to the quality of life for older adults is their ability to remain independent and in their homes for as long as possible. Home-based case management is increasingly used in the community and allows older adults to delay institutionalization (Boult, Boult, & Pacala, 1998; Schore, Brown, & Cheh, 1999). Although community-based case-management programs are still diverse and somewhat fragmented (Quinn, 1995), there is a growing consensus that in-home care yields positive outcomes and is cost-effective. According to a Genworth Cost of Care Study (2016), the median annual cost of care in a skilled nursing home varies between $82,125 and $92,378. However, the cost of in-home care is approximately $46,000. Not only is home-based care more economical, it also allows older adults to remain in a familiar environment with their social support structures (family, friends, religious institutions, etc.) in close proximity. Researchers such as Goldstein (1983) have highlighted the importance of an alternative to institutionalized or long-term care for frail older adults. But the choice to live at home with assistance is predicated on the ability of the individual to function somewhat independently. The activities of daily living (ADLs)—the basic tasks of independent care such as eating, ambulating or transferring, dressing, bathing, grooming/dental care, and toileting independently—are often assisted by professionals such as social workers or health care providers. Instrumental activities of daily living (IADLs) are considered more complex functions, but remain essential for living independently (McInnis-Dittrich, 2014). IADLs include activities such as shopping and food preparation, using a phone, taking and coordinating medications, financial management, and use of independent transportation. Social workers need to have strong clinical skills to conduct comprehensive biopsychosocial assessments, evaluate risks, and connect the older adults with vital services that will enable them to live safely and comfortably in their own homes. Care coordination, consistent monitoring, and networking skills are critical to ensuring that the changing needs of the consumer are addressed in a timely and effective manner.

Adult Day Programs

Adult day programs are geared toward older adults with multiple chronic conditions, disabilities, or cognitive impairment (National Care Planning Council, 2002). They range from social activity centers that allow a respite for the caregivers, to medically staffed day centers with a focus on health and wellness (Family Care America, 2016). These centers allow for older adults to remain in their own homes or with their caregivers, while receiving health and wellness programs in a supervised environment. Currently, more than 4,000 of these programs operate in the United States (Family Care America, 2016). Social workers frequently provide care coordination and socialization activities in these centers.

Caregiving

The average age of a caregiver in the United States is 69.4 years, and nearly half of all care recipients (47%) are older than 75 (National Alliance for Caregiving & AARP, 2015). Many caregivers of older adults are themselves growing older. Of these caregivers, some report being in fair to poor health (Generations United, 2003). As mentioned earlier in the chapter, a significant number of caregivers provide unpaid service to older adults coping with dementia or AD. A diagnosis of a serious or terminal illness or a degenerative one like AD often pushes the older adult and his or her family into crisis mode. Lack of knowledge about services and interventions, anxiety about the progress of the illness, and the need for resources and psychosocial supports are critical at this juncture. Often these issues arise when the situation is already dire, as the individual or family has not planned ahead. Social workers can help families become aware of such realities before a crisis arises and plan accordingly in order to save time and resources and reduce strain on the caregiver. Furthermore, systematic and comprehensive planning can ensure a higher quality of care for all involved. With few geriatricians in the United States, and the increased numbers of older adults, social workers will be essential in bridging the gap between generalized and specialized knowledge within other health professions. Becoming familiar with nursing and allied health service professionals, medication and treatment regimens, durable medical equipment needs, and other practical skills will advance the on-the-job knowledge of social workers.

Case Example 12.1

John (88) and Sarah (85) have been married for nearly 65 years. They have two sons, Maxwell (63) and Herbert (61). Both sons are married, have two children each, and live in the same city as their parents. The adult children are close to their parents and visit them about four times a year, usually during holidays.

About 2 years ago, Sarah started to show signs of memory loss. She could not remember names or familiar places and grew increasingly confused and agitated in social situations. After a round of tests, she was diagnosed with Alzheimer's-related dementia. John was warned that Sarah's condition would grow increasingly worse and she would eventually need assistance with ADLs and IADLs. John refused all outside help and insisted that he would take care of Sarah on his own.

At first, things seemed to be going well. Sarah loved the idea of being in her own home surrounded by familiar objects and spaces. She appreciated that she and John could still

(continued)

Case Example 12.1   *(continued)*

socialize with their friends and attend church weekly. However, while visiting their parents on Mother's Day, Maxwell and Herbert noticed that Sarah had declined considerably. She needed assistance with eating, showering, and going to the bathroom and needed constant vigilance so that she did not wander away. The sons noticed that John had grown quite frail himself and was unable to provide the care necessary for Sarah without endangering her or himself. The house was in complete disarray and had not been cleaned in a while. Maxwell broached the subject with his father but John refused any help. He insisted that he was fine and could take care of both of them. Herbert suggested that they should move their mother to a nursing home and John grew very agitated. He asked his sons to stop interfering in their lives and reminded them that he was their father.

Both sons are very worried about their parents but are not sure how to proceed. They respect their father's right to make his own decisions but do not believe that they are in the best interests of their mother or himself. They decide to contact a social worker (you) at the community senior center. How could you assist this family?

The practice issues in Case Example 12.1 are complex and multilayered. On one hand, the social worker needs to assist Sarah in getting connected with comprehensive health care and social services to help her cope with her declining cognitive and functional abilities. This would ensure that she receives integrated care in a safe environment. Additionally, the social worker must also work with John and his children to educate them about Sarah's condition, address John's resistance to seeking assistance, inform them about the services and resources available to them, and assist them in accessing those critical services. It also appears that John may himself need social, emotional, and physical supports to ensure his continued well-being.

Advance Planning

It may be hard to believe that in 2017 discussion about planning for an aging family member or friend's health needs, money, and death is still considered taboo, but it is. It may coincide with the perspective that when people are well, children don't want to interfere with personal matters and suggest any impending decline. Also, parents often don't want to burden their children with care, or even the idea of dependency. The majority of adults, as many as 75%, have not had a discussion about care needs and living and dying arrangements or finances for their aging parent. Consequently, when care is actually needed, very few plans or structures are in place to aid in this transition (Lustbader & Hooyman, 1994). See Advance Care Planning Tips from the National Institute on Aging at nia.nih.gov/health/publication/advance-care-planning.

People generally prefer autonomy over their lives without interference, but the paradox is that not interfering or failing to plan can create even more hardship for families when a change in health occurs. Despite the fact that the majority of people—nine out of 10—believe that health care preferences and end-of-life discussions are important, few broach the subject with an older family member, waiting until the elder raises the topic first (The Conversation Project, 2017). And even a third of spouses haven't discussed these key features of end of life with one another (Moorman, Hauser, & Carr, 2009). Social workers can help raise critical awareness, educate, and facilitate communication and advance planning. Social workers are often called upon to discuss living wills, care preferences, and end-of-life decisions aligned with the Patient Self Determination Act of 1990. Taking a central role in organizations that are often led by physicians, nurses, administrators, and other health professionals is a key skill that gerontological social workers are called to do. Social work has fortunately changed from being "guests in a host setting" in most places, but the legacy of social work still has challenges not just to be present at the table, but to be at the head of the table alongside clients, and not just be seen as the coordinator of admissions and discharges, durable medical equipment needs, home care, psychological service consults, and transportation (as is the case in some facilities). See Chapter 9 for a discussion of palliative care.

Physical and Behavioral Health

The way people feel physically and emotionally can largely dictate how they interact with the outside world—which leads to issues like social isolation, loneliness, and declines in overall well-being (McInnis-Dittrich, 2014). The most disabling and prevalent health issues for individuals age 65 and over are heart disease, cancer, and stroke, and these are even more prevalent in the African American/Black community, Hispanics, and Native Americans. The psychological conditions that may increase with age include dementia, depression, anxiety, substance addiction and/or dependency, and suicide. Despite risks, older adults are often more reluctant than younger people to seek care and treatment (American Psychological Association, 2017).

In the absence of a national health care system, older adults must navigate a complex network of medical providers that include primary care physicians, specialists, surgeons, nurse coordinators, physical therapists, occupational therapists, pharmacies, and mental health counselors. Depending on the nature of their health insurance (in addition to Medicare or Medicaid), they may be able to access specific professionals with differing parameters. In addition to medical offices and counseling centers, often older adults must also engage with hospitals, rehabilitation centers, assisted living residences, and skilled nursing facilities. This complex array of providers and services can be overwhelming. Getting the service one needs is predicated on the knowledge of these providers, access to them, resources available for utilization, and other systemic barriers. Social workers are critical in helping educate older adults and families about their choices and assist them in making informed decisions. Advocating on behalf of their consumers and facilitating systems integration are core skills necessary to serve effectively.

Prevention

While the overall health of older adults may be improving with advances in health care and treatment, diet and exercise are still challenges that may lead to premature death. As many as 70% of persons over 65 do not meet the current recommended standards of 150 weekly minutes of moderate aerobic exercise plus strength training, which reduce such health issues as obesity, cardiovascular conditions, and certain cancers (U.S. Department of Health and Human Services [USDHHS], Office of Disease Prevention and Health Promotion, 2008). Just over 20% of the adult population meets the minimum recommendations (Centers for Disease Control and Prevention [CDC], 2014). Based on 2015 statistics, an estimated 17% of the 65 and over U.S. population participated at levels that met the recommendations (Maberry, 2016). Certain groups appear to be particularly at risk of sedentary lifestyles, including racially and ethnically diverse, less-educated persons, and socioeconomically challenged older adults (CDC Morbidity and Mortality Weekly Report, 2001). Data indicate that these older adults demonstrate the highest rates of disablement and they are less likely to be involved in physical activity programs (CDC, 2014; Maberry, 2016). Social workers can and should learn effective strategies and referrals to activity programs or individual activities just as they would refer to programs for mental health, home care, and coordination of durable medical equipment.

Engaging older adults in physical activity and socialization and finding creative ways for people to engage in such behavioral change (diet, exercise, etc.) is helpful to promote health and wellness. Similarly, many prevention efforts are critical to the health of older adults. Regular health screenings for blood pressure, cancer, diabetes, physical impairments (vision, hearing, etc.) and mental health allow for timely and effective intervention. Change is hard for everyone, especially those who have lived their lives a certain way for decades. Cultural preferences (food, activities, utilization of mental health services, etc.) also may influence decision making. Furthermore, even when made aware of the importance of health prevention, some older adults may choose not to engage in any interventions. Social workers must utilize their negotiation and empathic skills to evaluate the concerns of the reluctant older adults and figure out innovative ways to assist them. While balancing the right to self-determination, social workers must assess risk and take the necessary steps to prevent harm to their clients.

In the community, social workers are often involved with complex cases. They have the knowledge and skills to address complex situations given their person-in-environment perspective. Social workers may propose solutions by finding alternative avenues that can help to improve patient outcomes to best fit the varied needs of older adults and their families. Even with a hip fracture, the most common injury requiring hospitalization, a social worker is more likely to be involved when the intersect of the environmental, physical, psychological, and economic issues requires further input to navigate the process (Sims-Gould, Bryne, Hicks, Franke, & Stolee, 2015). Social work practice done right can maximize independence, quality, and decisional capacity of the older population while supporting the caregivers and moving toward more intentional and empowered practice in the decades to come.

Elder Abuse

The National Center on Elder Abuse defines elder abuse as "any knowing, intended or careless act that causes harm or serious risk of harm to an older person—physically, mentally, emotionally, or financially" (2017). A national study showed that nearly 11% of Americans 60 years old and older faced some type of elder abuse in a 1-year period (Acierno, Hernandez-Tejada, Muzzy & Steve, 2008). Elder abuse can occur in private homes, hospitals, assisted living residences, or skilled nursing facilities. However, it is far more difficult to observe and address when an older adult lives at home. Often, the victims are abused by family or others close to them either in home settings or in care facilities. Some older adults may not even be aware that they are being abused by their family members, caregivers, or service providers because they suffer from cognitive impairments. In other cases, an older adult may be ashamed to report abuse because they think they should have known better. Additionally, some care recipients may fear losing their source of support if they report the abuser, assuming they are even aware of how to do so. Social workers must be trained in assessing for abuse and providing access and advocacy for the individual. Maintaining the client's safety is paramount and skills in conflict resolution, working with legal authorities, and managing family dynamics are essential.

Institutional Living

Individuals need institutional or supervised care when a chronic condition, trauma, or illness limits their ability to carry out basic self-care tasks, called ADLs, such as eating, bathing, toileting, dressing, walking or transferring, or IADLs, such as household chores, meal preparation, or managing money. Depending on the severity of impairment, individuals can be served in their own home or in institutional settings. Institutional care often involves the most intimate aspects of people's lives—what and when they eat, personal hygiene, getting dressed, using the bathroom. The two most common types of institutional care settings are assisted living residences and skilled nursing facilities. Assisted living is congregate living, almost exclusively funded by private pay sources (i.e., the older adult or his or her family) in private homes in a gated community, townhouses, apartment buildings, or commercial residences. The residents receive a wide variety of assistive and supportive services such as meals, transportation, recreational activities, case management, exercise, and health promotion programs. They may also receive assistance with ADLs and IADLs if required. This arrangement allows individuals to live semi-independently in a safe environment. Skilled nursing facilities or nursing homes are medical facilities that serve older adults with significant impairment (dementia, AD, physical illnesses, etc.) who need a higher degree of health care.

There is no question that older adults want to remain in their own homes—it may be the single most important factor and concern for people who are declining. Most older people do live at home with the help of individuals who provide unpaid caregiving support. However, about 5% of the population lives in the skilled nursing home level at any one time, and those who live to be 80 have a 50% chance of spending some time in a nursing home, including short-term rehabilitation care (Federal Interagency Forum on Aging-Related Statistics, 2004). The CDC (2013) estimated that there were approximately 1.38 million older adults living in nursing homes, and another 713,000 residing in assisted living facilities in 2012. Although almost everyone wants to age in place, most people die in the hospital; however, this is changing with even higher numbers of older adults opting to use hospice care in the home setting and in facilities. The strongest predictor of spending time in an institution is the absence of caregivers coupled with advanced age, being female and White, and living alone prior to placement—single people, those never married, and those without offspring are at a disproportionate risk of requiring help as they do not have the same access to resources. However, race and culture often influence caregiving and institutional use for many reasons, including the expressed and internalized mistrust of health care systems and policies and the preference of known versus unknown care providers.

Demand for elder care, including institutional care, will be fueled by a steep rise in the number of Americans living with AD, which could nearly triple by 2050 to 14 million, from 5 million in 2013 (Hebert, Weuve, Scherr, & Evans, 2013). The caregiving burden for people with AD can be profoundly taxing on the caregiver's physical, psychological, and financial status, requiring social work knowledge of a holistic and multidisciplinary approach to buffer profound stress to both the caregiver and care recipient (Wennberg, Dye, Streetman-Loy, & Pham, 2015).

Social workers serving in skilled nursing facilities or assisted living programs are tasked with clients who have significant impairments and chronic conditions. Specialized skills are needed to engage the residents in healthy activities. Additionally, they must work with family members and other health professionals to ensure consistency and quality of care.

POLICY

Several social policies influence the design, implementation, and accessibility of health care services and programs. Funding for such programs comprise a complex array of federal, state, local, and private resources. This chapter focuses on four federal social policies that have guided the development of health care in the United States. These policies have had a substantial impact on who is eligible for services, the type of services one is entitled to, the quality of services provided, and ultimately the lives of individuals affected by them. In many ways, the guidelines and standards created by these policies have influenced the very structure of the continuum of care for older adults. The four major social policies that affect the health of older adults are Medicare, Medicaid, the Older Americans Act (OAA), and the Supplemental Nutritional Assistance Program (SNAP).

Medicare

Medicare is the federal health insurance program for people who are 65 or older, certain younger people with disabilities, and people with end-stage renal disease (permanent kidney failure requiring dialysis or a transplant). To be eligible for Medicare, older adults must be a citizen or permanent resident of the United States, be 65 years of age, and be eligible for Social Security or Railroad Retirement Board benefits. In other words, these individuals have contributed to Medicare through taxes levied on their employment income. Currently, 46.3 million older adults receive health insurance through Medicare (National Center to Preserve Social Security and Medicare, 2017). There are four components (parts) of coverage for health care:

- Medicare Part A, which covers inpatient hospital stays, care in a skilled nursing facility, hospice care, and some home health care. A monthly premium (approximately $100 is deducted from the social security payment each month for this coverage.
- Medicare Part B, which covers certain doctors' services, outpatient care, medical supplies, and preventive services (screenings, vaccinations, etc.). Recipients pay a monthly premium for this component of the health coverage.
- Medicare Part C, which is an optional health plan offered by a private company that contracts with Medicare to provide the Part A and Part B benefits (also called Medicare Advantage plans). These health plans may also help cover other services not reimbursed by Parts A and B.
- Medicare Part D is an optional program that offers prescription drug coverage to Medicare recipients. These plans are offered by insurance companies and other private companies approved by Medicare.

Medicaid

Medicaid is a joint federal and state program that, together with the Children's Health Insurance Program, provides health coverage to over 74.6 million Americans, including children, pregnant women, parents, seniors, and individuals with disabilities (Centers for Medicare and Medicaid Services [CMS], 2017). Medicaid provides health coverage to more than 4.6 million low-income seniors who receive Supplemental Security Income (SSI) instead of Social Security benefits (CMS, 2017). These individuals have a limited working history and have low incomes. Eligibility based on income varies from state to state; however, most older adults who do not qualify for Medicare are eligible for Medicaid. The recipients must be U.S. citizens or permanent residents. Medicaid covers all components (Parts A through D) offered by Medicare for older adults who are eligible (Paying for Senior Care, 2016). Medicare enrollees who have limited income and resources may get help paying for their premiums and out-of-pocket medical expenses from Medicaid (Paying for Senior Care, 2016).

Medicaid also covers skilled nursing facility care beyond the 100-day limit of skilled nursing facility care that Medicare covers (Paying for Senior Care, 2016). There are income and asset requirements in order to be qualified for Medicaid reimbursement for long-term care. In fact, Medicaid, through its state affiliates, is the largest single payer for nursing home care. While estimates vary, it is estimated that Medicaid pays at least 40% of the total nursing home costs in the United States (Paying for Senior Care, 2016).

Older Americans Act

In 1965, Congress enacted the OAA, which established the U.S. Administration on Aging (AoA) and state agencies on aging to address the social services needs of older people. The Act helped create a vast network for the delivery of social services to the aging population. "The broader goal of OAA is to help older people maintain maximum independence in their homes and communities and to promote a continuum of care for the vulnerable elderly" (National Health Policy Forum, 2012, p. 1).

The Act comprises seven titles that include a series of formula-based and discretionary grants. The federal government calculates grants to each state and territory based on the proportion of adults age 60 and over residing in those states or territories. Thus, states/territories with a higher proportion of older adults receive a greater allocation each year. Additionally, there are other grants that are based on services provided or specific target populations that are deemed vulnerable. Eligibility for programs funded by OAA is limited to age—all individuals have to be age 60 and older, and "most services do not require means testing or copayments, but donations may be requested and some newer programs may have cost sharing on a sliding scale" (National Committee to Preserve Social Security and Medicare, 2017).

- Title I: This title highlights the major goals of the social policy and its intended outcomes for older adults (adequate nutrition, improved mental and physical health, opportunity for employment, and delay in institutionalization).
- Title II: This title establishes the AoA within the USDHHS as the chief federal agency that is the primary advocate for older people. The AoA is charged with coordinating national efforts on health and long-term services and support activities that would enable older people to live independently in their homes and communities and prevent/delay institutionalization. As a result of this title, Aging and Disability Resource Centers (ADRC) have been set up in states and territories to serve as clearing houses for information about benefits, entitlements, health care, and social services.
- Title III: This title provides funds for supportive and nutrition services, family caregiver support, disease prevention, and health promotion activities. The funds are distributed through the State Agencies on Aging and the local Area Agencies on Aging to private, nonprofit service providers. Supportive services include access services (such as transportation and information and assistance), home care, and legal assistance and senior center programs. The nutritional component of the title provides meals and socialization to older people in congregate settings (senior centers, retirement communities, etc.), or home-delivered meals to less ambulatory, frail older people. The goal of the nutrition program is to address hunger and food insecurity and to promote socialization and health through nutritional education. The National Family Caregiver Support Program, also under this title, provides grants for caregiver-related programs such as information and referrals, individual counseling, support groups, caregiver training, and respite services for caregivers.

A very small but significant component of this title focuses on providing physical fitness and diabetes control classes, chronic disease management, and prevention efforts such as medical and dental screening, nutrition counseling, pharmacology consultation, and immunizations.

- Title IV: This title provides support for training, research, and demonstration projects in the field of aging. Research and training grants are awarded to a wide range of public and private organizations, state and area agencies on aging, and institutions of higher learning to design, implement, and/or evaluate innovative interventions.
- Title V: This title provides part-time jobs for unemployed, low-income people age 55 and older, who need assistance in finding and applying for employment. Under the Service Community Senior Employment Program (SCSEP), individuals are assisted by various contracted organizations to find employment in community services such as hospitals, schools, and senior centers.
- Title VI: This title provides funds for supportive and nutrition services for older Native Americans. Indian tribal organizations, Alaskan Native organizations, and nonprofit groups representing Native Hawaiians are eligible under this title.
- Title VII: This title funds programs to prevent elder abuse, neglect, and exploitation. It also provides for an Ombudsman program to investigate complaints of residents of nursing facilities, board and care facilities, and other adult care homes. (National Health Policy Forum, 2012)

It is estimated that nearly 3 million older adults received services funded by the OAA in 2012, such as home-delivered meals, home care, or case management services. Almost 8 million older adults (14% of the older population) used services such as transportation, information and assistance, or congregate meals, on a less regular basis (National Health Policy Forum, 2012).

Supplemental Nutrition Assistance Program

The Supplemental Nutrition Assistance Program (SNAP) offers nutrition assistance to low-income individuals and families, including older adults age 60 and over. If an older adult qualifies for SSI, they are most likely eligible for food assistance. The goal of SNAP is to promote food security and improve the health of its recipients. The allocations to individuals and families are determined by the states. Recipients receive a fixed amount of cash assistance each month that can be used toward the purchase of food produce and products (U.S. Department of Agriculture, 2017). In 2016, more than 44 million individuals received SNAP benefits (U.S. Department of Agriculture, 2017). The NCOA (2016) reports that more than 4.8 million low-income older adults rely on SNAP to stay healthy, and on average, they receive $108 per month in assistance. NCOA (2016) also estimates that an additional 5 million older adults could benefit from this program but have not been able to access it. Nutrition is one of the key factors in maintaining or improving the physical and mental health of older adults; thus, this program is a vital source of support for this population.

RESEARCH

The fields of health care and social services have moved toward program designs and services that are evidence based. In other words, programs and services must be guided by a theoretical framework and also have been tested for effectiveness. These scientifically evaluated interventions are increasingly being relied on by the network of health care providers. It is believed that providing research-tested and validated programs or services is ethical, responsible, and client focused. Furthermore, all providers are now required to document not just the types of services they provide (outputs) and the demographic characteristics of their consumers, but they must also evaluate the effect of their services (outcomes). In other words, providers must reach out to all in need, but must also be responsible for helping their consumers realize the expected goals of the specific service/program. This is where scientific research knowledge and skills becomes a critical tool for providers and funders.

Additionally, many health care programs and services are underfunded or there are emerging needs that are unmet by existing structures. Research is necessary to reach out to all individuals, especially those who belong to marginalized, oppressed, or vulnerable groups. Conducting comprehensive needs assessments is important to help document unmet needs and highlight barriers to access and utilization of health care. In order to advocate for changes in existing social policies, create new social policies, or develop resources for underfunded services, social workers and other professionals need data to inform their advocacy efforts. We need rigorous scientific studies that can demonstrate the positive health outcomes of various programs (community based and institutional) that exist currently or pilot projects that test a new intervention. The results of these studies can affect funding and policy decisions, thereby enhancing the quality of lives of older adults.

For instance, research into case management programs for homebound older adults has shown positive health outcomes, such as reduced isolation and depression (United Neighborhood Houses, 2005), lower frequency of hospitalizations (Shapiro & Taylor, 2002), a delay in degenerative disability and institutionalization (Stuck et al., 1995), and an increase in program or care satisfaction (Cummings et al., 1990). A more medically oriented version of case management has been shown to decrease mortality (Boult et al., 1994), increase care satisfaction (Morishita, Boult, Boult, Smith, & Pacala, 1998), and reduce caregiver burden (Weuve, Boult, & Morishita, 2000).

Only one large-scale study has evaluated the outcome of a social service–oriented case management program in New York City (Shapiro & Taylor, 2002). Those older adults who received the intervention had significantly higher subjective well-being and were less likely to be institutionalized or die than those in the comparison group across the 18-month period (Shapiro & Taylor, 2002).

Similarly, senior center participation has been shown to have positive health outcomes for older adults. Engaging in social activities has been associated with enhanced well-being among community-dwelling older adults (Everard, Lach, Fisher, & Blum, 2000; Lemon, Bengston, & Peterson, 1972), an increase in physical function and a slower decline in functional status (Ungar, Johnson, & Marks, 1997). Research has demonstrated that senior center participants have better psychological well-being than nonparticipants, including depressive symptoms (Choi & McDougall, 2007), friendship formations (Aday, Kehoe, & Farney, 2006), and stress levels (Farone, Fitzpatrick, & Tran, 2005, Maton, 1989). Skarupski and Pelkowski (2003) showed that health education and promotion offered at senior centers improved diet and nutrition among participants. Maton (2002) found that senior center participation contributed to a heightened perception of general well-being. Meis (2005) and Carey (2004) found that senior center members felt less isolated and experienced a greater level of social support than their nonparticipating counterparts. Senior centers also serve as critical information and resource centers for older adults and their families (Pardasani & Sackman, 2014).

Health promotion and prevention programs have also been shown to be effective in enhancing the lives of older adults. "Health promotion and disease prevention activities include primary prevention—the prevention of disease before it occurs—and secondary prevention—the detection of disease at an early stage" (Resnick, 2001). Some evidence suggests that older adults benefit from primary and secondary health promotion activities

(Resnick, 2001). Exercising, reducing cholesterol levels, and monitoring blood pressure improve overall health status and physical fitness of older adults. Engagement in health promotion activities or programs enhances strength and balance while reducing the incidences of fractures, myocardial infarctions, and cerebral vascular accidents (Ettinger, 1996; Goldberg & Chavin, 1997; Gregg, Cauley, Seeley, Enrud, & Bauer, 1998).

Similarly, evidence-based interventions such as Matters of Balance (to reduce falls), Active Choices (to engage older adults in exercise), Stanford University's suite of self-management programs (living with chronic disease, pain management, and diabetes management), Healthy IDEAS (identifying depression and seeking help), REACH II (targeting caregivers of individuals with AD) and BRITE (substance abuse screening and interventions) are some examples of evidence-based interventions that have been approved for funding under Title III of the OAA (NCOA, 2012). These interventions are offered by a diverse network of community-based providers in various settings and have documented positive health outcomes for older adults. However, more research is needed on culturally responsive and competent interventions that can engage and motivate individuals from various minority groups.

CONCLUSION

Health care for older adults is a complex and critical issue. As the population ages, innovative and effective practices are necessary to serve them comprehensively. It is important to think of health care service models along a continuum of care in order to meet the diverse needs of older adults in the United States. Service providers, professionals, and agencies (public and private) need to work in an integrated and coordinated fashion to ensure consistency and quality of services. While attention is being paid to designing effective and efficient health care services, we must not forget the interrelated social policy issues. As social workers we must continue to organize older adults and their families to advocate for safe and healthy communities. Finally, we must not forget our ethical responsibility to engage in evidence-based practice while simultaneously using research to highlight disparities and inequities in our health care system.

CHAPTER DISCUSSION QUESTIONS

1. What, in your opinion, are the most critical health care issues with regard to older adults today?

2. A large majority of older adults do not seek out or utilize mental health services. What do you think are the reasons for the low utilization? How would you address that?

3. What do you think are the unique health care and social service needs of LGBT older adults?

4. How could social workers ensure that services and programs are culturally competent?

5. Less than one third of all adults age 65 and older engage in regular exercise. We know that exercise and physical activity improve the health and well-being of older adults. How would you engage more older adults in such activities?

6. The funding for most programs and services aimed at improving the health of older adults is limited. This means that not all older adults have similar access to comprehensive and quality care. How would you change that?

CASE EXAMPLE AND DISCUSSION QUESTIONS

Case Example 12.2

You are a social worker at a case management agency that serves frail, homebound older adults. It is your responsibility to conduct a comprehensive assessment with every new client to ascertain the type of services they need, as well as the degree of home assistance required. Additionally, you make monthly home visits to all your clients to check in with them and monitor their well-being. As case manager, you coordinate the network of providers (home health aides, visiting nurses, home-delivered meals, etc.) who serve your client.

Yolanda is a 65-year-old widow who lives with her daughter, Juanita (40). Juanita, a single mother, also has two daughters—Geneshia (16) and Lyneshia (14). Yolanda suffered a stroke a couple of years ago and is now completely dependent on her daughter to provide care for her. Juanita is a full-time caregiver for her mother. Yolanda receives SSI, which amounts to approximately $700 per month. Additionally, she receives $120 in food stamps (SNAP). Juanita receives very little child support from the father of Geneshia and Lyneshia. She also receives $180 in food stamps (SNAP).

During your last home visit, you became very concerned for Yolanda. She had soiled herself and was lying in bed in her soiled clothes. She seemed more frail than usual and asked you for food. You started to ask her questions about her health, but she seemed very anxious and kept glancing at her daughter. Juanita actually answered all your questions. You noticed bruises on both of Yolanda's arms. Upon inquiry about these bruises, Yolanda teared up but refused to speak. Juanita, growing increasingly agitated, stated that her mother had tried to get up from the bed on her own and had fallen as a result. She continued to complain about how difficult and ungrateful her mother is. You believe that Yolanda is a victim of physical and emotional abuse at the hands of her daughter.

Questions for Discussion

1. What is the first step that you should consider doing?

2. How would you protect Yolanda?

REFERENCES

Acierno, R., Hernandez-Tejada, M., Muzzy, W., & Steve, K. (2008, March). *National Elder Mistreatment Study*. Final report to the National Institute of Justice, Washington, DC.

Aday, R., Kehoe, G., & Farney, L. (2006). Impact of senior center friendships on aging women who live alone. *Journal of Women Aging, 18*(1), 57–73. doi:10.1300/J074v18n01_05

Administration on Aging. (2016). *A profile of older Americans*. Washington, DC: Administration for Community Living, U.S. Department of Health and Human Services.

Allen, P. D., Cherry, K. E., & Palmore, E. (2009). Self-reported ageism among social work practitioners and students. *Journal of Gerontological Social Work, 52*(2), 124–134. doi:10.1080/01634370802561927

Alzheimer's Association. (2015). Alzheimer's disease facts and figures. Retrieved from https://www.alz.org/facts/downloads/facts_figures_2015.pdf

American Psychological Association. (2017). Mental and behavioral health and older Americans. Retrieved from http://www.apa.org/about/gr/issues/aging/mental -health.aspx

Bern-Klug, M. (2008). State variation in nursing home social worker qualifications. *Journal of Gerontological Social Work, 51*(3–4), 379–409. doi:10.1080/01634370802039734

Boult, C., Boult, L., Murphy, C., Ebbitt, B., Luptak, M., & Kane, R. L. (1994). A controlled trial of outpatient geriatric evaluation and management. *Journal of the American Geriatrics Society, 42*(5), 465–470.

Boult, C., Boult, L., & Pacala, J. T. (1998). Systems of care for older populations of the future. *Journal of American Geriatrics Society, 46*, 499–505.

Carey, K. (2004). The lived experiences of the independent oldest-old in community-based programs: A Heideggerian hermeneutical analysis. *Dissertation Abstracts International, A: The Humanities and Social Sciences, 65*(6), 2366-A (University of Chicago).

Centers for Disease Control and Prevention. (2013). Long-term care services. Retrieved from http://www.cdc.gov/nchs/data/nsltcp/long_term_care_services_2013.pdf

Centers for Disease Control and Prevention. (2014). Facts about physical activity. Retrieved from https://www.cdc.gov/physicalactivity/data/facts.htm

Centers for Disease Control and Prevention Morbidity and Mortality Weekly Report. (2001). Increasing physical activity: A report on recommendations of the Task Force on Community Preventive Service. Retrieved from https://www.cdc.gov/mmwr/preview/mmwrhtml/rr5018a1.htm

Centers for Medicare and Medicaid Services. (2017). July 2017 Medicaid and CHIP enrollment data highlights. Retrieved from https://www.medicaid.gov/medicaid/program-information/medicaid-and-chip-enrollment-data/report-highlights/index .html

Choi, N., & McDougall, G. (2007). Comparison of depressive symptoms between home-bound older adults and ambulatory older adults. *Aging Mental Health, 11*(3), 310–322. doi:10.1080/13607860600844614

Cummings, J. E., Hughes, S. L., Weaver, F. M., Manheim, L. M., Conrad, K. J., Nash, K., . . . Adelman, J. (1990). Cost-effectiveness of VA-based home-care: A randomized clinical trial. *Journal of the American Geriatrics Society, 46*, 499–505.

Espinoza, R. (2014). *Out and visible: The experiences and attitudes of lesbian, gay, bisexual and transgender older adults, ages 45–75*. New York, NY: Services and Advocacy for GLBT Seniors (SAGE).

Ettinger, W. (1996). Physical activity and older people: A walk a day keeps the doctor away. *Journal of American Geriatrics Society, 44*, 207–208.

Everard, K., Lach, H., Fisher, E., & Blum, M. (2000). Relationship of activity and social support to the functional health of older adults. *Journal of Gerontology: Social Sciences, 55B*(4), s208–s212.

Family Care America. (2016). What is adult day care? Retrieved from http://www .caregiverslibrary.org/caregivers-resources/grp-caring-for-yourself/hsgrp-support -systems/what-is-adult-day-care-article.aspx

Farone, D., Fitzpatrick, T., & Tran, T. (2005). Use of senior centers as a moderator of stress-related distress among Latino elders. *Journal of Gerontological Social Work, 46*(1), 65–83. doi:10.1300/J083v46n01_05

Federal Interagency Forum on Aging-Related Statistics. (2004). *Older Americans 2004: Key indicators of well-being.* Washington, DC: U.S. Government Printing Office, Federal Interagency Forum on Aging-Related Statistics.

Federal Interagency Forum on Aging-Related Statistics. (2016). *Older Americans 2016: Key indicators of well-being.* Washington, DC: U.S. Government Printing Office, Federal Interagency Forum on Aging-Related Statistics.

Generations United. (2003). A guide to the National Family Caregiver Support Program. Retrieved from http://www.gu.org/LinkClick.aspx?fileticket=P2DtwHlXt8w%3D&tabid=157&mid=606

Genworth Financial, Inc. (2016). Cost of care survey. Retrieved from https://www.genworth.com/dam/Americas/US/PDFs/Consumer/corporate/131168_050516.pdf

Goldberg, T., & Chavin, S. (1997). Preventive medicine and screening in older adults. *Journal of American Geriatrics Society, 45,* 345–354.

Goldstein, R. (1983). Psychotherapy of the elderly. Case #1: Institutionalizing a spouse: Who is the client? *Journal of Geriatric Psychiatry, 16*(1), 41–49.

Gregg, E., Cauley, J., Seeley, D., Enrud, K., & Bauer, D. (1998). Physical activity and osteoporotic fracture risk in older women. Study of Osteoporotic Fractures Research Group. *Annals of Internal Medicine, 129,* 81–88.

Hebert, L. E., Weuve, J., Scherr, P. A., & Evans, D. A. (2013). Alzheimer disease in the United States (2010–2050) estimated using the 2010 census. *Neurology, 80,* 1778–1783. doi:10.1212/WNL.0b013e31828726f5

Krout, J. (1998). *Senior centers in America* (5th ed.). New York, NY: Greenwood Press.

Leest, L. (1995). *Senior centers and life satisfaction* (Doctoral dissertation). Yeshiva University, New York, NY.

Lemon, B., Bengston, V., & Peterson, J. (1972). An exploration of the activity theory of aging: Activity types and life satisfaction among in-movers to a retirement community. *Journal of Gerontology, 27*(4), 511–523.

Lustbader, W., & Hooyman, N. (1994). *Taking care of aging family members, revised and expanded: A practical guide.* New York, NY: The Free Press.

Maberry, S. (2016). *Physical activity promotion from the social cognitive theory perspective: An examination of mobile fitness apps* (Unpublished doctoral dissertation), Louisiana State University School of Social Work, Baton Rouge, LA.

Maton, K. (2002). Community settings as buffers of life stress? Highly supportive churches, mutual help groups and senior centers. In T. Revenson, A. D'Augelli, S. French, D. Hughes, & D. Livert (Eds.), *A quarter century of community psychology: Readings from the American Journal of Community Psychology* (pp. 205–235). New York, NY: Kluwer Academic/Plenum.

Maton, K. I. (1989). Community settings as buffers of life stress? Highly supportive churches, mutual help groups, and senior centers. *American Journal of Community Psychology, 17*(2), 203–232.

McInnis-Dittrich, K. (2014). *Social work with older adults* (4th ed.). New York, NY: Pearson Higher Education.

Meis, M. S. (2005). Geriatric orphans: A study of severe isolation in an elderly population. *Dissertation Abstracts International, A: The Humanities and Social Sciences, 67*(5), 2766-A (Fielding Graduate Institute).

Moorman, S. M., Hauser, R. M., & Carr, D. (2009). Do older adults know their spouses' end-of-life treatment preferences? *Research on Aging, 31*(4), 463–491. doi:10.1177/0164027509333683

Morishita, L., Boult, C., Boult, L., Smith, S., & Pacala, J. T. (1998). Satisfaction with outpatient geriatric evaluation and management. *The Gerontologist, 38*(3), 303–308.

National Alliance for Caregiving and AARP. (2015, June). Caregiving in the U.S. Research Report. Retrieved from http://www.aarp.org/ppi/info-2015/caregiving-in-the-united-states-2015.html

National Association of Social Workers. (2015). Standards and indicators for cultural competence in social work practice. Retrieved from https://www.socialworkers.org/LinkClick.aspx?fileticket=7dVckZAYUmk%3D&portalid=0

National Association of Social Workers. (2017a). Aging. Retrieved from https://www.socialworkers.org/pressroom/features/issue/aging.asp

National Association of Social Workers. (2017b). Code of ethics. Retrieved from https://www.socialworkers.org/About/Ethics/Code-of-Ethics/Code-of-Ethics-English

National Care Planning Council. (2002). About adult day care. Retrieved from https://www.longtermcarelink.net/eldercare/adult_day_care.htm

National Center to Preserve Social Security and Medicare. (2017, February). Fast facts about Medicare. Government Relations and Policy. Retrieved from http://www.ncpssm.org/Medicare/MedicareFastFacts.aspx

National Committee to Preserve Social Security and Medicare. (2017). Older American Act. Retrieved from http://www.ncpssm.org/PublicPolicy/OlderAmericans/Documents/ArticleID/1171/Older-Americans-Act

National Council on Aging. (2012). Highest tier evidence-based health promotion/disease prevention programs. Retrieved from https://www.ncoa.org/resources/ebpchart/

National Council on Aging. (2015). Senior centers: Fact sheet. Retrieved from https://www.ncoa.org/wp-content/uploads/FactSheet_SeniorCenters.pdf

National Council on Aging. (2016). SNAP and senior hunger facts. Retrieved from https://www.ncoa.org/news/resources-for-reporters/get-the-facts/senior-hunger-facts/

National Health Policy Forum. (2012). *Older Americans Act of 1965: Programs and services.* Washington, DC: The George Washington University.

National Institute of Senior Centers. (2012). Senior centers. Retrieved from http://www.ncoa.org/national-institute-of-senior-centers/

Pace, P. (2014, February 24). Need for geriatric social work grows. *NASW News, 59*(2), p. 1.

Pardasani, M., & Sackman, B. (2014). New York City senior centers: A unique, grassroots, collaborative advocacy effort. *Activities, Adaptation & Aging, 38*(3), 200–219.

Paying for Senior Care. (2016). Medicaid and long-term care for the elderly. Retrieved from https://www.payingforseniorcare.com/longtermcare/costs.html

Population Reference Bureau. (2015). *Aging in the United States.* Washington, DC: Population Bulletin.

Quinn, J. (1995). Case management in home and community care. *Journal of Gerontological Social Work, 24,* 233–248.

Resnick, B. (2001). Promoting health in older adults: A four year analysis. *Journal of the American Association of Nurse Practitioners, 13*(1), 23–33.

Schore, J. L., Brown, R. S., & Cheh, V. A. (1999). Case management for high-cost Medicare beneficiaries. *Health Care Financing Review, 20,* 87–101.

Shapiro, A., & Taylor, M. (2002). Effects of a community-based early intervention program on the subjective well-being, institutionalization, and mortality of low-income elders. *The Gerontologist, 42*(3), 334–341.

Sims-Gould, J., Bryne, K., Hicks, E., Franke, T., & Stolee, P. (2015). When things are really complicated, we call the social worker: Post-hip-fracture care transitions for older people. *Health and Social Work, 40*(4), 257–265.

Skarupski, K., & Pelkowski, J. (2003). Multipurpose senior centers: Opportunities for community health nursing. *Journal of Community Health Nursing, 20*(2), 119–132. doi:10.1207/S15327655JCHN2002_05

Stuck, A. E., Aronow, H. U., Steiner, A., Alessi, C. A., Bula, C. J., Gold, M. N., . . . Beck, J. C. (1995). A trial of in-home comprehensive geriatric assessments for elderly people living in the community. *New England Journal of Medicine, 333*, 1184–1189. doi:10.1056/NEJM199511023331805

The Conversation Project. (2017). Your conversation starter kit. Retrieved from http://theconversationproject.org/wp-content/uploads/2017/02/ConversationProject-ConvoStarterKit-English.pdf

Torres-Gil, F., Spencer-Suarez, K., & Rudinica, B. (2014). The Older Americans Act and the nexus of aging and diversity. In K. Whitfield & T. Baker (Eds.), *Handbook on minority aging* (pp. 367–377). New York, NY: Springer Publishing

Ungar, J., Johnson, C., & Marks, G. (1997). Functional decline in the elderly: Evidence for direct stress-buffering protective effects of social interactions and physical activity. *Annals of Behavioral Medicine, 19*, 152–160.

United Neighborhood Houses. (2005). *Aging in the shadows: Social isolation among seniors in New York City.* New York, NY: Author.

U.S. Census. (2017, April 10). *Older Americans Month: May 2017.* Release Number: CB17-FF.08.

U.S. Department of Agriculture. (2017). *Supplemental Nutrition Assistance Program (SNAP).* Washington, DC: Food and Nutrition Service.

U.S. Department of Health and Human Services, Office of Disease Prevention and Health Promotion. (2008). 2008 Physical activity guidelines for Americans. Retrieved from http://www.health.gov/paguidelines/pdf/paguide.pdf

Wennberg, A., Dye, C., Streetman-Loy, B., & Pham, H. (2015). Alzheimer's patient familial caregivers: A review of burden and interventions. *Health & Social Work, 40*(4), 162–169. doi:10.1093/hsw/hlv062

Weuve, J. I., Boult, C., & Morishita, I. (2000). The effects of outpatient geriatric evaluation and management on caregiver burden. *The Gerontologist, 40*, 429–436.

Health for Immigrants and Refugees

Elaine P. Congress

The number of immigrants and refugees in the United States represents about 13% (40 million people) of the total U.S. population (Zong & Batalov, 2017), with 40% of those living in large urban areas, such as New York (37%), Los Angeles (35%), and Miami (40%) being immigrants (U.S. Census, 2010). An increasing number of immigrants also live in smaller cities, suburban, and rural environments (Cohen, 2017; Congress, 2016; Suro & Singer, 2002). Immigrants and refugees are a very diverse population with differing characteristics, resources, and backgrounds. Although immigrants come from over 140 different countries (Pew Hispanic Center, 2013) and speak 350 languages (Castillo, 2015), the following 10 countries are the most likely to be the country of origin of those who have migrated to the United States: Mexico (29%), China (5%), India (5%), Philippines (4%), El Salvador (3%), Vietnam (3%), Cuba (3%), Korea (3%), Dominican Republic (2%), Guatemala (2%) (Zong & Batalov, 2017).

Immigrants have lived in the United States from varying amounts of time and have differing degrees of assimilation. Some came when they were children and have lived in the United States for most of their lives. Many of these immigrants are undocumented and Deferred Action for Childhood Arrivals (DACA) has been a federal government policy to provide these children and young adults a way to move toward citizenship (Chang, 2016) and at the time this article was written remains as a policy that positively affects young people's access to health care (Shear & Yee, 2017). Legalizing young people's status has enabled many to access health care through insurance (if they work for an employer with over 50 employees) or to receive Medicaid if they are not employed and within Medicaid standards.

Other immigrants are recent arrivals and may have initially come as visitors, students, or with work permits. While some stay only for a short time, such as international students, others remain in the United States after their status has changed and enter the ranks of the undocumented. Although the undocumented receive the most attention, they are certainly not the majority of immigrants as most immigrants are either naturalized citizens or may be "green card holders" waiting to apply for citizenship (Passel & Cohn, 2016).

This chapter focuses on policy, practice, and research issues related to immigrant health because improving the health and well-being of the growing number of immigrants and refugees is an important goal for social workers in the health field. To further understand this special population, the following topics will be discussed: reasons for migrating, demographic characteristics of those who migrate, U.S. legal categories of migrants, as well as common misconceptions about migrants. Policies that affect their use and barriers to use of the health care system will follow. Policy and practice are closely connected in professional work with all clients but this is probably most true in work with immigrants where government and agency policies continually impact work with immigrant clients. In the practice section, two assessment tools—the Cultural Health Assessment Tool (CHAT) and the culturagram—are introduced to enhance understanding and support work with immigrants in the health care field. The chapter concludes with a discussion of existing research on immigrants and health care, as well as areas that need further research.

WHY DO PEOPLE MIGRATE?

Migration is not a new phenomenon as it has occurred since the beginning of time. Why do people migrate? The push–pull theory (Lee, 1966) proposes that migrants are often "pushed" from their country of origin by economic hardship or by political and social oppression, and "pulled" to the country of destination by hopes of better economic/ social opportunities, as well as security and freedom. People come to the United States because of both push and pull factors. Push and pull factors that contribute to migration can be considered on three levels: the macro (the political, economic, and environmental factors), the mezzo (social, community, and family relationships), and micro (personal characteristics that influence a person's decision to migrate). Macro conditions of poverty, extreme weather changes, and war often have led people to leave their countries of origin and migrate to the United States. Mezzo reasons often relate to people's decisions to immigrate if others from their community have traveled before. This is a familiar phenomenon where immigrants from a certain location may all settle in the same place in the United States. There are also micro personal decisions about migrating. Often people who are very connected with others in their countries of origin or have anxiety about learning a new language and culture may not want to migrate (Potocky-Tripodi, 2002).

DEFINITION OF IMMIGRANTS AND REFUGEES

Often the terms immigrants and refugees are used interchangeably, but there are many differences as the word "immigrants" is a broad general term used to apply to all people who have migrated to the United States after birth. Some are naturalized citizens, while others have documents—"green cards"—that make them eligible for citizenship. A smaller number of immigrants do not have the required documents to become a green card holder or citizen and thus are considered to be undocumented or illegal.

A subset of immigrants are refugees, a special group of immigrants who have had to leave their countries of origin because of fear of persecution or harm related to their nationality, race, religion, political origin, or social group. Their refugee status is protected through the United Nations (UNHCR Convention on Refugees, 1951/1967). In 2016, the United States took in 85,000 refugees but this number fluctuates from year to year (Krogstad & Radford, 2017). Those who are granted refugee status receive relocation services for 6 months and then they can progress toward citizenship. Their protected status enables them to apply for Medicaid in order to receive health care services or to receive it from their employers.

The UN-designated category of refugees does not include environmental refugees who are people who have migrated because extreme natural disasters of tsunami or earthquake or weather changes of floods or droughts have made it impossible to survive.

Unfortunately, those who become environmental refugees are not granted official refugee status and may be considered undocumented. Others have migrated because civil war or violence in their countries of origin make it dangerous to remain. Those who have made it to the United States often seek asylum here to secure their right to remain.

COMMON MISCONCEPTIONS ABOUT IMMIGRANTS

The many misconceptions about immigrants may unfortunately lead to prejudice, stigmatization, micro aggressions, and even acts of violence that negatively impact the physical and mental health of immigrants. A frequent belief is that immigrants take jobs away from native-born Americans, but cities with large immigrant populations such as Miami, Los Angeles, and New York report that this is not the case (Congress, 2017). Most immigrants work in construction, restaurants, and service positions, many of which are low paying and sometimes dangerous, while many native-born Americans do not take these jobs (Griswold, 2012). Another false belief is that immigrants contribute to crime. Cities with large immigrant population often report lower crime statistics than in other cities with fewer immigrants (Ingraham, 2017).

PRACTICE

Cultural Health Assessment Tool

A first step for a social worker's work with immigrant clients in a health setting is assessment. Too often, the only focus is on the current needs of clients who appear for service without learning about their experiences before coming to the health care facility.

A longitudinal approach that stressed learning about the health history of a patient was seen as the best way to learn about and plan for appropriate interventions with immigrants in a health care setting. This led to the development of the CHAT to understand the immigrant's current and past health and health care experiences (Congress, 2010; see Figure 13.1). The CHAT assessment grew out of the recognition of the value of Pine and Drachman's (2005) three-stage approach to immigrants that looked at immigrants before migrating, while in transit, and in their current situation.

The first part consists of a CHAT assessment of the health of clients before migrating to the United States. Did they endure food deprivations or malnutrition? Was health care

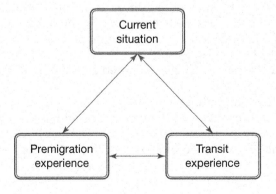

Figure 13.1 Cultural Health Assessment Tool (CHAT).

available in their country of origin? In terms of behavioral/mental health, did immigrants experience any traumatic events caused by violence, war, or natural disasters that led to their decision to migrate? Many clients come from developing countries where they may have endured famine or food shortages. Food in a country like the United States may not look or taste similar to what they had in their countries of origin. As much as 90% of food in an American grocery store may be different than what immigrants were familiar with in their countries of origin (personal communication). Also immigrants from developing countries may suffer from residual effects of tropical or infectious diseases unknown in the United States. In terms of mental/behavioral health, immigrants, especially those from rural environments, may have limited understanding of mental health symptoms and be reluctant to seek help.

Knowledge of prevention, medical assessment, and treatment, which is so familiar to those in the United States, may be minimal. Immigrant populations may be less likely to know about and use preventive services than the native-born population (Xu & Borders, 2008). Moving from a developing country with little attention paid to prevention may be a challenging experience for many immigrants as illustrated in Case Example 13.1.

Case Example 13.1

One night Gabriela with her very sick 2-year son appeared in the emergency room of a large public hospital. After noting that the child's temperature was 104, the doctor immediately asked where the child's immunization records were. The mother responded that she had never brought the child to a doctor before because he had not been sick. The doctor immediately called the social worker to discuss if this mother should be reported to child welfare because of medical neglect.

In the United States and in many other developed countries, there is a very involved system of health care for both mother and child. Pregnant women are seen regularly for prenatal assessment of both mother and unborn child. After birth, mothers are advised to bring their infants to well-baby clinics for regular checkups and immunizations. In this case example, Gabriela came from a rural section of her country of origin where the nearest health facility was over 50 miles away and only used for emergencies. That is why Gabriela did not bring her child for any medical care prior to the emergency room visit.

While the first part of a longitudinal assessment of immigrant health focuses on the immigrant's prior health condition before migrating, the second part involves an exploration of the transit experience. For those with legal status, migrating may only have involved a long plane ride. Others, especially those who arrive without proper papers, may have had a physically and/or emotionally challenging travel experience over water or desert. The stress of a dangerous, unhealthy transit may add to the trauma that immigrants may have originally experienced and that contributed to their decision to leave their country of origin.

The third part of a longitudinal assessment of immigrants in a health care setting involves an understanding of the physical-psycho-social-family-community factors that currently affect them. Are immigrants healthier now that they have migrated to the United States, which has a highly developed system of health care? As discussed previously, many, because of their immigration status or low income, may not be able to access health care.

Other threats to good health may affect immigrants after they have migrated. First, immigrants may experience work environments that are not conducive to good health.

Immigrants frequently are employed in dangerous occupations, such as farming and mining in rural areas or high-risk construction in cities (Bravo, 2017). Many immigrant women experience continual exposure to chemicals in nail salons (New York State Department of Health, 2016).

Despite the common belief that immigrants from developing countries may arrive with compromised health, there is some evidence that the health of immigrants is better when they first arrive than after years of living in the United States. The healthy immigrant effect indicates that often Latino immigrants arrive in the United States healthier than they become (Fennelly, 2007; McDonald & Kennedy, 2004). Being exposed to American's high-carbohydrate, high-sugar diet with limited access to exercise may contribute to the development of cardiovascular disease and diabetes (Koya & Egede, 2007; Misra & Ganda, 2007).

Most of the research on the healthy immigrant effect has been done with Latinos rather those of other ethnic backgrounds. However, there is also some evidence that Black immigrants from Africa and South America are initially healthier than American-born Blacks (Goel, McCarthy, Phillips, & Wee, 2004; New York Health Department, 2015; Read & Emerson, 2005). Similar to the study of Latinos who have migrated, this also suggests that American diet and lack of exercise may have a detrimental effect on immigrant health.

Immigrants may have little understanding of mental health services that are available. In the United States there has previously been a clear division between physical and mental health services that has been perpetuated by different financing stream (Stanek, 2014). Immigrants may have come from backgrounds with no mental health services and may fear that they will be considered "loco" upon mention of anxiety or depression.

Environmental Effects on Immigrant Health

Instead of placing the blame on immigrants for not taking proper care of themselves, it is important to look at environmental factors that contribute to poor health outcomes for immigrants. Food deserts in poor communities, as well as the lack of recreational facilities, may play a role in immigrants' non-healthy diet and lack of exercise. Fast food stores and restaurants may dominate, and parks for exercise are often nonexistent or unsafe to enter in communities where immigrants live. Many immigrant parents have to work at multiple low paying jobs and may have limited time to shop and cook nutritious food for their families or travel frequently to recreational facilities for exercise.

Because of poverty, many immigrants live in communities where there is continual risk of violence. Immigrants are much more likely to be the victim than the perpetuator of violent crimes (Ingraham, 2017). And the true number of immigrants who are victims of crime is probably unreported because of fear of deportation or lack of information and education about how to report crimes.

Language differences and education have been suggested as barriers to many legal immigrants receiving health care. Often children are kept out of school to interpret for parents, which interrupts their schooling and exposes them to parental health issues. This points to the ongoing need for bilingual, bicultural social workers or professional interpreters adequate to best service immigrant clients (Ortiz Hendricks, 2013).

Migration From Hot to Cold Environment

An area rarely addressed in understanding immigrants' experience is the impact of migrating from a warmer climate to a colder one. Many immigrants move from countries near the Equator with much higher temperatures to cities and other environments in the United States with much colder weather. This environmental change may require physical, psychological, social, and economic adjustments. Immigrant families are now exposed to new cold and flu viruses when parents and children spend so much more time in closed environments. Also, there may be additional financial burdens for poor immigrant families who for the first time must purchase winter coats and boots for growing children. Not only are there health concerns, but also social adjustment issues. When a number of Somali refugees were resettled in Manchester, New Hampshire, a mother sent her children to school without boots and heavy coats on a day when a heavy snowfall was predicted. The school staff debated about whether to call protective child welfare services because of the mother's apparent disregard for her children's well-being (Congress, Personal communication).

Psychological Effects on Immigrant Health

Family stress often detrimentally affects immigrants' psychological health when children want to be independent, while parents, fearful for their children's safety especially in a strange country, may insist that children stay close to home. There may be an expectation that children, especially daughters, come home after school to help with housework and care for younger siblings (Congress, 2011). Sometimes, there is more marital conflict when women are more able to find employment such as childcare and house cleaning that do not require legal documentation and men remain unemployed. This may be related to an increase in alcohol abuse, especially among Latino men (Galvan & Caetano, 2003).

A major psychological stress that many immigrants also experience is prejudice and discrimination. In the current political climate, anti–Middle East attitudes and behaviors may be very apparent in many neighborhoods where immigrants live. Unfortunately, the United States has a long history of racism, and immigrants with darker skin may encounter racial prejudice for the first time. Even if there is no major evidence of discrimination, micro aggressions can still negatively affect immigrants' experiences in America (Sue, 2010). Psychological stress caused by discrimination can also lead to physical health problems (Ryan, Gee, & Laflamme, 2006).

Culturagram

In health care settings social workers often lack specialized assessments skills needed to understand and work effectively with immigrant clients. They are aware that generalizations about clients based on their ethnicity often are not accurate, fail to capture the individual characteristics of immigrants and their families, and may encourage stigmatization of particular ethnic groups.

In order to work more effectively with immigrant clients, the *culturagram* was first developed in 1994, modified in 2000 and 2009, and used in work with culturally diverse people (Lum, 2010), battered women (Congress & Brownell, 2007), children (Congress, 2002), older people (Brownell, Fenley, & Kim, 2016), families in crisis (Congress, 2000), Mexican families (Congress, 2004a), Latino and Asian families (Congress & Kung, 2013), immigrant families with health problems (Congress, 2004b, 2013), refugees (Congress, 2012), and in family development theory (Congress, 2008).

This assessment tool, which grew out of practice experience, provides a visual representation of the cultural assessment of a family. Adapting a cultural humility approach, the culturagram provides for individual assessment of each family and thus avoids generalization and stereotyping that may detrimentally affect work with clients and families from different cultural backgrounds. While cultural competence implies that the social worker will develop knowledge to work effectively with culturally diverse families, a cultural humility approach implies that, given the power differentiation that exists between the client and the social worker as well as the diversity of individual clients, social workers must learn anew about each client they meet. In using the culturagram the client is always viewed as the best source for information about the cultural background of the family, as well as individual members.

The culturagram (2009) includes the following 10 elements that are seen as essential in understanding the cultural background of the client:

1. Reasons for immigrating
2. Immigration status
3. Length of time in the United States
4. Language spoken at home and in the community
5. Health beliefs, access, and care
6. Impact of trauma and crisis events in the past and in the present
7. Contact with cultural institutions and holidays, food, and dress
8. Past and current experiences with racism, discrimination, and bias
9. Values about education and work
10. Family values involving gender, age, myths, and rules

The 10 elements in the culturagram (1994) were initially identified as the most important characterizations to improve understanding of immigrant clients. Feedback from students and conference attendees from 1994 to 2009 led to some modification of these elements to include discrimination and bias (#8), as well as the impact of trauma past and present (#6).

The culturagram is the client's story about who he or she is, and using a diagram (see Figure 13.2) to understand an immigrant family has been seen as very effective. This cultural assessment tool can be applied to work with the immigrant family described in this case example.

Of particular interest and relevance to this chapter on health care is #5 of the culturagram that focuses on health status, beliefs, and access to the health care system. Some immigrants may have compromised health because of conditions related to premigration experiences of food deprivation or psychological trauma. The perilous and dangerous trip to the United States may have negatively affected their physical and psychological health. After migration to this country where food and exercise choices are different and limited by living in poor communities, their health may be further at risk.

In addition to access challenges, use of the health care system may vary for immigrants who come from countries where there may be limited focus on prevention and medical care is only available for emergencies. Treatment might consist of herbal medicines or practices that may be unfamiliar to the American social worker. Adopting a cultural humility approach, social workers strive to learn more about their clients' perceptions about health and well-being.

Some immigrants may have beliefs about health that seem very different from those of U.S. social workers in the health field. Despite the growing number of immigrants from other countries with differing beliefs, the literature on alternative types of treatment, although increasing, is still small. Some immigrants may prefer traditional medicine because there are barriers to access and discriminatory experiences that immigrants encounter in a health care setting (Ransford, Carrilo, & Rivera, 2010). Some alternative health practices, such as acupuncture and herbal medicines that might have seen initially to be antithetical to accepted medical practices, are now often an integral part of current health care (Congress & Lyons, 1992).

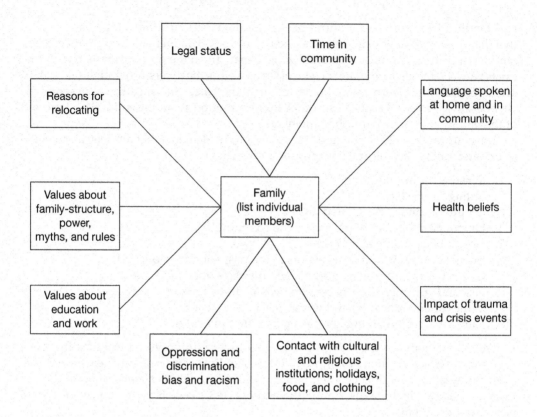

Figure 13.2 Culturagram.

Source: Reprinted from Chang-Muy, F., & Congress, E. (Eds.). (2016). *Social work with immigrants and refugees: Legal issues, clinical skills, and advocacy* (2nd ed., p. 75). New York, NY: Springer Publishing.

Intersectional Approach

In understanding cultural beliefs about health, the social worker needs to take an intersectional approach. In addition to ethnicity, gender, age, class, religious, socioeconomic, and educational differences may affect the client's overall heath, beliefs about heath treatment, and access to health care. Power and status differences also impact immigrants' interaction with social workers in the health field (see Chapter 4, Intersectionality, Social Work, and Health).

The social worker usually works with a health care establishment that subscribes to a Western model of health care involving a focus on prevention, physical examination, blood tests, x-rays, MRI, and surgery if needed. A challenge may emerge for clients who have very different ideas about health. For example, a woman with pneumonia believes that the best remedy for her illness is a special drink that her grandmother sent her from her home country.

POLICY

Policy issues around health continually affect practice with immigrants and refugees. Immigration laws prohibit people with certain health conditions such as a contagious disease of public health significance including infectious syphilis, gonorrhea, or active tuberculosis. Prior to 2010, those with AIDS were prevented from migrating (Centers for Disease Control and Prevention [CDC], 2017).

Because of the perceived quality of U.S. health care, many migrate to the United States for medical treatment. While a common perception is that health care in the United States is excellent, health statistics are disturbing. In a 2013 study conducted by the National Institutes of Health (NIH) of 17 high-income countries, the United States had almost the highest rates of maternal mortality, infant mortality, heart and lung disease, sexually transmitted infections, adolescent pregnancies, injuries, homicides, and rates of disability. Furthermore, life expectancy was at least 4 years less than that of the highest-ranking developed countries (NIH, 2013). And some of these negative outcomes may be related to the fact that a large number of immigrants may lack access to adequate health care.

Access to Health Care

What policies affect the access of immigrants for health care? With the Patient Protection and Affordable Care Act (ACA) many people including immigrants have been able to access health care. Yet it is disturbing to note that Hispanics, one of the largest ethnic groups in the United States, have not been able to take advantage of health care insurance as much as White or Black populations (Krogstad & Lopez, 2014). Health care insurance is very expensive for those who are slightly above Medicaid standards and many immigrants working in low paying service jobs fall into this category. Other immigrants work in small businesses with fewer than 50 employees where their employers are not required to provide health insurance for them. And neither health care insurance nor Medicaid coverage are available for the almost 12 million undocumented immigrants (Pew Research Center, 2013).

Hospitals provide emergency health care for all regardless of immigrant status and ability to pay. All who are in a life-threatening health situation such as an accident, heart attack, or stroke, as well as women who are in labor or giving birth receive free emergency medical care. Many, but not all, states provide health care for uninsured children, which often means that uninsured children rarely see doctors (Ku, 2006). This may have serious implications for children's current and future health. While adults often receive special free preventive health care programs such as cancer screening and blood pressure monitoring, a serious problem arises if, having identified a health care problem, a person lacks medical insurance to follow up with further evaluation and treatment.

Policy of Health Care Agencies

Policy and practice issues are inextricably related. A clinical social worker in health care cannot work with an immigrant client individually or as an administrator without becoming aware of government and agency policy and its impact on immigrant clients.

One of the most challenging issues for both practitioners and administrators has to do with immigration status. Professional social workers understand the ethical mandate of providing equal opportunity/nondiscrimination to all regardless of their nationality, race, religion, or immigration status (National Association of Social Workers, 2008). They are keenly aware of the challenges of counseling clients about their health concerns when these clients live in constant fear of deportation because of their immigrant status. Often social workers are not trusted as they are mistakenly thought to be associated with the government.

Those who administer agencies may have to struggle with the financial consequences of providing services to those for whom their institutions will not receive government or insurance payments. Social work administrators also have to ensure that interpreters are available for clients who speak different languages and that an agency atmosphere that is welcoming to new immigrant populations is created. As more and more health services are provided outside of the hospital, community-based programs that address the needs and increase accessibility of immigrant clients need to be developed.

RESEARCH

Although there is a growing increase in the number of immigrants in the United States, there is need for much more research on immigrants' health, as well as their use of the health care system. Immigrant status is often a major deterrent for immigrants accessing health care (Ransford, Carrillo, & Rivera, 2010; Xu & Borders, 2008). Some of this is related to the ability to pay, while at other times perception of real or perceived rejection, as well as reliance on traditional health care may prevent immigrants from using health care institutions. Also different populations visit health care facilities with differing incidence of illness and use of health facilities to treat these illnesses (Kao, 2009).

What type of health problems do immigrants bring to health care agencies? In the United States only recently has there been a recent attempt to integrate physical and mental health treatment. It has been pointed out that often physical and behavioral health problems are connected but in the past treatment has been very separate. Nardone, Snyder, and Paradise (2014) point out five ways in which Medicaid is seeking to integrate both physical and mental health care. They are:

1. Universal screening. Screening can be a valuable way to understand more about an individual's condition and risks. There are a number of evidence-based screening tools that can be used in this process.
2. Navigation. Navigators, such as social workers, can be used to help clients on Medicaid learn to navigate the complex, often-separated fields of physical and mental health.
3. Co-location. In the past, physical health facilities both in the hospital and in the community were often quite separated. Currently there is a movement to create co-located facilities so to coordinate treatment for physical and behavioral health symptoms.
4. Health homes. Under the ACA more states have created health homes to service people with serious mental illness. Community mental health centers provide care in an integrated manner to clients with serious mental illness, as well as physical problems.
5. System-level integration of care. This step is probably the most important but probably the most difficult to achieve. While certain facilities may have adopted an integrative approach to change, a whole system to adopt this approach is most challenging.

Although social workers have always believed in an integrated approach to assessing and treating people in a medical or behavioral health setting, funding streams and subsequently treatment have long remained separated into physical and mental health facilities. More research is needed on the most effective ways to do this. Also it should be noted that there has been no research on how immigrants will use new integrated health systems. Because many immigrants come from backgrounds in which physical and psychological difficulties are seen as connected, this current integrated approach to health care should appeal to immigrants. Research in this important area is needed.

Many immigrants have health beliefs that may differ from traditional ones and there is a paucity of research in this area. Part of this may be due to the fact that some immigrants may avoid the health care system completely or be reluctant to share their views as they feel it will not be acceptable. In order to learn more about the health beliefs of immigrants, more research is needed on what their beliefs are and what impact do they have on their lives.

Additional questions are what models have been used to integrate indigenous health practices with Western medical care and how effective are they? Also, does assimilation change the amount that immigrants use the health care system? While some literature has pointed out that the longer a person or family lives in the United States the more likely they are to use the American health care system (Kao, 2009), this is not always true. For example, even foreign-born Latino citizens use the health care system less than native-born Americans (Krogstad & Lopez, 2014). Language has been seen as one of the barriers, but this does not provide the full explanation. There is need for further exploration of immigrants' use of the health care system and the reasons for their use or failure to use.

Does the health of immigrants remain the same depending on how long the immigrant has lived in the United States? The healthy immigrant effect has also been used to describe the fact that the health of many immigrants is better initially than for many native-born Americans (Kennedy, Kidd, McDonald, & Biddle, 2015). This pattern has been found to be consistent for those in other English-speaking countries. Natural selection (healthy people are those most able to migrate) has been suggested as an explanation of why immigrants are often healthier than native born; however, the results are not conclusive. Much of the research has been conducted with Latino populations but this may not be true for other ethnic groups who have immigrated to the United States.

Guidelines for Effective Work With Immigrants

Social workers, whether they are employed in government, for-profit, or nonprofit agencies, will encounter challenges in working with immigrant clients in health care settings. Some guidance to help in navigating these issues include:

1. Recognize the ongoing connection between policy and practice.
2. Use an intersectional approach in understanding immigrants and refugees.
3. Strive to individualize immigrant clients.
4. Avoid workplace and professional micro aggressions against immigrants and discourage others from using them.
5. Explore ethical challenges, especially when professional ethical standards differ radically from current policy and practice in health care facilities.
6. Partner with colleagues within one's health care agency to provide better services for immigrant populations.
7. Participate with other stakeholders in the health care field and clients in advocating for fairer policies toward immigrants.

CONCLUSION

The focus of this chapter was on health and health care for immigrants and refugees. There is need for continued research on both the physical and behavioral health problems that immigrants encounter and how the length of time when seeking care may affect their health outcomes. There is much uncertainty about future government policies that will be in place to guide practice with immigrant clients in the health field. Thus, it behooves social workers to monitor closely current and changing government policies that impact immigrants as well as their access to health care. Professional organizations, like the American

Medical Association and the American Public Health Association, as well as migration policy and research organizations like the Pew Research Center, National Immigration Center, and National Immigration Legal Center, are keenly aware of how the right to health and well-being for all, and especially immigrants, have been challenged. Now more than ever there is a need to join with other like-minded organizations to advocate for our common shared mission of promoting the right to health and well-being for all.

CHAPTER DISCUSSION QUESTIONS

1. What are the health beliefs of immigrants when they first come to the United States? What has been the prior use of health care?

2. Has immigrants' health been affected by their premigration and/or transit experience? If so, how?

3. Does the health of immigrants deteriorate while living in the United States? If so, in what ways and for which populations?

4. How does the current health care policy affect immigrants?

5. What will be the impact of the proposed health care plans on immigrants who are citizens, who have green cards, or who are undocumented?

6. Since undocumented immigrants are usually not able to access health care, how can social workers strive to ensure that all immigrants receive the health care that they need?

CASE EXAMPLE AND DISCUSSION QUESTIONS

Case Example 13.2

Carmen is a 35-year-old Latina woman who saw the hospital social worker to discuss discharge plans for her 60-year-old mother, Rosa, who had been hospitalized for diagnostic tests for kidney disease. Rosa does not want to return to the hospital for subsequent tests and says that the spiritualist can provide the care that she needs. Carmen also has some health problems of her own. Because of excessive bleeding, she had recently gone to the emergency room. Carmen had brought Lucia to interpret and learned that she (Carmen) needed more tests and possible surgery. Because she is undocumented, Carmen is not eligible for Medicaid and does not have funds for this surgery or follow-up treatment.

The social worker learned that Carmen was having increasing conflicts with her 16-year-old son, Juan Jr., who had begun to cut school and stay out late at night. Her 14-year-old daughter, Lucia, who now weighs 200 pounds, has become very depressed, tearful, and did not want to go to school. Last week Carmen found that Lucia had hidden two bottles of aspirin in her room.

Carmen indicated Juan Jr., was the source of much family conflict, as he believed he did not have to respect Pablo, Carmen's boyfriend, who is not Juan's father. Because Pablo and Carmen are undocumented immigrants, they have been able to find only occasional "off the books" work. Carmen, however, has been able to work more regularly as a home care worker and babysitter, and Pablo is embarrassed that Carmen is the primary breadwinner. Recently, Pablo has started to stay out late with his friends and often arrives home after excessive drinking. (Adapted from Congress, 2013, *Immigrants and Health Care*, pp. 117–118.)

(continued)

Case Example 13.2 *(continued)*

Questions for Discussion

1. What are the barriers that this family has in seeking health care?

2. How should the social worker react to alternative health care beliefs that Rosa has?

3. What are the family conflicts and mental health issues in this example and how should the social worker address them?

REFERENCES

Bravo, D. (2017). 2 years, 31 dead construction workers: New York can do better. *The New York Times*. Retrieved from https://www.nytimes.com/2017/01/16/opinion/2-years-31-dead-construction-workers-new-york-can-do-better.html?_r=0

Brownell, P., Fenley, R., & Kim, J. (2016). Older adult immigrants in the United States: Issues and Services. In F. Chang-Muy & E. Congress (Eds.), *Social work with immigrants and refugees: Legal issues, clinical skills, and advocacy* (pp. 273–301). New York, NY: Springer Publishing.

Castillo, J. (2015). At least 350 languages spoken in US homes. Retrieved from http://www.cnbc.com/2015/11/04/at-least-350-languages-spoken-in-us-homes-new-report.html

Center for Immigration Studies. (2012). Profile of America's foreign-born populations; Table 5. Retrieved from http://cis.org/2012-profile-of-americas-foreign-born-population#3

Centers for Disease Control and Prevention. (2017). Immigration and refugee health laws and regulations. Retrieved from https://www.cdc.gov/immigrantrefugeehealth/laws-regulations.html

Chang, F. (2016). Legal classifications of immigrants. In F. Chang-Muy & E. Congress (Eds.), *Social work with immigrants and refugees: Legal issues, clinical skills, and advocacy* (2nd ed., pp. 43–66). New York, NY: Springer Publishing Company.

Chang-Muy, F., & Congress, E. (Eds.). (2016). *Social work with immigrants and refugees: Legal issues, clinical skills, and advocacy* (2nd ed.). New York, NY: Springer Publishing.

Cohen, P. (2017). In rural Iowa, a future rests on immigrants. *The New York Times*, 1. Retrieved from https://www.nytimes.com/2017/05/29/business/economy/storm-lake-iowa-immigrant-workers.html?_r=0

Congress, E. (2002). Using culturagrams with culturally diverse families. In A. Roberts & G. Greene (Eds.), *Social work desk reference* (pp. 57–61). New York, NY: Oxford University Press.

Congress, E. (2004a). Crisis intervention and diversity: Emphasis on a Mexican immigrant family's acculturation conflicts. In P. Meyer (Ed.), *Paradigms of clinical social work, Volume 3, Emphasis on diversity* (pp. 125–144). New York, NY: Brunner-Routledge.

Congress, E. (2004b). Cultural and ethnic issues in working with culturally diverse patients and their families: Use of the culturagram to promote cultural competency in health care settings. *Social Work in Health Care, 39* (3/4), 249–262.

Congress, E. (2008). The culturagram. In A. Roberts (Ed.), *Social Work Desk Reference* (2nd ed., pp. 969–975). New York, NY: Oxford University Press.

Congress, E. (2010, November 10). Advancing Social Justice for Immigrants and Refugees: Developing a Cultural Health Assessment. Presented at APHA, Denver, CO.

Congress, E. (2011). Culturagram use with culturally diverse families. In M. Craft-Rosenberg & S. Pehler (Eds.), *Encyclopedia of family health* (pp. 259–264.) Thousand Oaks, CA: Sage Publication.

Congress, E. (2012). Social work with refugees. In D. Elliott & U. Segal (Eds.), *Refugees worldwide: Law, policy and programs* (Vol. 4, pp. 197–218). Santa Barbara, CA: Praeger.

Congress, E. (2013). Immigrants and health care. In R. Keefe (Ed.), *Handbook for public health social work* (pp. 103–121). New York, NY: Springer Publishing.

Congress, E. (2016). Introduction: Legal and social work issues with immigrants. In F. Chang-Muy & E. Congress (Eds.), *Social work with immigrants and refugees: Legal issues, clinical skills, and advocacy* (2nd ed., pp. 3–41). New York, NY: Springer Publishing.

Congress, E. (2017). Immigrants and refugees in cities: Issues, challenges, and interventions for social workers. *Urban Social Work, 1*(1), 20–35.

Congress, E., & Brownell, P. (2007). Application of the culturagram with culturally and ethnically diverse battered women. In A. Roberts (Ed.), *Battered women and their families*. New York, NY: Springer Publishing.

Congress, E., & Kung, W. (2013). Using the culturagram to assess and empower culturally diverse women. In E. Congress & M. Gonzalez (Eds.), *Multicultural perspectives in working with families* (3rd ed., pp. 1–20). New York, NY: Springer Publishing.

Congress, E., & Lyons, B. (1992). Cultural differences in health beliefs: Implications for social work practice in health care settings. *Journal of Social Work Practice in Health Care, 17*(3), 81–96. doi:10.1300/J010v17n03_06

Fennelly, C. (2007). The healthy migrant effect. *Minnesota Medicine, 90*(3), 51–53.

Galvan, F., & Caetano, R. (2003). Alcohol use and related problems among ethnic minorities in the United States. *Alcohol Research & Health, 27*(1), 87–94.

Goel, M. S., McCarthy, E. P., Phillips, R. S., & Wee, C. (2004). Obesity among immigrant subgroups by duration of residence. *Journal of the American Medical Association, 292*(23), 2860–2867. doi:10.1001/jama.292.23.2860

Griswold, D. T. (2012). Immigration and the welfare state. *Cato Journal, 32*(1), 159–174. Retrieved from http://www.cato.org/pubs/journal/cj32n1/cj32n1-11.pdf

Ingraham, C. (2017). Trump says sanctuary cities are hotbeds of crime. Data say the opposite. *Washington Post*. Retrieved from https://www.washingtonpost.com/news/wonk/wp/2017/01/27/trump-says-sanctuary-cities-are-hotbeds-of-crime-data-say-the-opposite/?utm_term=.099096d40a21

Kao, D. (2009). Generational cohorts, age at arrival, and access to health services among Asian and Latino immigrant adults. *Journal of Health Care for the Poor and Underserved, 20*(2), 395–414.

Kennedy, S, Kidd, M., McDonald, J., & Biddle, N. (2015). The healthy immigrant effect: Patterns and evidence from four countries. *Journal of International Migration and Integration, 16*(2), 317–332. doi:10.1007/s12134-014-0340-x

Koya, D. L., & Egede, L. E. (2007). Association between length of residence and cardiovascular disease risk factors among an ethnically diverse group of United States immigrants. *Journal of General Internal Medicine, 22*(6), 841–846. doi:10.1007/s11606-007-0163-y

Krogstad, J., & Lopez, H. (2014). *Hispanic immigrants more likely to lack health insurance than U.S. born*. Washington, DC: Pew Research Center. Retrieved from http://www.pewresearch.org/fact-tank/2014/09/26/higher-share-of-hispanic-immigrants-than-u-s-born-lack-health-insurance/

Krogstad, J., & Radford, J. (2017). *Key facts about refugees to the U.S.* Washington, DC: Pew Research Center. Retrieved from http://www.pewresearch.org/fact-tank/2017/01/30/key-facts-about-refugees-to-the-u-s/

Ku, L. (2006). Why immigrants lack health care and health insurance. Migration Policy Institute. Retrieved from https://www.migrationpolicy.org/article/why-immigrants-lack-adequate-access-health-care-and-health-insurance/

Lee, E. (1966). A theory of migration. *Demography, 3*, 47–57.

Lum, D. (2010). *Culturally competent practice* (4th ed.). Belmont, CA: Brooks Cole.

McDonald, J. T., & Kennedy, S. (2004). Insights into the "Healthy Immigrant Effect": Health status and health service use of immigrants to Canada. *Social Science & Medicine, 59*(8), 1613–1637. doi:10.1016/j.socscimed.2004.02.004

Misra, A., & Ganda, O. (2007). Migration and its impact on adiposity and type 2 diabetes. *Nutrition, 23*, 696–708. doi:10.1016/j.nut.2007.06.008

Nardone, M., Snyder, S., & Paradise, J. (2014). Integrating physical and behavioral health care: Promising Medicaid models. Kaiser Family Foundation. Retrieved from https://www.kff.org/report-section/integrating-physical-and-behavioral-health-care-promising-medicaid-models-executive-summary

National Association of Social Workers. (2008). *Code of Ethics*. Washington, DC: Author.

National Institutes of Health. (2013). U.S. health in international perspective: Shorter lives, poorer health. Retrieved from https://www.nap.edu/resource/13497/dbasse_080620.pdf

New York State Department of Health. (2016). Review of chemicals used in nail salons. Retrieved from https://www.health.ny.gov/press/reports/docs/nail_salon_chemical_report.pdf

Ortiz Hendricks, C. (2013). The multicultural triangle of the child, the family and the school: Culturally competent approaches. In E. Congress & M. Gonzalez (Eds.), *Multicultural perspectives in working with families* (3rd ed., pp. 57–63). New York, NY: Springer Publishing.

Passel, J., & Cohn, D. (2016). *Overall number of unauthorized immigrants holds steady since 2009*. Washington, DC: Pew Research Center Retrieved from http://www.pewhispanic.org/files/2016/09/PH_2016.09.20_Unauthorized_FINAL.pdf

Passel, J., & Taylor, J. (2010). *Unauthorized immigrants and their U.S. born children*. Washington, DC: Pew Research Center. Retrieved from http://www.pewhispanic.org/2010/08/11/unauthorized-immigrants-and-their-us-born-children/

Pew Hispanic Center. (2013). Statistical portrait of the foreign-born population in the United States, 2011. Retrieved from http://www.pewhispanic.org/files/2013/01/PHC-2011-FB-Stat-Profiles.pdf

Pine, B., & Drachman, D. (2005). Effective child welfare practice with immigrant and refugee children. *Child Welfare, 84*(5), 537–562.

Potocky-Tripodi, M. (2002). *Best practices for social work with immigrants and refugees*. New York, NY: Columbia University Press.

Ransford, H. E., Carrillo, F., & Rivera, Y. (2010). Health care-seeking among Latino immigrants: Blocked access, use of traditional medicine, and the role of religion. *Journal of Health Care for the Poor and Underserved, 21*(3), 862–878. doi:10.1353/hpu.0.0348

Read, J., & Emerson, M. (2005). Racial context, black immigration and the U.S. black/white health disparity. *Social Forces, 84*(1), 181–199.

Ryan, A., Gee, G., & Laflamme, D, (2006). The association between self-reported discrimination, physical health and blood pressure: Findings from African-Americans, Black immigrants and Latino immigrations in New Hampshire. *Journal of Health Care for the Poor and Underserved, 17*, 116–132. doi:10.1353/hpu.2006.0092

Shear, M., & Yee, V. (2017, June 17). Dreamers to stay in U.S. for now, but their long-term fate is unclear. *The New York Times*, A17.

Stanek, M. (2014). Promoting physical and behavioral health integration: Considerations for Aligning Federal and State Policy. *National Academy for Promotion of State Health Policy.* Retrieved from http://www.nashp.org/sites/default/files/Promoting_Integration.pdf

Sue, D. W. (2010). *Microaggressions in everyday life: Race, gender, and sexual orientation.* Hoboken, NJ: John Wiley & Sons.

Suro, R., & Singer, A. (2002). *Latino growth in Metropolitan America: Changing patterns, New Locations.* Washington, DC: Center on Urban & Metropolitan Policy and the Pew Hispanic Center, The Bookings Institution, Survey Series.

UNHCR Convention on Refugees. (1951/1967). Retrieved from http://www.unhcr.org/3b66c2aa10.pdf

U.S. Census. (2010). Foreign born population of the United States 2010. Retrieved from http://www.census.gov/prod/2012pubs/acs-19.pdf

Xu, K. T., & Borders, T. (2008). Does being an immigrant make a difference in seeking physician services? *Journal of Health Care for the Poor and Underserved, 19*(2), 380–390. doi:10.1353/hpu.0.0001

Zong, J., & Batalov, J. (2017). *Frequently requested statistics on immigrants and immigration in the United States.* Washington, DC: Migration Policy Institute. Retrieved from http://www.migrationpolicy.org/article/frequently-requested-statistics-immigrants-and-immigration-united-states/

14

Health and HIV/AIDS

Julie A. Cederbaum, Erik M. P. Schott, and Jaih Craddock

In 2015, over 39,500 people were diagnosed with HIV in the United States with an estimated 1.2 million people living with HIV (PLWH; Centers for Disease Control and Prevention [CDC], 2016a). Of those 1.2 million PLWH, about one in eight are not aware they are infected with HIV (CDC, 2016a). HIV disproportionately affects minority groups in the United States (Kaiser Family Foundation [KFF], 2017a). Men who have sex with men (MSM) are more affected by HIV than any other group in the United States, with Black MSM experiencing disproportionate rates of HIV compared to other racial/ethnic groups (CDC, 2016b). Among women, more than 7,000 women were diagnosed with HIV in 2015. While HIV diagnoses among women have declined sharply in recent years, Black women continue to experience HIV at disproportionate rates (CDC, 2016c). Young people are also at increased risk; 22% of all new infections in the United States are among individuals 13 to 24 years (CDC, 2016d). Further, HIV-positive youth are the least likely to be linked to HIV-related care (CDC, 2016d). In this chapter, we discuss current practice, policy, and research for individuals living with HIV, with the goal of exploring the multisystemic ways in which social workers can make informed, empowered, and directive change in the lives of persons living with HIV/AIDS.

PRACTICE

Medical case management (MCM) is a highly coordinated provision of care (Liau et al., 2013) that, when delivered by a clinical social work professional, typically entails a range of client-centered services. These services link clients with primary medical care for the treatment of HIV/AIDS, psychosocial support (that may include group treatment), and other services such as nutrition and housing. Enhanced medical outcomes are in fact the output of this global goal of MCM and the rationale behind the Substance Abuse and Mental Health Services Administration (SAMHSA) framework for coordinated and integrated health care (Heath, Wise, & Reynolds, 2013; see Chapter 7, Integrated Behavioral Health Care). MCM is a core medical service under the most recent Ryan White reauthorization and a critical component of clinical practice with persons living with HIV (PLWH; Weiser et al., 2015).

Key activities in an HIV/AIDS MCM approach are:

1. Intake
2. Biopsychosocial assessment
3. Development of an individualized service plan (ISP)
4. Coordination of services
5. Client monitoring
6. Reevaluation and adaptation of the ISP (Weiser et al., 2015)

Intake

For many AIDS service organizations (ASOs), the focus of the initial intake is to determine program eligibility. The intake also serves to gather basic information from the client, including presenting needs, and helps the social worker gauge the client's levels of motivation. The tasks at intake may include: (a) gathering demographic information; (b) collecting basic information to determine eligibility; (c) documenting residency; (d) establishing the documentation of HIV infection (typically laboratory results or a certified letter); and (e) documenting income to establish eligibility based on financial need (most federal-funded and state-funded MCM programs require this documentation; Weiser et al., 2015). These initial tasks lay the groundwork for the full biopsychosocial assessment that typically follows intake.

Biopsychosocial Assessment

The purpose of the biopsychosocial assessment is for the social worker to gather relevant information. This relevant information collected during the biopsychosocial assessment will facilitate the creation of an ISP. Conducted in a collaborative fashion, which feels at times like a conversation, the assessment allows for the client and social worker to establish rapport and form a therapeutic alliance and working relationship. The strength of this connection is that it facilitates the sensitive and relevant data to be collected from the client that then, in turn, allows for the social worker to make an accurate assessment (Hepworth, Rooney, Dewberry Rooney, & Strom-Gottfried, 2013).

The biopsychosocial model refers to biological, psychological, and social domains. Engel (1980) provides an original framework that depicts how each of these three domains can influence and be influenced by a disease such as HIV/AIDS. There is a bidirectional influence with each of these domains. This influence within the biopsychosocial model is an essential feature in the conceptualization of the assessment and treatment of HIV/AIDS.

The biological domain can include physical, physiological, biochemical, nutritional, or genetic domains. The psychological domain can include emotional, affective, cognitive, behavioral, spiritual, and personality domains. Environmental, cultural, family, work, and interpersonal domains can be included in the social domain (Andrasik, Goodie, & Peterson, 2015).

It is essential to gather a baseline functioning to capture a client's general medical history. This is inclusive of general health, as well as the specifics of the client's HIV disease progression and any opportunistic illnesses they may have experienced. Additionally, the data will be helpful to assess for co-occurring physical health issues. These health problems may include, but are not specific to, tuberculosis, hepatitis, or any chronic or untreated sexually transmitted infections (STIs) such as chlamydia, gonorrhea, or syphilis. An assessment of the client's level of motivation for medication adherence (MA) is key at this point in treatment (Andrasik et al., 2015).

Psychological Domain

When assessing psychological functioning, it is important to include an in-depth mental health history as part of the ISP. It is also important to gather a substance use history as well. This self-report from the client may also include additional aspects of psychosocial support, such as prior mental health treatment experiences (e.g., individual, couples, or group therapy). The social worker should be interested in gathering information on a family history of mental health or substance-related treatment and outcomes. For the ISP, these data are essential for developing long-term goals and objectives (Hepworth et al., 2013).

Social Domain

For the assessment of a client's social domain, it is essential that the social work practitioner gather information on the client's immediate environment. The social worker often assesses for a *goodness-of-fit*. Germaine's (1973) definition of *goodness-of-fit* offers an understanding of the adaptive balance between organism and environment. This suggests a novel way of viewing the relationship of the person infected with HIV, which includes the family affected by HIV, to the environment.

Individualized Service Plan

Following the performance of an effective strengths-based assessment, the ISP is developed. An ISP contains the specific goals and unique objectives relating directly to the assessment data (Hepworth et al., 2013). There are suggested activities that provide guidance for medical social workers. Some appropriate activities in the development of an ISP include assistance with: (a) insurance and/or medical treatment payment programs; (b) accessing medical care for HIV/AIDS treatment; (c) assessment and resources for oral, nutritional, mental health, and substance abuse treatment and care; (d) housing; (e) transportation; (f) food; and (g) translation services (Health Resources and Services Administration HIV/AIDS Bureau, 2009).

Medication Treatment Adherence

During the medication treatment and adherence phase, the social worker's most important role becomes that of a liaison and advocate; the social worker communicates the client's progress and issues related to adherence to the interprofessional team. In this phase, the social worker coordinates and provides ongoing support for treatment compliance and MA. Assessing the client's readiness is key in this process of adherence monitoring, as this may change at various points in development based on the interplay of other factors such as social, cognitive, emotional, physical, behavioral, and environmental life domains (Andrasik et al., 2015).

As stated previously, a critical role of the medical social worker is the coordination of communication and services with the treatment team. This can be within a clinic or agency. Case conferences, access to client records, and use of written communication (e.g., emails, texts) are all examples of forms of this coordination. This important coordination on the part of the social work team member also promotes consistent service quality and allows for effective evaluation of interprofessional service delivery. Finally, it is essential that all social workers are mindful of their legal and ethical responsibilities to their clients (e.g., informed consent, limits to confidentiality, consent to release medical information; Ojikutu et al., 2014).

Of note are the following predictors of the positive or poorer likelihood of MA. Positive MA factors include: previous adherence, comprehension of information, high level of medical knowledge, treatment is believed to be effective, perceived benefits outweigh the inconvenience, trust in provider, belief in ability to follow regimen, and social support (e.g., spiritual community, friends, neighbors, family [biological or logical]). Poorer likelihood of MA for people living with AIDS (PLWA) include: poor comprehension of information, regimen interferes with lifestyle, side effects, treatment burden, depression, negative cognitions/schemas about HIV, negative cognitions/schemas about the ability to follow regimen, poor availability and differing expectations of staff or provider and client (Chesney, 2000).

ISP Reassessment

The ongoing process of reassessment is the final task for the medical social worker. A client's medical, interpersonal, and emotional well-being changes over time. Because of this, the MCM model suggests ongoing reassessment as a core activity. It is useful to conduct reassessment routinely, when clinically or programmatically appropriate, throughout the time the client is an active member with their ASO. It is essential that the medical social worker always takes a strengths-based approach to the continued processing of mutually agreed upon goals with the client. While we must address setbacks, providing ample positive reinforcement surrounding accomplishments will have a significant positive benefit on the client typically (Hepworth et al., 2013). An important goal of MCM to remember is to be mindful that meeting a goal of increased independence and autonomy from formal routine case management services benefits the client, ASO, and the more macro systems involved in the delivery of coordinated care (Ojikutu et al., 2014).

Case Example 14.1

Samantha is a 54-year-old Black (African American) cisgender heterosexual woman referred to the MCM program at her county's local ASO. Her husband of 25 years recently passed away from AIDS in the local hospital. He had been an intravenous crystal methamphetamine addict; he hid his HIV status from his wife until his last hospitalization. After an assessment that deemed Samantha "high-risk," and then testing positive for HIV in the hospital's emergency room (ER), the interprofessional team, consisting of a doctor, nurse, and social worker, made an immediate referral to the local ASO. Samantha was referred for services at the ASO for support regarding the death of her husband, concurrent with learning about his HIV status and her own. She presents for assessment and intervention at the ASO affiliated with the hospital where she was diagnosed. While at the ER, Samantha was given the news that she was HIV-positive, she has been informed that she in fact has an AIDS diagnosis due to her current T-cell count of 7 (an AIDS diagnosis is given when an individual's T-cells fall below 200 and they have experienced opportunistic infection; UCSF Medical Center, 2017). She is in possession of the laboratory result at the time of intake.

As discussed in Samantha's case, she presents at the ASO (with her daughter and granddaughter; social domain) for her biopsychosocial assessment in a state of crisis. She and her family are in a state of shock regarding the AIDS diagnosis, as well as in grief surrounding the loss of their husband, father, and grandfather (psychological domain). Samantha and her family know very little about HIV/AIDS (cognitive domain). Samantha's affect appears visibly shaken and she cries uncontrollably at times, with moments of clarity. Her mood is depressed and she is withdrawn (psychological domain). Samantha can insightfully acknowledge the need for counseling services, as well as the need to begin medical treatment for her AIDS diagnosis (psychological and cognitive domains). As her husband was the primary income earner in the household where she lived with her daughter and granddaughter, Samantha has been unable to pay the rent on their apartment; she has subsequently moved out. She presents with an immediate housing resource need (social domain). While supported by her daughter, Samantha's sister and other family members were highly discriminatory when she revealed her serostatus. She is also scared that someone from her religious community may find out her state of health (social and psychological domains).

It is the role of the social worker on the interprofessional team to review the assessment findings. Based on the review of Case Example 14.1, the social worker orders and then determines which clinical activities are most salient for Samantha. The client, in collaboration with the social worker, then develops a mutually agreed upon ISP that includes the goals with specific corresponding objectives, activities, and the anticipated timelines during the contracted treatment period. In subsequent sessions with her social worker, Samantha continues to review the goals in the ISP and refines strategies to meet these goals.

Based on Case Example 14.1, the ISP for Samantha is centered on her goals related to treatment adherence. There are multiple goals for the ISP which, if effective, should have a direct correlation with enhancing adherence. Samantha has successfully begun antiretroviral therapy (ART) and has managed the side effects with relative ease. She has continually met at the agreed upon times with her social worker. This goal was a priority due to her low T-cell count. Her T-cell count is now at 233; she no longer has an opportunistic infection. The secondary goal needing to be addressed is permanent housing. The social worker plans an objective with the client to apply for Housing Opportunities for Persons with HIV/AIDS (HOPWA) program and obtain permanent Section 8 housing. This goal correlates with enhancing MA in that Samantha requires a place of her own to prepare healthy meals and store medication that needs refrigeration. This is particularly important because her family's current temporary housing is limiting due to the hostile and discriminatory environment her sister has created.

POLICY

The federal government funds much of policy and programs related to HIV/AIDS in the United States. While states also provide funding for services, this chapter focuses on federal level policy as the variability within states (for many reasons including state budgets, prevalence of HIV/AIDS, among others) makes state-level data challenging to provide with any level of depth. The 2017 federal fiscal budget included $27.5 billion for domestic HIV efforts (KFF, 2016). These funds were designated in the following ways: 61% treatment and care; 9% cash and housing assistance; 8% research; and 3% prevention. Mandatory spending for HIV was $19.7 billion for fiscal year 2017 (the remaining being discretionary funding determined annually by Congress); these funds went to support Medicaid, Medicare, Social Security Disability Insurance (SSDI), Social Security Insurance (SSI), and Federal Employees Health Benefits Plan (KFF, 2016). However, much of the federal funding is distributed to states who allocate funds at the state level. Here we detail programs related to HIV testing and prevention programs, treatment and care, and housing to highlight ways that federal funds support prevention of HIV and intervention, and support for HIV-infected individuals and families.

Federal Testing and Prevention Programs

Federal funds partially support HIV counseling programs, a critical prevention and identification resource for individuals who are engaged in high-risk activity (e.g., unprotected sexual intercourse or IV drug use). Federal government agencies work with community organization (at a local level) providing support for HIV testing programs and prevention initiatives (U.S. Department of Health and Human Services/Secretary's Minority AIDS Initiative Fund [SMAIF], 2017a). Testing is considered part of prevention (controlling the spread of HIV) and provides the opportunity to engage in HIV counseling, testing, and referral to services for persons living with HIV/AIDS. Prevention efforts funded by the federal government are diverse. The CDC supports the National Prevention Information Network and provides links to prevention initiatives and resources funding by the government and nongovernmental organizations (see resources at npin.cdc.gov/disease/hiv). The CDC also offers access to prevention programs including: (a) Acts Against AIDS Campaign (to reduce incidence of HIV; CDC, 2017a); (b) a compendium of evidence-based interventions (EBIs) and best practices for HIV prevention (CDC, 2017b), including the Diffusion of Effective Intervention Initiative (DEBI) program (CDC, 2016c); and (c) a comprehensive listing of research through the Replicating Effective Programs Plus program (CDC, 2016f). For a full listing of federal prevention initiatives, visit the HIV.gov website (formerly AIDS.gov).

Treatment and Care Programs

There are a number of treatment and care programs funded by the federal government. Treatment and care programs include: (a) HIV/AIDS treatment guidelines, (b) behavioral health programs, (c) housing, and (d) Ryan White funding. In the following, we provide some information about treatment guidelines and behavioral health program efforts with greater emphasis placed on the HOPWA and Ryan White CARE programs.

Treatment Guidelines and Behavioral Health Services

The U.S. Department of Health and Human Services is responsible for publishing guidelines to assist medical providers who service persons with HIV. The guidelines, developed in collaboration with agencies across the federal government (and with input from clinicians and care providers), set the standard of care in HIV/AIDS (U.S. Department of Health and Human Services/AIDSInfo, 2017). Behavioral health services, particularly those targeting substance use and HIV are also supported by federal funds. These include: (a) the National Mental Health Information Center (operated by the SAMHSA); (b) the Safe Needle Disposal program (operated by NeedyMeds; formerly the CDC); and (c) AIDSOURCE, a resource clearinghouse (operated by the National Library of Medicine, National Institutes of Health; U.S. Department of Health and Human Services/AIDSInfo, 2017). The National Mental Health Information Center is a resource compendium that provides access to best practices and consumer guides related to topics of mental health and substance use for individuals living with HIV/AIDS. Many of the guides are available in multiple languages for use in clinical practice (SAMHSA, 2015). Established in 2002, the Safe Needle Disposal program (formerly Safe Community Needle Disposal program) is a resource to educate the public about the safe disposal of sharps and community-sponsored sharps disposal options (Safe Needle Disposal & NeedyMeds, 2017). Last, AIDSource is a comprehensive collection of HIV/AIDS-related resources (selected by experts and librarians). The goal of AIDSource is to provide access to quality-reviewed current HIV/AIDS information (U.S. National Library of Medicine, 2017). Resources are available in English and Spanish. Topics include, but are not limited to: (a) basic HIV/AIDS information, (b) policies and programs, (c) medical practice guidelines, (d) prevention, (e) resources, and (f) statistics/surveillance data (U.S. National Library of Medicine, 2017). These federally funded programs provide social workers with up-to-date information for planning, psychoeducation, EBIs, and resource connectivity.

Housing

There are several sources of support related to housing for persons living with HIV/AIDS. Federal funds support antidiscrimination measures, fair housing, and community planning and development (most significantly the HOPWA program). The goal of the Office of Community Planning and Development seeks to develop viable communities that provide housing, a suitable living environment, and expanded economic opportunities for low-income persons (U.S. Department of Housing and Urban Development [HUD], n.d.). HOPWA falls under the purview of this HUD program.

HOPWA is the only federally funded housing program for individuals living with HIV/AIDS. Overseen by HUD, states, local communities, and nonprofit organizations receive distributed funds for housing projects that benefit individuals and families living with HIV/AIDS (U.S. Department of Health and Human Services/SMAIF, 2017b). HOPWA includes a formula program in which eligible metropolitan cities (more than 500,000 residents) with 1,500 (or greater) cumulative AIDS cases (in the past 5 years) received funds. There are also competitive programs to which applicants (such as states, local governments, or nonprofit organizations) may apply and be awarded funding to create or sustain housing, social services, program planning or development of new housing for individuals or families living with HIV/AIDS. Beneficiaries of these programs must be low-income persons with a verified HIV/AIDS diagnosis. There are a number of services provided under HOPWA that include: (a) the short-term rent, mortgage, and utility program that provides financial assistance to maintain eligible clients in their housing when they are facing a financial or medical crisis (assistance available for up to 21 weeks in a 52-week period); (b) permanent housing placement which provides move-in grants for security deposit, first month's rents, utility turn on, and moving-related costs (available once every 3 years for individuals moving into permanent housing); (c) crisis housing that provides emergency and transitional housing for clients who are at risk of homelessness or are homeless; and (d) tenant-based rental assistance (up to 12 months; City of Los Angeles, 2016). Support services related to HOPWA can include housing specialists (who help clients locate and maintain affordable housing), resident services coordinator (individuals who provide support services within housing developments for individual and families with HIV/AIDS), benefits counseling, and legal services (particularly related to fair housing). While locations where social workers serve persons with HIV/AIDS may have limited resources related to HIV-specific housing, HOPWA resources should be explored to create opportunities for permanent (and if needed, supportive) housing for individuals and families with HIV.

Ryan White CARE Act

Established in 1990, the Ryan White Comprehensive AIDS Resources Emergency (CARE) Act is one of few disease-specific health programs in the United States and is the largest federally funded program for persons living with HIV/AIDS (Health Resources and Service Administration, n.d.). The program is a "payer of last resort," which means that it covers treatment when no other resources are accessible to an individual. This includes individuals without health insurance and those who are insured but have coverage gaps. It is estimated that about 500,000 individuals received at least one medical, health, or support service through the CARE program; 65% of these individuals have incomes at or below the federal poverty line (in 2017, this was $11,880 for a single individual and $24,300 for a family of four; KFF, 2017b). Of individuals served, one fifth are uninsured, 71% are male, 55% are between the ages of 40 and 59 years, 73% are individuals or racial/ethnic minority status, and 48% are men who identify as having sex with men or bisexual (KFF, 2017b).

The structure of Ryan White is such that 75% of dollars fund core medical services; the remaining funds bolster prevention and community-based programs. Five parts of the CARE Act are described here. Part A provides funding to eligible metropolitan areas (population of 50,000 or greater) with 2,000 (or greater) reported AIDS cases within the previous 5-year period. The funding establishes (a) planning councils and (b) tasks identified agencies/government groups in the locality to complete needs assessments, develop HIV care delivery plans, and set funding priorities (KFF, 2017b). Part B provides funding to states, territories, and Washington, D.C., to provide direct services to persons living with HIV/AIDS. This includes oversight and implementation of the AIDS Drug Assistance Program (ADAP) and supplemental ADAP (KFF, 2017b), which pay for HIV-related medication. Part C of the CARE Act funds early intervention services, including HIV testing, case management, risk reduction (RR) counseling, and capacity development and planning grants. These services help to support the HIV care continuum (also referred to as the treatment cascade), a model that outlines sequential steps for the medical care of individuals with HIV; the goal is to achieve viral load suppression (U.S. Department of Health and Human Services/SMAIF, 2017a). The four-stage treatment cascade model includes: (a) HIV testing and diagnosis, (b) receiving and remaining in care, (c) receipt and use of antiretroviral medications (ARTs), and (d) achieving viral load suppression (U.S. Department of Health and Human Services/SMAIF, 2017a). Ryan White programs ensure that all individuals, regardless of insurance status, can work toward the goal of viral suppression. Part D of the CARE Act provides funds for family-centered and community-based services to children, youth, and women living with HIV and their families. Activities are outreach, prevention, primary and specialty medical care, and psychological services (KFF, 2017b). Last, Part F funds provide supplemental support to AIDS education and training centers, for dental programs, to minority AIDS initiatives, and to special projects of national significance. To explore your state's Ryan White programs profile, go to hab.hrsa.gov/stateprofiles/.

In the current political climate, many of the core health resources are at risk. For now, funding for HIV/AIDS policies and programs remains stable, with cuts not yet planned. However, social workers must remain advocates to ensure that the policies that support the well-being of HIV-positive people remain a national and global priority.

Regardless of their ability to pay, clients of most ASOs receive top quality integrated health care. U.S. residents who are infected and affected by HIV disease can seek services at the local ASO in their county of residence (if available). As detailed in the policy section, funding for ASOs comes from federal, state, and county grants (along with private donations). A comprehensive ASO, like the one Samantha accessed, provides a full spectrum of services. These include: (a) treatment, support, and education for the newly diagnosed, to care for long-term survivors; (b) HIV medical services; (c) an onsite pharmacy; (d) mental health, case management, and support groups; and (e) supportive services for benefits including ADAP enrollment and HOPWA enrollment. Using SAMHSA's framework for levels of integrated health care (refer to Chapter 7, Integrated Behavioral Health), most ASOs are a Level 2 (basic collaboration at a distance) or Level 3 (basic collaboration onsite; Heath et al., 2013). Often, it is the more intensive behavioral health component that is missing that keeps many ASOs from being a Level 5 or 6. Level 3 ranking indicates *basic collaboration onsite*. This means that services are provided in the same facility but not the same offices. When two programs, like an ASO and behavioral health organization, do not share the same physical facility, they would rank between a Level 2 or 3 for an integrated health care setting in SAMHSA's framework (Heath et al., 2013). In this case, because the ASO is not a Level 5 or 6, we would want to utilize the MCM knowledge and skills discussed to increase communication, collaboration, and provide effective care coordination for the patient/client. In doing so, we not only meet the client's immediate needs, but provide a supportive system that meets the varied needs that may arise.

RESEARCH

Research and prevention efforts in the United States include behavioral and biomedical interventions at the individual and community levels (CDC, 2016g). Individual-level biomedical interventions have included ART, pre-exposure prophylaxis (PrEP), and post-exposure prophylaxis (PEP; CDC, 2016g). For individual-level behavioral preventions, research and prevention efforts have focused on increasing condom use, HIV testing, and HIV disclosure among PLWH.

Individual-Level Behavioral Preventions

Condom Use

Both laboratory and epidemiologic studies have demonstrated that consistent and correct use of condoms reduces the risk of STIs and HIV (CDC, 2013). However, changing condom use behaviors have proven to be challenging, due to condom use involving negotiations among sexual partners (Ricks et al., 2014). This is why, along with promotion of condom use, HIV testing has been emphasized as another paramount HIV prevention for community health.

HIV Testing

In recent years, emphasis has been placed on HIV testing to increase individual awareness of personal HIV status. The CDC recommends that everyone between the ages of 13 and 64 years get tested for HIV annually and for high-risk individuals every 3 to 6 months (CDC, 2016h). Studies have shown that individuals who know their HIV status can protect other sexual partners from being infected and decrease their viral load by engaging in ART (CDC, 2017d; National HIV/AIDS Strategy [NHAS], 2016a; Venkatesh et al., 2010). However, unlike other health disparities (i.e., diabetes, cancer, hypertension), HIV is highly stigmatized (Pellowski, Kalichman, Matthews, & Adler, 2013). HIV stigma has been shown to be a barrier to HIV testing and seeking HIV-related care after testing positive. Due to the stigmatizing nature of HIV, many people avoid or opt out of testing for HIV, even if they are aware of the benefits (NHAS, 2016a).

Disclosure of HIV Status

In an effort to bolster health outcomes for PLWH and decrease transmission rates, HIV disclosure is critical (Obermeyer, Baijal, & Pegurri, 2011). While there is a link between disclosure and positive outcomes, disclosing one's HIV status can be a challenging decision. Individuals living with HIV may not disclose their status because of privacy concerns, self-blame, fear of rejection, and protecting the other person (Elopre et al., 2016; Geiger, Wang, Charles, Randolph, & Boekeloo, 2017). Further, individuals who disclose their serostatus may face discrimination and stigmatization due to the behaviors that are associated with HIV, such as drug addiction, prostitution, sexual identity, and promiscuity (Sauceda, Wiebe, Rao, Pearson, & Simoni, 2013; Vyavaharkar et al., 2011). While negative outcomes of disclosure are more often present in the literature, there are also positive outcomes associated with disclosing one's HIV serostatus including increased discussions of safer sex, increases in safer sexual activities and condom use (Mayfield-Arnold, Rice, Flannery, & Rotheram-Borus, 2008). Furthermore, disclosure is associated with better health outcomes and social support, as well as reduced HIV transmission to sexual partners and improved MA (Elopre et al., 2016; Geiger et al., 2017).

Individual-Level Biomedical Interventions

Antiretroviral Therapy

Due to the increasing number of PLWH, there has been an increased focus on both health promotion and HIV prevention for PLWH, such as ART (KFF, 2017a). ART is a combination of HIV medications (HIV regimen) that prevents HIV from multiplying in the body (NHAS, 2016a). ART is not a cure but can control the virus through suppression so that people can have healthier and longer lives, and so that people can reduce the risk of transmitting HIV to others (NHAS, 2016a). Optimal ART adherence is critical in achieving both clinical and preventive benefits through viral load suppression. Helping PLWH enter and remain in HIV primary care is pivotal in the HIV care continuum, which begins with the diagnosis of HIV infection, entry into and retention in HIV medical care, access and adherence to ART and viral load suppression (NHAS, 2016a).

Pre-Exposure Prophylaxis and Postexposure Prophylaxis

PrEP and PEP are biomedical preventive interventions for HIV-negative individuals that involve taking medication to prevent the acquisition of HIV (CDC, 2016i). PrEP is an HIV prevention medication (Truvada) that an HIV-negative person can take daily before being exposed to HIV to help prevent the acquisition of HIV (NHAS, 2016b). However, it does not protect from other STIs (e.g., gonorrhea, chlamydia, herpes, syphilis). PEP is an HIV prevention medication that involves taking an anti-HIV drug within 24 to 72 hours after possible exposure to HIV to try to reduce the chances of becoming HIV-positive (CDC, 2016j). The longer a person waits to start PEP, the less effective PEP becomes (NHAS, 2016c). PrEP and PEP have been shown to be highly effective in preventing HIV, if taken correctly, and can be prescribed by a health care provider upon request (CDC, 2016g).

Individual-level behavioral preventions and biomedical interventions have been shown to be effective methods of reducing incidence of HIV and are promoted by the CDC and the NHAS (resources can be found by visiting the HIV.gov website [formerly AIDS.gov] at https://www.hiv.gov/hiv-basics). To promote these preventions and interventions in an effective and efficient manner, the CDC has put together a list of recommended evidence-based HIV interventions to assist with decreasing sexual risk behaviors and increasing HIV prevention behaviors.

Evidence-Based HIV Interventions

CDC's Recommended Evidence-Based HIV Interventions

The CDC provides recommendations for EBIs for health departments and community-based organizations to implement (CDC, 2016k). Health care and prevention providers can use these recommended best practices identified as resources when making decisions to meet the needs of high-risk populations and PLWH. The CDC's list of EBI recommendations, also known as the HIV/AIDS Prevention Research Synthesis (PRS) Project was initiated in 1996 (CDC, 2016k). Initially, the PRS Project systematically reviewed and summarized the cumulative body of HIV prevention literature to identify EBIs, best practices, and public health strategies for reducing HIV transmission and infection, what is called RR interventions. Over the years, the HIV/AIDS PRS Project expanded the scope of systematic review efforts to include the identification of EBIs for improving HIV MA and viral load suppression among PLWH; and identifying best practices for linkage to, retention in, or re-engagement in HIV care (LRC) (CDC, 2016k).

Systematic reviews are continuously taking place to identify EBIs that show evidence of efficacy. Based on the overall quality of the study, evidence-based RR behavioral interventions are classified as either *best-evidence* or *good-evidence* for the RR and MA interventions and evidence-based and evidence-informed for the LRC interventions. See Table 14.1 for details of inclusion criteria. Currently there are 59 evidence-based HIV RR interventions, 12 MA interventions, and 13 LRC interventions deemed "best" or "good" (CDC, 2016i). For the full list of EBIs recommended by the CDC, visit the Compendium of Evidence-Based Interventions and Best Practices for HIV Prevention at www.cdc.gov/hiv/research/interventionresearch/compendium.

Table 14.1 Inclusion Criteria for Inclusions as a "Best Practice" Intervention

Type of EBIs	Grading Criteria	Review Process (A Priori Criteria)	Inclusion Criteria Not Currently Included
Risk reduction	Best evidence Good evidence	• Systematic search • Screened to determine eligibility	(a) Focus on an HIV, AIDS, or STD behavioral intervention (b) Outcome evaluation with a comparison arm (c) Published or accepted for publication in a peer-reviewed journal (d) Conducted in the United States or a U.S. territory, and (e) Focus on a target population of PLWH, MSM, or transgender persons (beginning with publications dated 2015 or later) Studies must also report: • Sex risk behaviors (e.g., abstinence, mutual monogamy, number of sex partners, negotiation of safer sex, condom use, refusal to have unsafe sex), • Drug injection behaviors (e.g., frequency of injection drug use, needle sharing), • Biologic measures of HIV or other STD infections (e.g., prevalence or incidence measures of hepatitis, HIV, or other STDs)

(continued)

Table 14.1 Inclusion Criteria for Inclusions as a "Best Practice" Intervention (*continued*)

Type of EBIs	Grading Criteria	Review Process (A Priori Criteria)	Inclusion Criteria Not Currently Included

MA	Best evidence Good evidence	• Quality of study design
		• Quality of study implementation and analysis
		• Strength of evidence of efficacy
			• HIV MA Intervention with:
			  • Educational/behavioral component OR
			  • Treatment delivery methods or monitoring devices to facilitate adherence
			• Published or accepted for publication in a peer-reviewed journal
			• Conducted in the United States or a U.S. territory
			• Outcome evaluation report with a comparison arm
			• Report any of the following relevant outcome data:
			  • Behavioral measures of adherence: electronic monitoring device (e.g., MEMs caps), pill count, pharmacy refill, self-report
			  • Biologic measure of adherence: HIV viral load

LRC	Evidence based Evidence informed	• Quality of study design • Quality of study implementation and analysis • Strength of evidence of findings	• Published or accepted for publication in a peer-reviewed journal • Conducted in the United States or a U.S. territory and has a comparison arm or if one group study design, has pre-post intervention data • Conducted outside of the United States and is a randomized controlled trial • Exclusively focus on persons diagnosed with HIV • Report any relevant LRC outcome data (i.e., linkage to HIV care, retention in HIV care, re-engagement in HIV care) • Use relevant measures for LRC outcomes (i.e., HIV medical visits documented in medical or agency records or surveillance reports; HIV viral loads and/or CD4 counts as proxies for HIV medical visits in above reports; self-reports validated by medical or agency records or surveillance reports)

EBI, evidence-based intervention; LRC, linkage to, retention in, or re-engagement in HIV care; MA, medication adherence; MEMs cap, Medication Event Monitoring System bottle cap; MSM, men who have sex with men; PLWH, people living with HIV; STD, sexually transmitted disease.

In addition to the CDC's Compendium of Evidence-based Interventions, the CDC has also developed the High Impact HIV/AIDS Prevention Project (HIP), which aims to maximize the effectiveness of current HIV preventions. The HIP project provides user-friendly kits with the materials and training information necessary to implement interventions in order for service providers to increase their ability to conduct effective intervention programs in their community (CDC, 2017c). For more information regarding HIV intervention trainings and toolkits, visit the Effective Interventions' website at effectiveinterventions.cdc.gov.

CONCLUSION

We are in the fourth decade of HIV; during this timeframe, we have seen numerous changes related to prevention, treatment, and care. These efforts have been supported by national and global efforts, recognizing the need for culturally responsive strategies to combat HIV. This chapter provided an overview of evidence-based practices and the federal policies and programs that support individuals living with HIV. Specifically, the work highlighted the vast array of medical and social support services provided by these critical funds. As with other important health programs, much of the determination of funds to prevent HIV and provide support to those who are HIV-infected is at the discretion of Congress and the U.S. president. During challenging political times, social workers must raise their voices and advocate for the critical services that can increase an HIV-positive person's access to medical and psychological care, accessible and affordable housing, and programs that increase awareness and reduce stigma for individuals living with HIV/at high risk of HIV exposure.

Social workers must continue to consider the structural barriers that place individuals at increased risk of HIV infection; these same structural barriers can also become barriers to service utilization. In general, structural barriers can be viewed as fourfold: (a) having access to the product or item of interest, (b) the physical structures in the environment, (c) the community social structures, and (d) messages derived from media and community culture (Cohen, Scribner, & Farley, 2000). Health behaviors are predicted by perception of neighborhood safety, housing, employment, and other opportunities. As such, we need to think about individuals in their contextual environment to assess risk and intervene most effectively. Social workers must work collectively with their interprofessional partners to meet the needs of the whole person, considering multisystem factors that influence well-being for individuals. By taking a person-centered approach to care, we respect the mutuality of behavioral and medical decisions and honor a client's right to self-determination.

CHAPTER DISCUSSION QUESTIONS

1. Given that HIV remains a highly stigmatized chronic condition, what strategies might you implement in your clinical practice to best meet the needs of individuals living with HIV?

2. Medical case management is an effective evidence-based intervention used to increase adherence and enhance service connectivity for individuals living with HIV. How might you utilize the elements of this case management intervention outside of an AIDS Service Organization to create a treatment and service coordination plan?

(continued)

3. There are a number of policies that benefit individuals with HIV including HOPWA, ADAP, and the Ryan White CARE funding. Discuss why you believe HIV has received such a high level of federal funding (compared to other chronic conditions) and the benefits and challenges that may come from these policies.

4. Research in HIV has primarily targeted two areas: medication adherence and individual behavior change. What systems-level interventions might work well to reduce risky behaviors?

5. HIV, which was once highly associated with mortality, is now designated a manageable chronic condition. How do you think this impacts individual-level interventions aimed at reducing risky sexual behaviors?

CASE EXAMPLE AND DISCUSSION QUESTIONS

Case Example 14.2

John is a 46-year-old White male who was diagnosed with HIV in 2007 and with AIDS in 2014. He is prescribed ARTs but his MA is inconsistent. In 2012, John was hospitalized; there he was diagnosed with cirrhosis of the liver and declining kidney function. In 2013, John's medication regiment stopped working due to nonadherence to the medication prescribed to him. John is an alcoholic and has been for the past 15 years, having been a hard liquor drinker in the past, but currently drinking exclusively beer; he has a long history of substance abuse but is not currently using illicit drugs. John has been recently housed in a community-based Section 8 apartment near your ASO; he is a new client to your organization that provides behavioral health services.

Questions for Discussion

1. Upon completion of an assessment, what might your treatment plan with John look like? Describe what you would prioritize in the treatment plan and why you made this choice.

2. How might you work with John to better adhere to his medication? Where would you begin? What therapeutic techniques would you use?

3. Given the negative interaction of many medication and alcohol, how might you use a harm reduction approach in your work with John?

4. Alcohol may be used by John because he is isolated. What might you do to influence his social connectedness?

REFERENCES

Andrasik, F., Goodie, J. L., & Peterson, A. L. (2015). *Introduction to biopsychosocial assessment in clinical health psychology.* New York, NY: Guilford Publications, Inc.

Centers for Disease Control and Prevention. (2013). Condom fact sheet in brief. Retrieved from https://www.cdc.gov/condomeffectiveness/brief.html

Centers for Disease Control and Prevention. (2016a). Basic statistics. Retrieved from https://www.cdc.gov/hiv/basics/statistics.html

Centers for Disease Control and Prevention. (2016b). Gay and bisexual men. Retrieved from http://www.cdc.gov/hiv/group/msm/index.html

Centers for Disease Control and Prevention. (2016c). HIV among women. Retrieved from http://www.cdc.gov/hiv/group/gender/women/index.html

Centers for Disease Control and Prevention. (2016d). HIV among youth. Retrieved from http://www.cdc.gov/hiv/group/age/youth/index.html

Centers for Disease Control and Prevention. (2016f). Intervention research. Retrieved from https://www.cdc.gov/hiv/research/interventionresearch/index.html

Centers for Disease Control and Prevention. (2016g). Effectiveness of prevention strategies to reduce the risk of acquiring or transmitting HIV. Retrieved from https://www.cdc.gov/hiv/risk/estimates/preventionstrategies.html

Centers for Disease Control and Prevention. (2016h). HIV testing. Retrieved from http://www.cdc.gov/hiv/testing/index.html

Centers for Disease Control and Prevention. (2016i). PrEP. Retrieved from https://www.cdc.gov/hiv/basics/prep.html

Centers for Disease Control and Prevention. (2016j). PEP. Retrieved from https://www.cdc.gov/hiv/basics/pep.html

Centers for Disease Control and Prevention. (2016k). Compendium of evidence-based interventions and best practices for HIV prevention. Retrieved from https://www.cdc.gov/hiv/research/interventionresearch/compendium/index.html

Centers for Disease Control and Prevention. (2017a). Act against AIDS. Retrieved from https://www.cdc.gov/actagainstaids/

Centers for Disease Control and Prevention. (2017b). Compendium of evidence-based interventions and best practices for HIV prevention. Retrieved from https://www.cdc.gov/hiv/research/interventionresearch/compendium/index.html

Centers for Disease Control and Prevention. (2017c). Effective interventions. Retrieved from https://effectiveinterventions.cdc.gov/en/HighImpactPrevention.aspx

Centers for Disease Control and Prevention. (2017d). Prevention benefits of HIV treatment. Retrieved from https://www.cdc.gov/hiv/research/biomedicalresearch/tap/

Chesney, M. A. (2000). Factors affecting adherence to antiretroviral therapy. *Clinical Infectious Diseases, 30*(Suppl. 2), S171–S176. doi:10.1086/313849

City of Los Angeles. (2016). Services of people living with HIV/AIDS. Retrieved from http://hcidla.lacity.org/people-with-aids

Cohen, D. A., Scribner, R. A., & Farley, T. A. (2000). A structural model of health behavior: A pragmatic approach to explain and influence health behaviors at the population level. *Preventive Medicine, 30*(2), 146–154. doi:10.1006/pmed.1999.0609

Elopre, L., Westfall, A. O., Mugavero, M. J., Zinski, A., Burkholder, G., Hook, E. W., & Van Wagoner, N. (2016). Predictors of HIV disclosure in infected persons presenting to establish care. *AIDS and Behavior, 20*(1), 147–154. doi:10.1007/s10461-015-1060-8

Engel, G. L. (1980). The clinical application of the biopsychosocial model. *American Journal of Psychiatry, 137*(5), 535–544. doi:10.1176/ajp.137.5.535

Geiger, T., Wang, M., Charles, A., Randolph, S., & Boekeloo, B. (2017). HIV serostatus disclosure and engagement in medical care among predominantly low income but insured African American adults with HIV. *AIDS and Behavior, 21*(1), 163–173. doi:10.1007/s10461-016-1479-6

Germaine, C. (1973). An ecological perspective in casework. *Social Casework, 54*, 323–330.

Health Resources and Service Administration. (n.d). History leading to the Ryan White CARE Act. Retrieved from https://hab.hrsa.gov/about-ryan-white-hivaids-program/history-leading-ryan-white-care-act

Health Resources and Services Administration HIV/AIDS Bureau. (2009). HAB HIV performance measures: Medical case management. Retrieved from https://careacttarget.org/library/hab-hiv-performance-measures-medical-case-management

Heath, B., Wise, R. P., & Reynolds, K. A. (2013). *Review and proposed standard framework for levels of integrated health care.* Washington, DC: SAMHSA-HRSA Center for Integrated Health Solutions.

Hepworth, D. H., Rooney, R. H., Dewberry Rooney, G., & Strom-Gottfried, K. (2013). *Direct social work practice: Theory and skills* (9th ed.). Belmont, CA: Brooks/Cole.

Kaiser Family Foundation. (2016). U.S. federal funding for HIV/AIDS: Trends over time. Retrieved from http://kff.org/global-health-policy/fact-sheet/u-s-federal-funding-for-hivaids-trends-over-time/

Kaiser Family Foundation. (2017a). The HIV/AIDS epidemic in the United States: The basics. Retrieved from http://kff.org/hivaids/fact-sheet/the-hivaids-epidemic-in-the-united-states-the-basics/

Kaiser Family Foundation. (2017b). The Ryan White HIV/AIDS program: The basics. Retrieved from http://kff.org/hivaids/fact-sheet/the-ryan-white-hivaids-program-the-basics/

Liau, A., Crepaz, N., Lyles, C. M., Higa, D. H., Mullins, M. M., DeLuca, J., . . . HIV/AIDS Prevention Research Synthesis Team. (2013). Interventions to promote linkage to and utilization of HIV medical care among HIV-diagnosed persons: A qualitative systematic review, 1996–2011. *AIDS and Behavior, 17*(6), 1941–1962. doi:10.1007/s10461-013-0435-y

Mayfield-Arnold, E., Rice, E., Flannery, D., & Rotheram-Borus, M. J. (2008). HIV disclosure among adults living with HIV. *AIDS Care, 20*(1), 80–92. doi:10.1080/09540120701449138

National HIV/AIDS Strategy. (2016a). Overview of HIV treatments. Retrieved from https://www.aids.gov/hiv-aids-basics/just-diagnosed-with-hiv-aids/treatment-options/overview-of-hiv-treatments/

National HIV/AIDS Strategy. (2016b). PrEP. Retrieved from https://www.aids.gov/hiv-aids-basics/prevention/reduce-your-risk/pre-exposure-prophylaxis/

National HIV/AIDS Strategy. (2016c). PEP. Retrieved from https://www.aids.gov/hiv-aids-basics/prevention/reduce-your-risk/post-exposure-prophylaxis/

Obermeyer, C. M., Baijal, P., & Pegurri, E. (2011). Facilitating HIV disclosure across diverse settings: A review. *American Journal of Public Health, 101*(6), 1011–1023. doi:10.2105/AJPH.2010.300102

Ojikutu, B., Holman, J., Kunches, L., Landers, S., Perlmutter, D., Ward, M., . . . Hirschhorn, L. (2014). Interdisciplinary HIV care in a changing health care environment in the USA. *AIDS Care, 26*(6), 731–735. doi:10.1080/09540121.2013.855299

Pellowski, J. A., Kalichman, S. C., Matthews, K. A., & Adler, N. (2013). A pandemic of the poor: Social disadvantage and the US HIV epidemic. *American Psychologist, 68*(4), 197–209. doi:10.1037/a0032694

Ricks, J. M., Geter, A., McGladrey, M., Crosby, R. A., Mena, L. A., & Ottmar, J. M. (2014). "I don't have a problem with it, but other guys do": An exploration of condom negotiation among young black men who have sex with men in the South. *Journal of Black Sexuality and Relationships, 1*(2), 1–14. doi:10.1353/bsr.2014.0003

Safe Needle Disposal & NeedyMeds. (2017). Safe needle disposal. Retrieved from http://www.safeneedledisposal.org/

Sauceda, J. A., Wiebe, J. S., Rao, D., Pearson, C. R., & Simoni, J. M. (2013). HIV-related stigma and HIV disclosure among Latinos on the US-Mexico border. In *Stigma, discrimination and living with HIV/AIDS* (pp. 187–203). Dordrecht, The Netherlands: Springer Netherlands.

Substance Use and Mental Health Services Administration. (2015). SAMHSA's efforts to address HIV, AIDS, and viral hepatitis. Retrieved from https://www.samhsa.gov/hiv-aids-viral-hepatitis/samhsas-efforts

UCSF Medical Center. (2017). AIDS diagnosis. Retrieved from https://www.ucsfhealth.org/conditions/aids/diagnosis.html

U.S. Department of Health and Human Services/AIDSInfo. (2017). Clinical guidelines. Retrieved from https://aidsinfo.nih.gov/guidelines

U.S. Department of Health and Human Services/Secretary's Minority AIDS Initiative Fund. (2017a). Federal testing programs. Retrieved from https://www.hiv.gov/federal-response/federal-activities-agencies/hiv-prevention-activities

U.S. Department of Health and Human Services/Secretary's Minority AIDS Initiative Fund. (2017b). HIV/AIDS care continuum. Retrieved from https://www.aids.gov/federal-resources/policies/care-continuum/

U.S. Department of Housing and Urban Development. (n.d.). Community planning and development. Retrieved from https://portal.hud.gov/hudportal/HUD?src=/program_offices/comm_planning

U.S. Department of Housing and Urban Development. (2017). Housing for persons living with HIV/AIDS. Retrieved from https://www.hudexchange.info/programs/hopwa/

U.S. National Library of Medicine. (2017). AIDSource. Retrieved from https://aids.nlm.nih.gov/

Venkatesh, K. K., de Bruyn, G., Lurie, M. N., Mohapi, L., Pronyk, P., Moshabela, M., . . . Martinson, N. A. (2010). Decreased sexual risk behavior in the era of HAART among HIV-infected urban and rural South Africans attending primary care clinics. *AIDS, 24,* 2687–2696. doi:10.1097/QAD.0b013e32833e78d4

Vyavaharkar, M., Moneyham, L., Corwin, S., Tavakoli, A., Saunders, R., & Annang, L. (2011). HIV-disclosure, social support, and depression among HIV-infected African American women living in the rural Southeastern United States. *AIDS Education and Prevention, 23*(1), 78–90. doi:10.1521/aeap.2011.23.1.78

Weiser, J., Beer, L., Frazier, E. L., Patel, R., Dempsey, A., Hauck, H., & Skarbinski, J. (2015). Service delivery and patient outcomes in Ryan White HIV/AIDS Program–funded and–nonfunded helth care facilities in the United States. *JAMA Internal Medicine, 175*(10), 1650–1659. doi:10.1001/jamainternmed.2015.4095

15

LGBT Health

Derek Brian Brown and Peggy L. Kelly

The lesbian, gay male, bisexual, transgender, queer, and questioning (LGBTQ) population is a diverse community that has historically been brought together to cope with an oppressive society. In the United States, lesbians, gays, and bisexuals represent approximately 3.4% of the total population (Gates & Newport, 2012; Ward, Dahlamer, Galinsky, & Joestl, 2014). Transgender persons represent approximately 0.6% of the population (Flores, Herman, Gates, & Brown, 2016). The LGBTQ community is as diverse as their heterosexual counterparts. For example, in terms of race and ethnicity, Gates (2014) found that lesbian, gay, and bisexuals do not significantly differ from heterosexual communities. However, when referring to age, LGBTQ persons are often younger than heterosexuals. In the 2013 National Health Interview Survey, heterosexual adults' average age was 47.0 years compared to 41.5 years for lesbians and gay men and 34.3 years for bisexuals. The younger age of persons who identify as LGBTQ is not surprising as individuals were raised in a more accepting society, which may account for their increasing percentage of the U.S. population (Gates, 2014). As society has become more accepting, younger sexual and gender minorities may feel safe and more comfortable disclosing their sexual orientation and gender identity.

In order to understand the lack of attention and the health care needs of this population, social workers first must understand the LGBTQ community. Terminology surrounding the LGBTQ community has produced widespread discussion, with different acronyms and definitions emerging. Four extensive resources that have been developed include: (a) Definitions related to sexual orientation and gender diversity (American Psychological Association [APA], n.d.); (b) Guidelines for psychological practice with transgender and gender-nonconforming people (TGGNC; APA, 2015); (c) The health of lesbian, gay, bisexual, and transgender people: Building a foundation for a better understanding: Glossary (Institute of Medicine [IOM], 2011); and (d) Glossary of LGBT terms for health care teams, created by the National LGBT Health Center of the Fenway Institute (2016). Links to these useful resources can be found in the reference section at the end of this chapter. Drawing upon these resources, the following is a brief discussion.

Sexual and gender minorities have often been used to describe health disparities among different groups (Alexander, Parker, & Schwetz, 2016). Sexual minorities are individuals whose sexual orientation is not heterosexual. The dimensions of sexual orientation are attraction, identification, and sexual behavior (IOM, 2011). Lesbians and gay men are sexual minorities, who may engage in same-sex behavior, be attracted to persons of the same sex, and/or identify as part of the sexual minority community. An important factor to consider is that individuals may or may not meet these three dimensions of sexual orientation. For example, a woman may be attracted to other women and identify as a lesbian but not have sex with other women.

Similarly, bisexuals are sexual minorities with an orientation toward both sexes. Bisexuals are persons who are emotionally and sexually attracted to people of their own gender and people of other genders (National LGBT Health Education Center, 2016) and how people self-identify. Queer is referred to as "an umbrella term that individuals may use to describe a sexual orientation, gender identity or gender expression that does not conform to dominant societal norm" (APA, n.d., p. 5). As the term had a negative connotation, people who identify as queer reclaimed this term in the 1990s as a form of empowerment. Last, individuals who are questioning their sexual orientation may identify as such and may or may not move toward an identification, attraction, and/or sexual behavior with the same sex.

Gender minorities are a heterogeneous group. The dimensions of gender are gender identity and expression, and transgender persons are gender minorities. Transgender persons identify and/or express their gender as different from their assigned sex. For example, a person who is assigned a birth sex of male may identify and express herself as a woman. As one cannot tell whether or not an individual is transgender, an important consideration in working with this population is asking all of your clients regardless of perceived gender for their preferred pronoun. Another important consideration is that sexual orientation and gender are different social categorizations. For example, a person can identify as transgender and be heterosexual. As a matter of fact in the U.S. Transgender Survey 2015 (James et al., 2016), more (41%) respondents than any others identified their sexual orientation as heterosexual.

As with all social group memberships, it is not easy to label someone's sexual orientation as bisexual, homosexual, or heterosexual. The important consideration when social workers work with members of the LGBTQ community is to practice client- and task-centeredness. Social workers can collaborate with their clients by asking how they wish to define their orientation.

HISTORY OF LGBT HEALTH

Lesbians and gay men have experienced tremendous gains in acceptance during the past decade. In 2016, 60% of people in the United States were satisfied with the acceptance of lesbians and gay men, which is a 28% increase from 2006 (McCarthy, 2016). Society's movement toward majority acceptance has been a shift since the major LGBTQ demonstrations of the 1960s, including the riots at Compton's Cafeteria in San Francisco in 1966, at the Black Cat Tavern in Los Angeles in 1967, and at the infamous Stonewall Inn in New York City in 1969.

The need for LGBTQ-specific health emerged in the 1970s. Attention to the LGBTQ population started as an endemic crisis colloquially known as the "gay plague" ravaged the urban sexual minority male population in the 1970s and early 1980s. The disease was first termed gay-related immune deficiency syndrome (GRID) and now is known as AIDS. Due to the stigmatization of this population and homosexual behavior, the nation did not respond to this crisis but instead blamed gay men for acquiring the disease. Gay men effectively organized into advocacy groups, such as the AIDS Coalition to Unleash Power (ACT UP), to demand equity in health care access and health services to address the AIDS crisis. A health care system of support emerged in the 1980s and 1990s to support persons with HIV, the virus that causes AIDS. The HIV system of care developed to serve first and mostly White gay and bisexual men and then transgender women. Unfortunately, the other physical health needs of gay and bisexual men and other groups within the LGBTQ community were largely ignored by the traditional health care system. LGBTQ persons had their broader health care needs served at community-based, LGBT health organizations in large urban centers, which arose in the 1970s. The behavioral health system aligned itself with the gaining acceptance of sexual minorities, as homosexuality was removed from the *Diagnostic and Statistical Manual of Mental Disorders* as a classified disease in 1986.

The U.S. health care system was able to move from a reactive to a proactive and supportive one of sexual and gender minorities in the 2000s. For example, the IOM (2011) released *The Health of Lesbian, Gay, Bisexual, and Transgender People: Building a Foundation for Better Understanding* as a compendium of the current state of knowledge of LGBT health and directs the health community of what is needed. The document clearly details how the LGBTQ population has persistent and pervasive health disparities when compared to heterosexuals.

LGBT HEALTH DISPARITIES

LGBTQ persons experience unique disparities in health risk behaviors, medical conditions, and behavioral health when compared to heterosexuals (IOM, 2011). LGBTQ individuals are also more likely to rate their health as poor, to suffer from chronic conditions, and have an elevated risk for mental health and substance abuse disorders (Ward et al., 2014).

These differences in stress-related health conditions have been identified in broad areas, including asthma, diabetes, headaches, allergies, osteoarthritis, gastrointestinal problems, cardiovascular disease, disability, and some forms of cancer, such as anal, breast, colorectal, and lung. Sexual and gender minorities also have a higher prevalence of health risk behaviors and disabilities than heterosexual people. The health needs of the LGBTQ community are further complicated by significant barriers to health care, such as cost, discrimination, and underutilization of services (Kates, Ranji, Beamesderfer, Salganicoff, & Dawson, 2016). These health disparities are a concern as each medical condition, psychiatric disorder, or health risk behavior can impact a person's quality of life and are associated with comorbid conditions and mortality.

LGBTQ POPULATION GROUPS

The LGBTQ population is diverse and it is important to examine the health concerns of specific groups. For example, from a life course perspective, LGBTQ youth and young adults have different health-related needs and experiences than older adults. Racial and ethnic minorities, persons living in poverty, persons living in rural areas, and other demographic considerations also have distinct health care concerns that warrant particular attention.

Youth

Youth is often perceived as a period of health and vitality. But among the LGBTQ population, young people can face inordinate and serious health concerns when compared to their older counterparts. For instance, according to a report by the IOM (2011) on the health of LGBTQ people, young Black men who have sex with men have a disproportionate share of the burden of HIV. Compared to heterosexual youth, lesbian, gay, and bisexual youth may have higher rates of smoking, drinking, and substance use. Homelessness among LGBTQ youth is also a serious health-related concern. A study by Ray (2006) concluded that between 20% and 40% of homeless youth identify as LGBTQ. Youth identifying as LGBTQ also report higher levels of violence, victimization, and harassment than heterosexual youth (IOM, 2011). Moreover, Heyman et al. (2017) found that 43.3% of youth and young adults ages 14 to 29 reported being treated poorly in the past year because they were LGBTQ, and 60.0% of respondents said they had been bullied in school. In addition, they also found that 42.9% of respondents had spent the night in the hospital for emotional reasons and 28.6% for both emotional and physical injury and illness.

Older Adults

Older adults who are LGBTQ face a number of challenges, as many also have experienced discrimination, stigma, and violence throughout their lives but, in addition, many losses associated with AIDS (IOM, 2011). LGBTQ older adults can experience age-related hardships such as social isolation and financial stress. However, they also face social inequities, which can compound their medical and mental health problems. Moreover, the risk of suicide among this population is estimated to be two to four times that of heterosexuals (Erdley, Anklam, & Reardon, 2014). Another concern is that LGBTQ older adults are less likely to have children who could provide them care as they age. As a result, they are more likely to live alone and rely on informal caregivers such as friends to provide them with care later in life (Stein, Beckerman, & Sherman, 2010).

Of particular concern to LGBTQ older adults is a distrust of the health care system stemming from years of discrimination. These persons came of age at a time when there was much less societal acceptance of sexual and gender minorities. As a result, a perceived fear of discrimination from health care providers, as well as perceptions of a lack of understanding from them, can pose barriers to older LGBTQ adults accessing care. A study by MetLife Mature Market Institute (2006) on the LGBTQ community found that 19% of respondents reported "little or no confidence that medical personnel would treat them with dignity and respect as LGBT individuals in old age" (p. 14).

Racial/Ethnic Minorities and the Poor

There are limited data on the economic status of LGBTQ persons and its implications for their health. A New York State (NYS) report on LGBT health (Frazer & Howe, 2016) indicated that 36% of respondents had incomes below 200% of the poverty line, 40% reported being food insecure in the past year, and 36% had trouble paying for housing or utilities. These figures were even more striking for persons of color, as 46% of these individuals were below 200% of poverty, 52% were food insecure, and 47% were housing insecure. Homelessness is also a pressing concern among the LGBTQ population. Although 18% of all respondents to the NYS survey said that they had been homeless at some point in their lives, the figure rose to 30% among people of color and 28% among transgender persons. The transgender population is also more likely to live in poverty and to lack health insurance than the general population. One survey of transgender individuals reported that 48% of respondents had to forego care when they were sick because they could not afford it (Kates et al., 2016). Relatedly, studies (U.S. Department of Health and Human Services [USDHHS], 2016) have shown that young Black gay and bisexual men and transgender women are at significantly higher risk of acquiring HIV/AIDS. These subpopulations also are less likely to have health insurance coverage (USDHHS, 2016).

Rural Populations

LGBTQ persons residing in rural settings may experience health disparities when compared to those living in urban areas. In a study by Fisher, Irwin, and Coleman (2014), which examined the differences in health disparities between rural and urban LGBTQ populations, they found that rural LGBTQ individuals tended to be younger, have lower educational attainment, make less money, have higher rates of monogamous relationships, and be more inclined to live with family. Furthermore, rural participants were more likely to describe themselves as bisexual, experienced more binge drinking, smoked tobacco more frequently, and reported lower rates of health insurance coverage than those in urban areas.

DETERMINANTS OF HEALTH

There may be many factors related to these differential health outcomes of LGBTQ persons when comparing them to heterosexuals or when contrasting subgroups within the sexual and gender minority communities. These factors may include sociodemographic ones, such as race, age, geography, and income. However, as the health disparities noted herein are all stress-related conditions, there may be other factors that may be related to LGBT health (see Chapter 3, Social Determinants of Health).

There are several factors, or determinants, of health for all people. These determinants of health include behavioral, biological, environmental, and health care factors. When social workers serve the LGBTQ population, they are most attuned to factors of human behavior and the social environment. As exemplified by Minority Stress Theory (Meyer, 1995, 2003) in Figure 15.1, discrimination is a significant factor of the social environment impacting the behavioral health of LGBTQ persons.

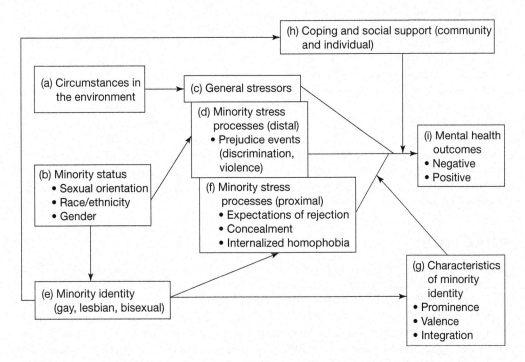

Figure 15.1 Minority Stress Theory. Conceptual model depicting the minority stress experienced by sexual and gender minorities and its relationship with mental health outcomes, general stressors, identity, and coping.

Source: Adapted from Meyer, I. H. (2003). Prejudice, social stress, and mental health in lesbian, gay, and bisexual populations: Conceptual issues and research evidence. *Psychological Bulletin, 129*(5), 674–697. Copyright 2016 by the American Psychological Association.

LGBT health disparities may be due to minority stress. Minority stress is defined as, "The excess (social) stress to which individuals from stigmatized social categories are exposed as a result of their social, often a minority, position" (Meyer, 2003, p. 675). Meyer (1995, 2003) developed this conceptual model termed minority stress theory. Meyer (1995, 2003) explains in the model how prejudice, discrimination, and the resultant stress experienced by LGBTQ persons affect their psychological health. In other words, the psychological health outcomes of LGBTQ people, such as depression and anxiety, are dependent on their environmental stressors or intrapsychic conflict surrounding their same-sex behavior, attraction, or identity. As with heterosexuals, Meyer (2003) further details in the model that LGBTQ persons can experience general stressors from environmental situations, such as poverty, that compound the impact of minority stress on their psychological health. He also describes that LGBTQ people cope with minority and general stressors to foster positive psychological health outcomes. For example, social support is a coping resource, and sexual minorities may congregate at community centers, bars, clubs, and other LGBTQ venues to cope with discriminatory experiences. Minority stress theory exemplifies a framework for understanding a societal factor of oppression and its relationship to behavioral health outcomes and possibly to health disparities of sexual minorities.

Similar to heterosexuals, LGBTQ persons may engage in behaviors that put themselves at risk of adverse physical and psychological health outcomes. For example, studies of lesbian and bisexual women reveal high rates of cigarette smoking, behaviors contributing to obesity such as inactivity and excessive caloric intake, and alcohol misuse (IOM, 2011). Ward et al. (2014) found group differences in respect to health behaviors, whereas 19.4% of heterosexual adults were current cigarette smokers, 27.2% were gay or lesbian, and 29.5% were bisexuals. Sexual minorities also reported higher rates of alcohol misuse than heterosexuals, as 35.1% of gay men and lesbians and 41.5% of bisexuals reported having five or more drinks in 1 day in the past year as opposed to 26.0% of heterosexual adults. These behaviors can be associated with stress-sensitive health conditions such as cancer, coronary disease, diabetes, and hypertension. Dearing and Hequembourg (2014) assert that one reason LGBTQ persons engage in these risky behaviors is to cope with the stigma of being a sexual minority and the concomitant stress. LGBTQ persons can internalize the negative reactions from individuals and cultural biases surrounding sexual orientation from society, which can result in feelings of low self-worth that can increase the propensity for risky behaviors such as excessive alcohol consumption (Dearing & Hequembourg, 2014).

PRACTICE

In collaboration with their clients, social workers can develop goals to increase coping and problem-solving skills to help address stressors. Following assessment, social workers can support their LGBTQ clients by understanding what strategies and processes this population uses to cope with and remain resilient against general and minority stressors. In regard to coping, McLaughlin, Hatzenbuehler, and Keyes (2010) suggest that some minorities who experience stigma suppress their emotions and do not discuss their feelings with others, are deprived of social support. Consequently, social support is a coping resource that can buffer the adverse effects of sexual orientation discrimination. Lehavot and Simoni (2011) also found that social support and, in addition, spirituality minimized the impact of minority stress on the behavioral health of lesbian and bisexual women. In regard to resiliency, two processes that are common among LGBTQ persons are positive LGB identity and emotional openness. Hill and Gunderson (2015) affirm that personal characteristics, such as optimism and positive LGB identity are characteristics in resilient LGBTQ persons. It may be that the majority of LGBTQ persons possess these personal characteristics and use these coping resources, as studies (Brown, 2012; McLaughlin et al., 2010) affirm that the majority of LGBTQ persons do not develop adverse health outcomes.

Social workers are often at the frontlines of providing services that support the health needs of LGBTQ persons; thus it is critical that they have the skills, knowledge, and attitudes necessary to provide culturally competent and responsive care. Yet stigma remains an overriding problem. LGBTQ individuals report that they often don't disclose their sexual orientation to health care workers due to the fear of stigma, to the discomfort and uncertainty about how the providers will react, and to the fear that they may receive substandard care as a result (Durso & Meyer, 2013).

Fredriksen-Goldsen, Hoy-Ellis, Goldsen, Emlet, and Hooyman (2014) proposed a set of core competencies and align them with strategies to improve professional practice and promote the well-being of LGBTQ older adults and their families. Among the competencies, which can be applied to working with LGBTQ individuals of all ages, is to "critically analyze personal and professional attitudes toward sexual orientation, gender identity, and age, and understand how factors such as culture, religion, media, and health and human service systems influence attitudes and ethical decision-making" (Fredriksen-Goldsen et al., 2014, p. 84). Unaddressed biases, they point out, can be manifest as micro-aggressions such as insults and invalidations, which can have profound effects on the mental and physical health of LGBTQ persons. Social workers need to work to overcome any biases in an effort to engage diversity and difference in practice with respect to LGBTQ issues. Social workers who openly engage diversity and difference are also better positioned to advocate for practice modalities and policies that advance the dignity and worth of LGBTQ individuals.

Engaging diversity and difference can foster trust between health care workers and clients. Building trust between social workers and the LGBTQ community is essential for the effective delivery of care. Whereas LGBTQ individuals may prefer to disclose their sexual identity to social workers, a client may avoid doing so if she, he, or ze (a gender-neutral pronoun) is assumed to be heterosexual (Mercier, Harold, Dimond, & Berlin, 2013). LGBTQ patients can respond with silence and withdrawal health care providers if they feel that trust has not been established. To help build this trust, Mercier et al. (2013) suggest that health care providers improve their knowledge and understanding about LGBT health, work on their communication skills, reflect on their personal attitudes about sexual minorities, and establish a welcoming practice environment. As specialists in communication, social workers can help to train other health care staff to communicate without judgment, to react appropriately to patient information, and ask the affirming follow-up questions.

Language can be a useful lexicon to communicate diversity and difference. Social workers need to be aware of their use of language and whether it reflects positive or negative values, attitudes, and beliefs about the LGBTQ community. Although terms such as "homosexual" and "transsexual" are used within the medical community, social workers should seek alternative vocabulary that are more validating of the realities of gender and sexual minorities. Alternatives such as "gay," "lesbian," and "transgender" are often considered more affirming, although the best practice for social workers is to respectfully ask clients what identifiers they would like to use (Kia, MacKinnon, & Legge, 2016).

A tool that can be very useful in ensuring that social workers engage diversity and difference in practice care when working with LGBTQ individuals is the Gay Affirmative Practice (GAP) scale, developed by social work scholar, Dr. Catherine Crisp. GAP requires practitioners to "celebrate and validate the identities of gay men and lesbians and actively work with these clients to confront their internalized homophobia and to develop positive identities as gay and lesbian individuals" (Crisp, 2006, p. 116). The 30-item GAP scale is intended to assess social workers' behaviors and beliefs when working with gay and lesbian individuals. It can be used as a self-assessment tool to evaluate whether social workers practice affirmatively when working with lesbian and gay individuals, or to assess the effectiveness of training programs geared toward helping practitioners work with this population. In both cases, the GAP can be instrumental in promoting more culturally competent practice with LGBTQ individuals.

Case Example 15.1

Monica is a 31-year-old African American, transgender woman who was born biologically male. She has five siblings but is estranged from all of her family members, as they have rejected her gender identity and expression. She lives in a moderately sized city and receives public assistance including SNAP and Medicaid. Off the books, Monica also supports herself by being an online prostitute.

Monica, formerly Maurice, identified herself as a gay male in her early 20s but felt as though a woman resided within her. She began transitioning to a woman at age 27. She started by taking hormones she received from another transitioning friend, Diane, who also taught her how to apply makeup and find suitable clothing. Diane told her of parties that she and other girls could attend. At these parties, the women obtained access to hormones, needles, and other items, such as collagen. Monica decided to attend these parties. She used shared needles and injected collagen into her lips to feminize them.

One day, Monica was on her way to another injection party and ran into an HIV testing and counseling mobile site. She knew one of the outreach workers, and he persuaded her to take a rapid HIV test. Monica was concerned that a client, who requested unprotected sex, may have been lying about his serostatus. Monica received her test results 15 minutes later, and she received a preliminary positive test result. Monica was distraught to learn that she was likely to be HIV+. As she processed her feelings with the counselor/tester, she told him she still planned to go to her party and would engage in risky behaviors such as needle sharing. The counselor explained what a risk this action would be to other people and referred her to primary care. Monica ignored the counselor's cautions but did later attend her medical appointment for a confirmatory test and care. A few weeks later after her primary care appointment and confirmatory test results were received, Monica was referred to the city's HIV/AIDS department and to you, a social worker employed there.

Advocacy

Given their work throughout the health care system, in hospitals, homecare, long-term care facilities, clinics, rehabilitation centers, and community agencies, among others, social workers have numerous opportunities to advocate on behalf of LGBTQ individuals. Social workers can also work collaboratively with institutions, other health care professionals, and clients to advocate for, and advance the health care needs of, the LGBTQ population. Social workers can also advocate for social change that seeks to reduce stigma and social oppression against LGBTQ individuals (Silvestre, Beatty, & Friedman, 2013).

Advocating on behalf of LGBTQ individuals is in line with the provisions of the National Association of Social Workers (NASW) Code of Ethics, which calls upon social workers to "challenge social injustice" and "pursue social change, particularly with and on behalf of vulnerable and oppressed individuals and groups of people" (NASW, 2017, p. 5). Through their advocacy efforts, social workers can makes strides toward eliminating health disparities among LGBTQ persons.

Organizations that provide LGBT health and social services should be supported, because they are often the entry point for other services, including health insurance, primary health care, mental health counseling, public benefits, and food pantries (Frazer & Howe, 2016). These organizations can also offer support groups, which can be of great assistance to LGBTQ individuals. There are a growing number of such organizations that social workers can partner with. To mention but a few, there are SAGE (Services and Advocacy for GLBT Elders), the Williams Institute, the Center for LGBT Health Research, the Family Acceptance Project, the National Coalition for LGBT Health, the National LGBTQ Task Force, and Fenway Institute.

Leadership/Administration

Organizational-level barriers to equitable health care for LGBTQ individuals include a lack of engagement of diversity and difference by health care providers, insufficient or nonexistent nondiscrimination policies, and the displaying of discriminatory behaviors. According to the Council of Social Work Education (2015), the dimensions of diversity are understood as the "intersectionality of multiple factors including but not limited to age, class, color, culture, disability and ability, ethnicity, gender, gender identity and expression, immigration status, marital status, political ideology, race, religion/spirituality, sex, sexual orientation, and tribal sovereign status" (p. 7). As a result of difference, people can either experience oppression, marginalization, and alienation, or privilege, power, and acclaim, with those in the LGBTQ community more likely to experience the former. Problems still exist in health care with explicit homophobia, along with a refusal to provide an accepted standard of care, with some health care providers admitting that they are sometimes or often uncomfortable providing care to LGBTQ patients (Khalili, Leung, & Diamant, 2015). One way to overcome these deficits is through training and education of health care staff about nondiscrimination policies and LGBTQ-inclusive procedures.

Diversity and difference training for health care providers, including social workers, as well as sensitive and inclusive clinical education, is a critical step in ensuring that LGBTQ populations receive quality health care services. As mentioned previously, stigma from health care providers was seen as a significant barrier to care among surveyed LGBTQ individuals. Training can be integrated into curricula for health care providers, at their initial training as well as in continuing education efforts. As Erdley et al. (2014) point out: "Effective competency training should address the importance of service delivery that provides for a safe and comfortable environment promoting trust and meaningful communication between provider and patient" (p. 375). Effective training will increase access among LGBTQ individuals to qualified health care professionals, especially for TGGNC individuals who perhaps have faced the greatest level of stigma and discrimination in health care.

Social workers have access to an increasing number of continuing education opportunities. The continuing education opportunities have been designed to increase social workers' knowledge about the unique needs of LGBTQ individuals, so as to enhance quality treatment of this population (Dearing & Hequembourg, 2014). In line with the provision of culturally competent care called for by the NASW, all social workers have a responsibility to improve their knowledge and sensitivity to sexual minority clients.

In order to increase participation in continuing education efforts that can improve the level of cultural competency, the trainings need to be engaging, easily accessible, and affordable, and ideally, mandatory (Dearing & Hequembourg, 2014).

Other ways to address disparities in health care access is for providers to use more sensitive and inclusive language in verbal and written communication, including on forms. Patients also need a comfortable and welcoming environment so that they feel safe to discuss their sexual and gender identity (Wilkerson, Rybiki, Barber, & Smolenski, 2011). Some suggestions offered by the Gay and Lesbian Medical Association include posting rainbow stickers in offices and providing pamphlets from LGBTQ nonprofits in medical clinics, which could improve the comfort level of LGBTQ clients (Erdley et al., 2014). Having gender-neutral bathrooms is also another way to signal that the health care environment is welcoming and free from discrimination and judgment (McClain, Hawkins, & Yehia, 2016).

POLICY

The increasing societal acceptance of LGBTQ persons has influenced corresponding shifts in the policy and legal landscape that have increased access to care and insurance coverage for sexual and gender minorities. These gains include the implementation of the Patient Protection and Affordable Care Act (ACA), the Supreme Court ruling in *Obergefell v. Hodges*, which legalized same-sex marriage nationally, and the efforts by the Obama administration to promote equal treatment of LGBTQ individuals in the health care system (Kates et al., 2016).

Although the future of the ACA remains uncertain as of this writing, it is nonetheless useful to highlight some of the changes it made with respect to LGBT health. One area is the increase of insurance coverage, either through the expansion of Medicaid or through coverage in insurance marketplaces. As a result of the ACA, the share of uninsured LGBTQ adults is estimated to have declined from 21.7% in 2013 to 11.1% in 2015. The ACA also contains important nondiscrimination provisions, as it prohibits discrimination on the basis of sex, which is defined to include sex stereotypes and gender identity, for any health program receiving federal funds, including Medicaid and Medicare. Federal regulations also bar discrimination in insurance plans based on sexual orientation and gender identity. Finally, the ACA requires expanded data collection efforts, such as the inclusion of questions on sexual orientation in national surveys, as discussed (Kates et al., 2016).

The Obama administration also took proactive steps to promote greater equity in health care for LGBTQ individuals. In June 2016, the announcement was made of a new Senior Advisor for LGBT health within the Office of the Assistant Secretary for Health (OASH). And a few months later, the National Institutes of Health (NIH) officially designated sexual and gender minorities as a health disparity population for purposes of research, as mentioned. The USDHHS also established an LGBT Policy Coordinating Committee (https://www.hhs.gov/programs/topic-sites/lgbt/reports/index.html) to help harmonize efforts with respect to LGBTQ policies among a number of agencies and departments (USDHHS, 2016).

Since 2010, the USDHHS has implemented a number of strategies to improve the health status of LGBTQ individuals, including: (a) increasing nondiscrimination protections in health care; (b) improving awareness of LGBT health and human services in communities and the workplace; (c) increasing capacity to serve LGBTQ communities; (d) collecting better data; and (e) coordinating research efforts to close information gaps on health disparities. With respect to nondiscrimination, for example, the Centers for Medicare and Medicaid Services issued a rule stating that patients have the right to have visitors of their choice, including "same sex domestic partners," and that advance directives are equally available to LGBTQ families (USDHHS, 2016).

Throughout this book, access to health care has been identified as a barrier for many individuals. This is even more prominent for the LGBTQ population. For example, Ward et al. (2014) found differences in health care access among adult women with 85.5% of heterosexuals reporting a usual place to go for medical care compared to just 75.6% of lesbians and 71.6% of bisexuals. Similarly, in a study of LGBTQ persons in NYS, Frazer and Howe (2016) found that nearly 23% of respondents had no primary health care provider and 22% had not been to a health care provider in the past year due to cost. Consequently, health care costs may be a factor related to health care barriers. Ward et al. (2014) similarly found that more women, who identified as lesbian (15.2%), did not obtain needed medical care due to cost than women who identified as heterosexual (9.6%). As there were no significant differences in uninsurance rates by sexual orientation, medical insurance coverage is likely not a factor in these differential outcomes. Besides cost, the cultural incompetence of health care providers may be another reason why LGBTQ persons may not access or may experience barriers to health care services. Frazer and Howe (2016) found that 31% of all LGB and 56% of transgender respondents reported that a health care barrier was not having health professionals trained in LGBTQ cultural competency. Nearly 10% of respondents also reported that they were denied health care services.

Transgender persons face similar and unique barriers to care including health insurance coverage and identity documents with information that may not be consistent with their current gender identity and/or expression. Frazer and Howe (2016) found that only 18% of transgender respondents had tried to change their identity documents while 36% wanted to change their documents but had not yet done so. Transgender respondents (43%) also noted issues that included not having confirmation-related care co-located with primary health care services (43%) and that insurance did not cover hormone therapy (62%). Kates et al. (2016) noted that many health plans specifically exclude coverage for vitally important health care services, such as sex confirmation surgery, mental health services, and hormone therapy (Kates et al., 2016), which are all necessary for the gender confirmatory process.

Social workers can help to ensure that policies are implemented in a way that ensures that LGBTQ individuals have access to high quality health care that engages diversity and difference, and is accepting and affirming. Social workers also needed to advocate for the LGBTQ community's health needs and for health care equity. For example, bullying has been identified as a major problem encountered by LGBTQ youth, and the development of effective anti-bullying interventions is necessary to prevent adverse health outcomes such as depression and suicidality. Moreover, particular attention is needed for TGGNC individuals, who can encounter additional challenges with respect to health care. Among these challenges is having identity documents that may not match their gender identity or expression. Changing these documents can be problematic, especially for public benefits such as Medicaid, and social workers are needed to assist TGGNC individuals navigate the often convoluted process of aligning their identity documents with their gender identity and expression.

RESEARCH

It is estimated that the existing literature on LGBT health represents only one tenth of one percent of the total peer-reviewed literature (Boehmer, 2002). There is limited research on the LGBTQ community, especially for bisexual and transgender populations. Furthermore, much of the research that has been conducted to date has been on HIV prevention and treatment, with most of this research examining gay men or men who have sex with men, a term used to describe males who engage in same-sex behavior but may not identify as a gay or bisexual. Since 1984, articles on men who have sex with men outnumber articles on other LGBTQ-related issues by at least two to one (Snyder, 2011). Moreover, this research has focused on factors affecting risk behaviors such as substance use and sexual risk, whether a person gets tested for HIV, insufficient health care utilization, and poor treatment adherence. As a result, it has had a tendency to overshadow other LGBTQ research, as well as led to a focus on disease and risk (Bogart, Revenson, Whitfield, & France, 2014).

An important consideration when looking at LGBT health research is that data on health disparities have only recently begun to be collected on a national level. The first time that the federal government made available nationally representative data on sexual orientation was in 2013. With the historic lack of national data on sexual orientation and gender identity, the majority of LGBT health research has been conducted with small, nonrepresentative samples (Kates et al., 2016). These respondents are also disproportionately focused on sexual minorities, such as lesbian, gay men, and bisexuals with less attention to transgender persons. The knowledge gap is beginning to be addressed, as the ACA now requires data collection on health disparities, including LGBTQ ones. The federal government also recently approved the addition of sexual orientation and gender identity questions in a key, national, and annual investigation, the Behavioral Risk Factor Surveillance System surveys (Kates et al., 2016).

A report issued by the IOM in 2011 on the state of research and science regarding the health of LGBTQ people was the first comprehensive overview of the field, and its recommendations have spurred further work on LGBT health. The NIH also established the Sexual and Gender Minority Research Office (SGMRO), which coordinates sexual and gender minority-related research and activities (USDHHS, 2016). The NIH designated sexual and gender minorities as a health disparity population, which will encourage researchers to collect and analyze data to better understand health disparities among LGBTQ populations (USDHHS, 2016).

Although these steps have helped to close the research gap on the health of LGBTQ individuals, additional research by social workers is still needed, particularly on special populations, including youth, older adults, racial and ethnic minorities, the poor, and rural populations. For example, there remains limited information about LGBTQ older adults' access to health care, although what is known suggests that they are medically underserved and more likely to experience health problems than heterosexual older adults (Morrison & Dinkel, 2012). Similarly, limited research has been conducted on rural LGBTQ persons, as the majority of literature contains samples of urban sexual and gender minorities. What little research that has been done on rural populations has focused on their mental health needs, access to services, and gender identity in conservative rural areas (Fisher et al., 2014).

Social workers can be at the forefront of efforts to improve LGBT health research. Social work researchers guided by our professional values can address the gaps in knowledge through their own investigations of LGBTQ persons, their health, and the contextual factors such as oppression that impact morbidity and mortality. As Mercier et al. (2013) point out, additional research can help social workers in improving policy, creating training programs to reduce homophobia among practitioners, and promoting culturally competent practice. Research can also promote more effective education and advocacy efforts, and can raise awareness of where change is needed in institutional and professional contexts.

CONCLUSION

The LGBTQ community has experienced gains in societal acceptance, especially during the last decade. Despite these advances, health disparities persist among this population when compared to heterosexuals and when subpopulations are contrasted. LGBTQ people are disproportionately represented in stress-related medical conditions, psychiatric disorders, and emotional problems, which can be compounded by health care access issues and barriers. A significant, contributing factor to these disparities and outcomes is minority stress. Guided by our professional code, social workers possess the capabilities to serve the LGBTQ community in a culturally competent and responsive manner. By affirming the identity, expressions, and behaviors of sexual and gender minorities as equal to heterosexuals, social workers can employ the various practice methods of research, policy, advocacy, leadership, and direct practice to empower LGBTQ persons and help them achieve equity in health care.

CHAPTER DISCUSSION QUESTIONS

1. Why is it important to understand LGBT health disparities for social work practice?

2. What are factors that social workers should be aware of when working with LGBTQ subpopulations, such as older adults, racial/ethnic minorities, and the poor?

3. What areas of LGBT health research can social workers become involved with?

4. Describe ways in which social workers can advocate for policies that advance LGBT health. You may use current and pending policies to inform your explanations.

5. Do you think that continuing education to improve LGBTQ diversity and difference practice among health care workers should be mandatory? Why or why not?

6. What are ways that social workers can help to make health care settings more welcoming and affirming to LGBTQ individuals?

7. How can social workers engage in self-reflection of their own biases in preparation for working with LGBTQ individuals?

CASE EXAMPLE AND DISCUSSION QUESTIONS

Case Example 15.2

Crystal is an 11-year-old White girl, who is questioning her sexual orientation. She is the youngest of three children to her parents, Chuck and Debbie. Crystal and her family live in a small town near a national park in a southwestern state. Chuck and Debbie are devout Mormons, and they along with their children attend their meetinghouse every Sunday. Chuck is a plumber, and Debbie works as a teacher in the public school in their town. Crystal attends the same school where her mother works.

Crystal has been a strong student in school where and usually earns all "A" grades on her report cards. She has been active in class and is generally well-liked by her peers. You are the school social worker, and Crystal's homeroom teacher, Amanda, has

(continued)

Case Example 15.2   *(continued)*

referred Crystal to you. Amanda has observed that Crystal has become withdrawn in class and has not completed her homework for the past month. Amanda mentioned that she told Debbie her concern, but she dismissed it. She also noted that Crystal's classmates have begun teasing her, and Amanda had to break up a fight between Crystal and her friend, Jenny. You begin to meet regularly with Crystal. After several meetings, Crystal confides that she has developed a crush on her classmate, Jenny, and Jenny has spread a rumor to all of her classmates that Crystal is a lesbian. Crystal is worried that her mother, Debbie, will find out and has expressed suicidality should her parents know of her crush.

Questions for Discussion

1. As the school social worker, how would you begin to engage and build a relationship with Crystal?

2. What contextual factors are likely associated with Crystal's feelings and behaviors?

3. How could you foster an affirming school environment for Crystal?

REFERENCES

Alexander, R., Parker, K., & Schwetz, T. (2016). Sexual and gender minority health research at the National Institutes of Health. *LGBT Health, 3*(1), 7–10. doi:10.1089/lgbt.2015.0107

American Psychological Association. (2015). Guidelines for psychological practice with transgender and gender nonconforming people. *American Psychologist, 70*(9), 832–864. doi:10.1037/a0039906

American Psychological Association. (n.d.). Definitions related to sexual orientation and gender diversity in APA documents. Retrieved from http://www.apa.org/pi/lgbt/resources/sexuality-definitions.pdf

Boehmer, U. (2002). Twenty years of public health research: Inclusion of lesbian, gay, bisexual, and transgender populations. *American Journal of Public Health, 92*(7), 1125–1130.

Bogart, L., Revenson, T., Whitfield, K., & France, C. (2014). Introduction to the special section on lesbian, gay, bisexual, and transgender (LGBT) health disparities: Where we are and where we're going. *Annals of Behavior Medicine, 47*, 1–4. doi:10.1007/s12160-013-9574-7

Brown, D. B. (2012). Effects of distal minority stress on lesbian, gay and bisexual psychological health and context (Doctoral dissertation). Retrieved from ProQuest Dissertations Publishing. (UMI No. 3544981)

Council on Social Work Education. (2015). Educational policy and accreditation standards. Retrieved from https://www.cswe.org/getattachment/Accreditation/Standards-and-Policies/2015-EPAS/2015EPASandGlossary.pdf.aspx

Crisp, C. (2006). The gay affirmative practice scale (GAP): A new measure for assessing cultural competence with gay and lesbian clients. *Social Work, 51*(2), 115–126. doi:10.1093/sw/51.2.115

Dearing, R., & Hequembourg, A. (2014). Culturally (in)competent? Dismantling health care barriers for sexual minority women. *Social Work in Health Care, 53*(8), 739–761. doi:10.1080/00981389.2014.944250

Durso, L., & Meyer, I. (2013). Patterns and predictors of disclosure of sexual orientation to health care providers among lesbians, gay men, and bisexuals. *Sexuality Research and Social Policy, 10*(1), 35–42. doi:10.1007/s13178-012-0105-2

Erdley, S., Anklam, D., & Reardon, C. (2014). Breaking barriers and building bridges: Understanding the pervasive needs of older LGBT adults and the value of social work in health care. *Journal of Gerontological Social Work, 57*(2–4), 362–385. doi:10.1080/01634372.2013.871381

Fisher, C., Irwin, J., & Coleman, J. (2014). LGBT health in the midlands: A rural/urban comparison of basic health indicators. *Journal of Homosexuality, 61,* 1062–1090. doi:10.1080/00918369.2014.872487

Flores, A. R., Herman, J. L., Gates, G. J., & Brown, T. N. T. (2016). How many adults identify as transgender in the United States? Retrieved from The Williams Institute website: https://williamsinstitute.law.ucla.edu

Frazer, M., & Howe, E. (2016). LGBT health and human services needs in New York State: A report from the 2015 LGBT health and human services needs assessment. New York, NY: The Lesbian, Gay, Bisexual & Transgender Community Center. Retrieved from https://gaycenter.org/thenetwork

Fredriksen-Goldsen, K., Hoy-Ellis, C., Goldsen, J., Emlet, C., & Hooyman, N. (2014). Creating a vision for the future: Key competencies and strategies for culturally competent practice with lesbian, gay, bisexual, and transgender (LGBT) older adults in the health and human services. *Journal of Gerontological Social Work, 57*(2–4), 80–107. doi:10.1080/01634372.2014.890690

Gates, G. J. (2014). LGBT demographics: Comparisons among population-based surveys. Retrieved from The Williams Institute website: https://williamsinstitute.law.ucla.edu

Gates, G. J., & Newport, F. (2012). Gallup special report: The U.S. adult LGBT population. Retrieved from https://williamsinstitute.law.ucla.edu

Heyman, J., Kelly, P., White-Ryan, L., Koch, D., Gregory, R., & Farmer, G. (2017). *Westchester Building Futures (WBF): LGBTQI2-S Report*. West Harrison, NY: Author.

Hill, C. A., & Gunderson, C. J. (2015). Resilience of lesbian, gay, and bisexual individuals in relation to social environment, personal characteristics, and emotion regulation strategies. *Psychology of Sexual Orientation and Gender Diversity, 2*(3), 232–252. doi:10.1037/sgd0000129

Institute of Medicine. (2011). The health of lesbian, gay, bisexual, and transgender people: Building a foundation for a better understanding. Retrieved from http://www.nationalacademies.org/HMD/Reports/2011/The-Health-of-Lesbian-Gay-Bisexual-and-Transgender-People.aspx

James, S. E., Herman, J. L., Rankin, S., Keisling, M., Mottet, L., & Anafi, M. (2016). The report of the 2015 U.S. transgender survey. Retrieved from National Center for Transgender Equality website: http://www.ustranssurvey.org/report

Kates, J., Ranji, U., Beamesderfer, A., Salganicoff, A., & Dawson, L. (2016). Health and access to care and coverage for lesbian, gay, bisexual, and transgender individuals in the U.S. Menlo Park, CA: The Henry J. Kaiser Family Foundation. Issue Brief, November 2016.

Khalili, J., Leung, L., & Diamant, A. (2015). Finding the perfect doctor: Identifying lesbian, gay, bisexual, and transgender-competent physicians. *American Journal of Public Health, 105*(6), 1114–1119. doi:10.2105/AJPH.2014.302448

Kia, H., MacKinnon, K., & Legge, M. (2016). In pursuit of change: Conceptualizing the social work response to LGBTQ microaggressions in health settings. *Social Work in Health Care, 55*(10), 806–825. doi:10.1080/00981389.2016.1231744

Lehavot, K., & Simoni, J. M. (2011). The impact of minority stress on mental health and substance use among sexual minority women. *Journal of Consulting and Clinical Psychology, 79*(2), 159–170. doi:10.1037/a0022839

McCarthy, J. (2016, January 18). Satisfaction with acceptance of gays in U.S. at new high. Retrieved from Gallup website: http://www.gallup.com/poll/188657/satisfaction-acceptance-gays-new-high.aspx

McClain, Z., Hawkins, L., & Yehia, B. (2016). Creating welcoming spaces for lesbian, gay, bisexual, and transgender (LGBT) patients: An evaluation of the health care environment. *Journal of Homosexuality, 63*(3), 387–393. doi:10.1080/00918369.2016.1124694

McLaughlin, K. A., Hatzenbuehler, M. L., & Keyes, K. M. (2010). Responses to discrimination and psychiatric disorders among black, Hispanic, female, and lesbian, gay, and bisexual individuals. *American Journal of Public Health, 100*(8), 1477–1484. doi:10.2105/AJPH.2009.181586

Mercier, L., Harold, R., Dimond, M., & Berlin, S. (2013). Lesbian health care: Women's experiences and the role of social work. *Journal of Social Service Research, 39*, 16–37. doi:10.1080/01488376.2012.730905

MetLife Mature Market Institute. (2006). *Out and aging: The MetLife study of lesbian and gay baby boomers.* Westport, CT: Author.

Meyer, I. H. (1995). Minority stress and mental health in gay men. *Journal of Health and Social Behavior, 36*(1), 38–56.

Meyer, I. H. (2003). Prejudice, social stress, and mental health in lesbian, gay, and bisexual populations: Conceptual issues and research evidence. *Psychological Bulletin, 129*(5), 674–697. doi:10.1037/0033-2909.129.5.674

Morrison, S., & Dinkel, S. (2012). Heterosexism and health care: A concept analysis. *Nursing Forum, 47*, 123–130. doi:10.1111/j.1744-6198.2011.00243.x

National Association of Social Workers. (2017). Code of Ethics. Retrieved from https://www.socialworkers.org/About/Ethics/Code-of-Ethics/Code-of-Ethics-English

National LGBT Health Education Center, a program of the Fenway Institute. (2016). Glossary of LGBT terms for health care teams. Retrieved from https://www.lgbthealtheducation.org/wp-content/uploads/LGBT-Glossary_March2016.pdf

Ray, N. (2006). *Lesbian, gay, bisexual and transgender youth: An epidemic of homelessness.* New York, NY: National Gay and Lesbian Task Force Policy Institute and the National Coalition for the Homeless. Retrieved from http://www.thetaskforce.org/static_html/downloads/HomelessYouth.pdf

Silvestre, A., Beatty, R., & Friedman, M. (2013). Substance use disorder in the context of LGBT health: A social work perspective. *Social Work in the Public Health, 28*, 366–376. doi:10.1080/19371918.2013.774667

Snyder, J. E. (2011). Trend analysis of medical publications about LGBT persons: 1950–2007. *Journal of Homosexuality, 58,* 164–188. doi:10.1080/00918369.2011.540171

Stein, G. L., Beckerman, N. L., & Sherman, P. A. (2010). Lesbian and gay elders and long term care: Identifying the unique psychosocial perspectives and challenges. *Journal of Gerontological Social Work, 53,* 421–435. doi:10.1080/01634372.2010.496478

U.S. Department of Health and Human Services. (2016). Advancing LGBT health and well-being: 2016 report. HHS LGBT Policy Coordinating Committee.

Ward, B., Dahlhamer, J., Galinsky, A., & Joestl, S. (2014). *Sexual orientation and health among U.S. adults: National Health Interview Survey, 2013.* National Health Statistics Reports No. 77. Hyattsville, MD: National Center for Health Statistics.

Wilkerson, J.M., Rybicki, S., Barber, C.A., & Smolenski, D.J. (2011). Creating a culturally competent clinical environment for LGBT patients. *Journal of Gay & Lesbian Social Services, 23*(3), 376–394. doi:10.1080/10538720.2011.589254

Health Care and Disability

Jeanne Matich-Maroney, Ralph Gregory, and Vincent Corcoran

While definitions of disability vary, virtually all now emphasize functional status over diagnostic category. According to the World Health Organization (WHO, 2017),

> Disabilities is an umbrella term, covering impairments, activity limitations, and participation restrictions. An impairment is a problem in body function or structure; an activity limitation is a difficulty encountered by an individual in executing a task or action; while a participation restriction is a problem experienced by an individual in involvement in life situations.
>
> Disability is thus not just a health problem. It is a complex phenomenon, reflecting the interaction between features of a person's body and features of the society in which he or she lives. Overcoming the difficulties faced by people with disabilities requires interventions to remove environmental and social barriers. (www.who.int/topics/disabilities/en)

To measure disability prevalence rates, conceptual definitions such as that noted by the WHO must be operationalized for the purposes of data collection. The annual American Community Survey (ACS) conducted by the U.S. Census Bureau is considered the most current and accurate measure of disability prevalence rates. The ACS captures disability data based on functional limitations in six domains including, vision, hearing, cognitive, ambulatory, self-care, and independent living (Erickson, Lee, & von Schrader, 2017).

In 2015, the annual ACS estimated 12.6% of the U.S. population was living with a disability (Erickson et al., 2017). ACS data indicate that disability rates increase by age cohorts. Among children and adolescents, ages 5 to 15, the rate was 5.3%, 10.2% for persons aged 16 to 64, and 35.5% for persons aged 65 and older (Erickson et al., 2017). Overall, the 2015 ACS estimated that approximately 40 million Americans are living with a disability.

While the ACS collects some data relative to disability among young children (i.e., those under 5), its primary focus is on those 5 years of age and older, and thus, actually underrepresents the prevalence of disability among children. Nonetheless, data for children under age 5 were reported for hearing and visual disabilities. For children under age 5, 0.4% reported a visual disability and 0.5% reported a hearing disability (Erickson et al., 2017). For hearing disability, 3.6% of the population identified as having hearing impairments, but this increased by age, "rising to 2.0% of 18–64 year olds, and to 14.8%

of those ages 65 and over" (Kraus, 2017, p. 12). Visual disabilities were reported in 2.3% of the population. Interestingly, cognitive disabilities and ambulatory disability saw the greatest differences by age. For cognitive disability, children and adolescents represented 4.1% of the population, and 4.5% for persons aged 18 to 64; however, 9.0% of older adults had cognitive disabilities (Kraus, 2017). Ambulatory disabilities for children ages 5 to 17 represent 0.6%, 5.1% for persons aged 18 to 64, and 22.6% for older adults (Kraus, 2017). Self-care limitations were reported by 2.5% while limitations in independent living were reported by 4.5% of the survey respondents (Kraus, 2017).

Racial and ethnic disparities as well as income disparities are prevalent in the census data relative to people with disabilities. The Centers for Disease Control and Prevention (CDC) found differences among racial and ethnic groups, with American Indian/Alaska Native, biracial and multiracial groups, and Black/African Americans having the highest percentages of disabilities (CDC, 2016a, 2016b). In addition, a direct association between disability and higher levels of poverty were observed in the data; as income increased, reported disability decreased (CDC, 2016a, 2016b). As can be gleaned from these data, a number of social and physical determinants of health appear to have a disproportionately negative impact on people with disabilities.

BACKGROUND

"From the earliest recorded history, people with disabilities have been ostracized, rejected, and discriminated against in society" (Mackelprang & Salsgiver, 1996, p. 7). Indeed, in the United States, individuals with disabilities have historically been demonized, imprisoned, shunned, and subjected to forced dependence within a disempowering medical model of health care and social service. Societal values and attitudes about people with disabilities have evolved over time, in large measure due to the efforts of pioneering disability activists, and eventually, the collective advocacy of the Disability Rights Movement that emerged in the latter part of the 20th century.

In the mid-late 1800s, Dorothea Dix, an early advocate for persons with psychiatric and other disabilities, spent her life investigating the squalid conditions of jails where many with disabilities were warehoused. Gollaher (1995) recounts how Dorothea Dix explored the conditions in jail throughout the country; the following is a brief excerpt regarding one of her visits to a Massachusetts jail:

> When she entered the jail and asked to examine it—the story goes her presence caused the jailer considerable consternation. Unable to fathom why a genteel-looking lady would want to walk through the dirty stinking facility, he at first suggested she must be deranged herself and perhaps ought to be under his control and not inquiring into the condition of those who were (p. 126).

Dix's work documented the conditions of individuals housed in jails, prompting the establishment of public asylums as an alternative to prison, and, at least on the face of it, a more humanitarian approach to the care of those with disabilities.

In the ensuing years, the philosophy of social Darwinism and eugenics came into prominence (Mackelprang & Salsgiver, 1996, p. 7). Premised on beliefs in genetic superiority, selection, and breeding, eugenics is often associated in the minds of many with the practices of Nazi Germany. In actuality, the Eugenics Movement got its start in the United States (Black, 2003). American eugenics practices included the forced sterilization of those deemed "inferior" so as to prevent their ability to reproduce. Many corporate foundations in America funded the movement and a number of universities included education and training in eugenics (Black, 2003). An initial legal challenge against involuntary sterilization was mounted in 1927 with the *Buck v. Bell* Supreme Court case, and a second challenge came in 1942 in *Skinner v. Oklahoma.* However, it wasn't until the 1974 *Relf v. Weinberger* case that informed consent for sterilization was mandated and the use of federal funds for involuntary sterilization discontinued (Singleton, 2014).

For much of the 20th century, American society continued to warehouse people with disabilities in large public institutions (Trattner, 1999). However, by mid-century, the increasingly expansive reach of television began to reshape public perceptions of people with disabilities, essentially by bringing them out of the shadows and into people's living rooms. Celebrities such as comedian Jerry Lewis hosted annual telethons introducing the nation to children with muscular dystrophy in the hope of raising funds to find a cure. Television news broadcasted the toll of Vietnam War casualties, many of whom were returning home as individuals with disabilities. It also contributed to raising awareness by exposing the squalid living conditions, neglect, and abuse in state institutions designed to serve people with disabilities. The heightened collective consciousness spurred by TV news images fueled action prompting both the deinstitutionalization of people with intellectual and developmental disabilities as well as the gradual and incremental expansion of health and other support services offered by the Veterans Administration.

The Mental Retardation and Community Mental Health Centers Act signed into law by President John F. Kennedy in 1963 initiated the move away from the common practice of institutionalizing those with psychiatric, developmental, or intellectual disabilities (formerly known as mental retardation). People with psychiatric disabilities living in state mental health facilities were the first to be discharged to the community under the mandates of this legislation. While it was an important piece of legislation that authorized considerable redirection of resources to community-based services and supports, the crucial element of planning for the full range of services and the timing of their rollout was not well executed and resulted in the unintended consequence of patients falling through the cracks, many of whom were subsequently lost to homelessness.

The Rehabilitation Act of 1973 constituted a galvanizing force in the disability rights movement as it represented the first time that people with disabilities were collectively recognized as a minority group and thus entitled to certain protections under the law. This act supported individuals as they transitioned from institutions to community living through the provision of a range of services, such as home modifications, support for personal care, and the pursuit of rehabilitation goals and gainful employment. Section 504 also called for local school districts to provide a "free appropriate public education" (FAPE) for all students with disabilities registered within their jurisdictions (U.S. Department of Education, 2015).

Community-based living for people with disabilities was further supported by the 1975 Willowbrook Decree. Willowbrook was a state-supported school for children with intellectual and developmental disabilities in New York State. Conditions at the Willowbrook State School, and quality of life for its residents spurred the battle for millions of dollars to be redirected to community-based services and residential options for people with intellectual and developmental disabilities (Peele, 1985). Moreover, the active engagement of families of individuals with intellectual/developmental disabilities in the design and planning for the shift from institutional to community-based care yielded far greater success than that experienced in the discharge of residents of state mental health institutions.

The Americans with Disabilities Act (ADA) is a landmark in civil rights legislation for people with disabilities, signed into law by President George H. W. Bush in 1990 (ADA, 1990, 2008). This civil rights law prohibits discrimination against persons with disabilities, and advanced the access agenda of the Disability Rights Movement by codifying equal opportunities in employment, public facilities, and commercial facilities and other areas (ADA, 1990). Through the provisions of this act, opportunities for people with disabilities to work, live independently, and participate in their communities have been significantly enhanced.

In 2008, the ADA Amendments Act further clarified both the meaning and interpretation of disability to ensure that its original, intentionally broad definition would be applied. On July 15, 2016, Attorney General Loretta Lynch signed a Final Rule incorporating the requirements of the ADA Amendments Act into the ADA Title II and Title III regulations. The Final Rule took effect in October 2016.

PRACTICE

Considering the broad definition of disability, social workers have historically been engaged in service to people with disabilities and their families in a myriad of capacities—as early intervention providers, school social workers, youth development counselors, medical social workers, clinical social workers, and substance abuse counselors. However, the consistency of the profession's commitment to the collective population of people with disabilities has not always been so evident. "From the beginning, social work has viewed itself as the profession with primary responsibility toward people who are subjected to discrimination and oppression. However, the profession has not embraced the causes of people with disabilities as it has other oppressed groups" (Mackelprang & Salsgiver, 1996, p. 7). Although the Disability Rights Movement has achieved a great deal with the passage of the ADA in 1990 and its subsequent amendments, considerable work remains (Bean & Hedgpeth, 2014; Dunn, Hanes, Hardie, & MacDonald, 2006; Meekosha & Dowse, 2007). The social work profession, guided by its ethical imperative to pursue social and economic justice, and informed by its strengths, empowerment, and ecological systems perspectives, is uniquely situated to support the rights of people with disabilities, particularly in relation to advancing consumer-driven approaches to care.

As noted, social workers have occupied a myriad of roles in their work with people with disabilities over the years. Typically, these roles are defined by practice setting and specific populations served, but generally involve both direct and indirect service provision. In the context of those roles, they "wear many hats," often functioning as advocates, brokers, mediators, educators, and facilitators adjunctive to their primary responsibilities.

The spirit and language of the ADA (as written in 1990 and amended in 2008 and 2016) echo and validate the strengths, empowerment, and ecological systems perspectives of social work practice. Moreover, the recent emphasis on addressing the social and physical determinants of health is uniquely suited to the wheelhouse of the social work profession. Collaboratively tackling health inequalities and disparities, promoting access and accommodations for people with disabilities in concert with those directly impacted by them are opportunities for the profession to make broad and meaningful contributions to enhancing the health and well-being of people with disabilities.

Children and Youth

Working with children and youth with disabilities requires that the social worker engage with their families, and particularly their parents. Parents have characterized their varied experiences interacting with professionals in disability services from extremely positive to dishearteningly negative (Hiebert-Murphy, Trute, & Wright, 2008). Social workers must recognize the heterogeneity in parental responses to their child's disability diagnosis, assess how the parental perception impacts family functioning, and tailor interventions to dually address emotional support and concrete service needs (Hiebert et al., 2008).

Family-centered approaches have long helped guide social work practice in child welfare, child mental health, and early intervention (Strock-Lynskey & Keller, 2007). As highlighted by Strock-Lynskey and Keller (2007), there are many strengths to this model when effectively implemented:

> *Family-centered practice is flexible, individualized, collaborative, and acknowledges the longevity of the family's involvement with the child (Mahoney, Boyce, Fewell, Spiker, & Wheeden, 1998) with the goal of providing services and support to families in order for them to support and maintain family functioning (Dunst, 2002). A family-centered model not only values the participation of the family in the development of the individualized family service plan (IFSP), but also supports family partnerships in program and policy development in the early intervention system and in other educational settings as well. (Dunst, 2002, as cited in Strock-Lynsky & Keller, 2007, p. 115)*

Recognizing the need for improved service to youth with disabilities, Strock-Lynskey and Keller (2007) constructed a conceptual family-centered framework focused on the understanding that youth with disabilities and their families may present with a host of different experiences. Within the context of this framework, Strock-Lynskey and Keller (2007) offer guidance for social workers. These guidelines are briefly summarized in the following. For more detail please see Strock-Lynskey and Keller (2007, pp. 129–130).

- Approach each family as unique
- Establish genuine collaboration with the family as a whole
- Actively engage the child, parents, and family as partners in the planning and implementation of care
- Promote maximal family participation through the provision of information, skills training, and resources
- Adopt a person-centered planning model to address the needs of the child/adolescent with a disability
- Recognize and continually assess the needs of siblings
- Support the family's rights to make choices, determine their own priorities, and identify the resources or supports necessary to promote optimal family functioning
- Empower families to become disability advocates or work as an advocate for the family
- Facilitate the full participation of the child and family as members of the interprofessional team serving the child/adolescent's needs
- Continually enhance one's knowledge and understanding of the intersectionality of diverse identities including that of disability and infuse it into the family-centered approach to work with children/adolescents with disabilities and their families

Adults

People with disabilities have different needs that vary by age, location, type and duration of disability, nature of support systems, as well as other factors that may impact their lives. Meaningful employment is an important opportunity for almost all adults. Individuals with disabilities tend to remain unemployed for longer periods of time than persons without a disability, and when they are employed, they typically earn less (Erickson et al., 2016). An early national longitudinal study of disability found that consumers of vocational rehabilitation services were more likely to obtain employment (Hayward & Schmidt-Davis, 2003). This is an important research finding as it has implications for the economic self-sufficiency and social interactions of people with disabilities, both of which are identified as significant health determinants. Thus, social workers need to be aware of the important role employment may play in health promotion for people with disability and conversely, the potential implications its absence may impose.

Older Adults

Aging often exacerbates previously diagnosed disabilities, whether cognitive or physical, and may also lead to the diagnosis of newly formed disabilities that are often consequences of the aging process alone (e.g., hearing loss, mobility problems). With the aging population increasing in the United States, social workers need to equip themselves with knowledge of care practices and interventions for this population.

One area of assessment critical to working with aging populations is mobility. Parker, Baker, and Allman (2002) promote the use of their Life-Space mobility assessment in elder care populations. Life space is defined as the capacity of the person to meaningfully move within their home environment and beyond. The assessment is comprised of six categorical levels that may constitute an elderly individual's environment: bedroom, home, outside home, neighborhood, town, and unrestricted. Parker et al. (2002) explain how this type of assessment may be beneficial to social work practice:

> Each level of Life-Space represents the person-in-environment, a theoretical approach widely used in social work practice. This allows the social worker to get a good impression of how the person has adapted to aging by observing an overview of where he/she might fit in the distribution range. In addition, it provides a "snap shot" of a person's routine. (p. 41)

The Life-Space assessment improves the ability of geriatrics social workers to emphasize the necessity of particular services and facilitate more efficacious supports or interventions for mobility deficits (Parker et al., 2002).

Older adults include those who have aged while diagnosed with a severe mental illness (SMI). Frequently individuals aging with SMI experience increased physical illness, functional impairment, cognitive deficits, and social disability (Cummings & Kropf, 2011). Unfortunately, there remains a scarcity of age-targeted services available for older individuals with serious psychiatric illnesses. However, Cummings and Kropf (2011) highlight the importance of positioning social workers at the forefront of program development:

> Social workers can play a vital role in the development of mental health programs tailored to the needs of an aging SMI population. It is critical that such programs focus not only on the psychological needs of older clients, but also on their social and medical needs as well. Training in the biopsychosocial model enables social workers to take a more holistic approach in framing programs to meet complex client needs. (p. 183)

As noted previously, some disabilities emerge as part of the aging process. However, there may be preventive strategies that can be promoted to forestall or delay the emergence of some disabilities in older adulthood. For example, Janke, Payne, and Van Puymbroeck (2008) found in a sample of 535 adults aged 65 and older that engagement in informal and formal leisure activities was associated with lower cognitive deficits, less functional impairment, and decreased self-perceptions of disability. Given this, social workers should be mindful of the potential importance of continued leisure activity and initiate discussion with older adult clients about it.

Living arrangements and/or housing may pose a challenge for adults as they age. As older adults proceed through the life course, there may be a need to acknowledge emerging challenges, and to reassess priorities, including that of living situations (Lawton, 1986), which may be closely associated with changes in their physical and cognitive functioning (Ewen, Hahn, Erickson, & Krout, 2014).

Case Example 16.1

Rebecca is a 60-year-old woman with a mild intellectual disability and epilepsy, who has just moved into a supervised apartment in a suburban community. As a young child, Rebecca was placed in a state-supported institution on the recommendation of her pediatrician. When the state institution was closed, Rebecca returned home to live with her family. She is generally self-sufficient and has been able to hold a job in a local retail store where she has worked for the last 25 years. Rebecca's parents are older now and they are concerned about what will happen to her as both they and she age. Rebecca seemed happy in her first few days in the apartment, and expressed the desire to start working in the new community, ride the bus on her own, and go shopping. Rebecca told the social worker that she finds it difficult to budget her money, prepare nutritious meals for herself, and to remember to take her medications. She is often anxious about being on her own, but at the same time, very much wants to be an "independent woman."

The social worker first needs to engage with Rebecca to gain a full understanding of her goals and values. A biopsychosocial assessment will allow the social worker to ascertain further insights about her initial adjustment to the supervised apartment including her feelings about leaving her family home and being on her own. Rebecca's parents are older now, but the social worker should collaborate with Rebecca to engage the family so as to further understand their concerns about Rebecca's future. When conducting the biopsychosocial assessment, the social worker needs to capture information related to family structure, current relationships, employment and educational status, medical diagnoses, mental health issues and symptom presentation, and other risk and protective factors. Upon completion of the biopsychosocial assessment, the social worker can collaborate with Rebecca to strategize as to how they can best work together to advance her self-defined goals.

POLICY

Policies related to people with disabilities have evolved significantly over the past half century. Institutions have steadily given way to community-based services. Inclusion has replaced isolation. The "normalization" of the lives of those with disabilities has become the goal (Chapin, 2014).

As discussed earlier, the passage of the ADA, which was originally signed in 1990, and amended in 2008 and 2016, represents a major departure from past policy directions in three ways:

1. It reflects a much stronger commitment to civil rights—a recognition that many of the fundamental rights of this population have been largely overlooked, ignored, or withheld in the past (Stern & Axinn, 2012).
2. It was not developed solely by policy leaders and elected decision makers, but was one of the first pieces of legislation in this area that fully involved those with

disabilities and their families in its development (Chapin, 2014). Such involvement in any policy arena can often lead to a much greater understanding of the most critical challenges faced by those being helped as well as provide new insights into ways that such challenges can be successfully overcome.

3. It moved from a focus on an individual's disability to a view that our society has an obligation to create an environment that is much more sensitive to the needs of the disabled. Chapin observes that "disability is no longer viewed as occurring solely in the individual but rather in the interface between personal capacity and environmental demands" (2014, p. 287).

This act, which promotes equal opportunity and access, places significant responsibility on employers to make reasonable accommodations (Chapin, 2014). Largely a "bricks-and-mortar" policy, a similar change in perspective about this population was introduced in the educational field in 1975. The Education for All Handicapped Children Act acknowledged that each child, although having some form of disability, is unique in terms of both their strengths and challenges. The act called for an individualized education plan (IEP) for each child, based on the philosophy that learning and socialization can be most effectively advanced in the least restrictive environment. The IEPs are developed by multidisciplinary teams in collaboration with the families and students (Chapin, 2014). This legislation, now called the Individuals with Disabilities Education Improvement Act (2004), seeks to ensure that the rights of children with disabilities and their parents are guaranteed and protected (Chapin, 2014).

In the larger sphere, the impetus for a less stigmatizing and oppressive approach to working with people with mental health challenges came about with the passage of The Mental Retardation and Community Mental Health Centers Construction Act, originally enacted in 1963, and amended in 1965 (Stern & Axinn, 2012). It brought about a significant reduction in the number of patients in mental hospitals and an increase in community mental health centers, offering a much less restrictive environment. Complementing this legislation, the State Comprehensive Mental Health Services Plan Act of 1986—a federal–state partnership—was enacted to encourage states, through flexible block grants, to budget more dollars of their own for community mental health centers (Chapin, 2014).

The Substance Abuse and Mental Health Services Administration (SAMHSA) was established within the U.S. Department of Health and Human Services in 1992. It administers an Alcohol, Drug Abuse, and Mental Health grant program that seeks to improve the lives of people with or at risk of mental and substance abuse disorders (Chapin, 2014). SAMHSA has been a leader in the development of community-level systems of care, nurturing formal collaborative efforts among service providers, on behalf of those served (Stroul & Blau, 2008).

Access is an important policy issue for people with disabilities. Mathis (2017) stated, "access to treatment had been the focus of many federal mental health efforts until President George W. Bush's New Freedom Commission on Mental Health laid out a far more ambitious vision in 2003—the goal of transforming service systems to facilitate 'recovery'" (p. 15). This effort continues today, helping people with disabilities to address issues, manage symptoms, build resilience, and promote independent living and choice (Mathis, 2017).

To what extent have the legislative initiatives highlighted achieved their goals? Most involved would say that some progress has been made in each of these policy areas. Many employers have made their facilities handicapped-accessible. But with only a few federal dollars available for this purpose, compliance with this largely unfunded mandate still falls short of the mark. The Individuals with Disabilities Education Act (IDEA) legislation faces a similar barrier. At a time when school budgets are strained, the cost to implement a child's IEP in the least restrictive environment is substantial, with school systems finding it very difficult to meet their obligations under this law. Competing for limited state and local funding with other often more attractive programs have kept many community centers operating at a "bare-bones" level. The cry of "Not in My Backyard" (NIMBY) has also been an enormous barrier to those organizations that are working to establish community-based housing for those being served. The lack of community-based services for those with mental health challenges has also been a factor in the rise of homelessness among this population. Efforts need to be expanded to address access to community-based services and enhancement of consumer-driven care.

Compounding these issues, the basic financial support systems utilized by most people with disabilities and their families to pay for living and health care costs are potentially facing some serious cutbacks. The linchpin of this financial support system is Social Security Disability Insurance, which was added to the core Social Security program in 1956. In 2010, over eight million disabled workers received benefits, including over two million spouses and children (Dolgoff & Feldstein, 2013). It is variously estimated that the Disability Insurance Trust Fund is expected to become insolvent within 2 to 10 years, resulting in an approximate 25% reduction in benefits, based on anticipated annual payroll collections that will continue. If this anticipated reduction is to be avoided, Congress will need to address the long-term viability of this fund (Dolgoff & Feldstein, 2013).

Enacted in 1965, Medicare, in addition to serving adults 65 and older, provides health care benefits to people with disabilities after they have received cash benefits for 24 months under the Social Security program (Dolgoff & Feldstein, 2013). Medicaid is a federal-state matching entitlement program that provides means-tested health-related services to low-income individuals and families. Among those eligible for Medicaid are people with disabilities, some of whom receive benefits from Medicare as well. Moreover, there is the Supplemental Security Income, a cash benefit, as well as block grants from Title XX of the Social Security Act for the provision of a range of social services, including many for individuals with disabilities (Dolgoff & Feldstein, 2013; see Chapter 12 for further discussion).

A national debate about the future of entitlements, including Social Security, Medicare, Medicaid, and Supplemental Security Income, as well as the extent of the role of government in the social welfare of its citizens, could lead to serious gaps in service and financial assistance for people with disabilities. Social workers have a strong role to play in this debate, especially because of our unique vantage point at the micro, mezzo, and macro practice levels.

RESEARCH

Disability-related research is vital to informing disability-related services at the micro, mezzo, and macro levels. Clarity about specific intervention, program, and policy effectiveness is important information for the social work practitioner so that appropriate/differential intervention selection can be made. One of the more compelling contemporary disability-related research issues is that of ensuring that the voices of people with disabilities are captured in the conduct of research about them. Increasing the voluntary participation of people with disabilities in research that has implications for their health and well-being is important if we are to fully honor their desire for self-directed lives.

Intervention research in disabilities appears to focus on several life domains, often dependent on the category of disability (e.g., cognitive, developmental, physical). Broadly speaking, intervention targets may include improvements in social participation, activities of daily living (ADLs), employment skills, health behaviors, or mobility. However, given the variability of disability categories, the wide age range of those with disabilities, and the numerous targeted life domains, social work practice is best served by tailoring interventions for their clients, grounded in evidence from research, based on the presenting disability, and the individual's current life circumstances. Nonetheless, this section will attempt to highlight a sample of research findings for interventions and programs used to increase specific functions for individuals with disabilities.

One area of particular importance in work with children living with disabilities is the concept of participation. Participation is most commonly defined by the WHO (2007) as "involvement in a life situation." A recent systematic review of the participation literature aimed to provide a uniform definition of this construct within the childhood disability literature (Imms et al., 2016). The review uncovered two emergent themes considered essential to the participation construct: attendance and involvement. Attendance and involvement are inextricably linked because attendance is a necessary prerequisite for involvement. "Once attendance has been achieved, involvement is possible, and the experience of involvement might include affect, willingness/motivation, and social aspects" (Imms et al., 2016, p. 35). The authors suggest that increased attendance and involvement may lead to shifts in perceived competence and self-confidence or self-esteem for the child with a disability.

A follow-up systematic review using the aforementioned definition of participation was conducted to assess how intervention studies have aimed to increase participation in children with disabilities (Adair, Ullenhag, Keen, Granlund, & Imms, 2015). Results of the review indicated that few intervention studies actually assessed for participation as a primary outcome. However, it was found that individualized education and mentoring programs did enhance participation outcomes. Nonetheless, the research is scarce, and Adair et al. (2015) suggest that future studies focus on individually tailored programs to increase participation among children with disabilities, while making sure to report methodically operationalized definitions of the participation construct.

Another area of research that is prominent for those living with disabilities, particularly among young adults, is the acquisition of employment and independent life skills. Parents often remain heavily involved in the life of their young adult child living with disability as they transition into adulthood. DiPipi and Jitendra (2004) therefore examined a parent-delivered intervention to teach purchasing skills to young adult children living with developmental disabilities. The study used a constant time delay procedure, which included the following steps in sequential order: task-direction, verbal prompt, 2-second delay, and feedback. After parents were trained in the constant time delay procedure, they were asked to teach their young adult child how to make a purchase in the community. Results indicated that parents were able to successfully teach purchasing skills to their children using the instructional procedure and that these skills were maintained when reexamined several weeks later (DiPipi & Jitendra, 2004).

In addition to developmental disabilities, many young adults may have work limitations due to a diagnosed mental disorder (Whiteford et al., 2013). Mattila-Holapp et al. (2016) examined the degree to which coupled psychotherapeutic and work-oriented interventions increased chances of employment for young adults with a mental disorder. In a sample of 1,163 young adult treatment and rehabilitation plans, they found that 22% had only a plan for psychotherapy, 23% had only a plan of work-oriented intervention, 46% had no proposal for either, and only 10% had proposal for both interventions in their rehabilitative plan. Results indicated that receiving coupled psychotherapy and work-oriented training predicted quicker entry into competitive employment (Mattila-Holapp et al., 2016).

Finally, recent research has explored the use of technology-mediated self-prompting interventions for adolescents and adults with disabilities. The use of technology-mediated self-prompting has been shown to be more effective relative to its low-tech equivalents (e.g., textual or picture prompts) for teaching daily living skills (Van Laarhoven et al., 2010). Given the emergence of these interventions and the increased availability of devices like tablets and smartphones, Cullen and Alber-Morgan (2015) performed a systematic review of technology-mediated self-prompting and the effect on increasing daily living skills. Results of the review indicated that technology-mediated self-prompting interventions have been effective for improving the adeptness of various living skills across a range of settings, client populations, and technologies (Cullen & Alber-Morgan, 2015). However, the authors note that several domains of daily living skills were underrepresented in the literature; no studies targeted caring for personal needs, demonstrating relationship responsibilities, or engaging in leisure activity.

CONCLUSION

Social work practitioners are uniquely positioned to work in different settings and at the intersection of multiple systems to address the needs of persons with disabilities. This chapter emphasized social work's contributions throughout the life span, in work with children and adolescents, as well as adults and older adults, to ensure that each receives age-appropriate, holistic, and disability-competent care that is increasingly self-driven and determined.

Policy advocates need to focus on the needs of individuals with disabilities across the life span, recognizing that such needs may change over time. The financing of health care and social services, as well as limited coordination of services across the continuum both continue to be in need of greater advocacy. Social workers need to collaborate with other professionals, families, and individuals with disabilities to advance the rights of persons with disabilities.

Social work research can help to inform decisions about intervention selection, program development, policy analysis, and new policy formulation. Social workers have long been on the front lines in service to people with disabilities; practice wisdom gained from this experience can be used to inform disability research. Moreover, collaborative partnerships with disability self-advocates present valuable opportunities to ensure their voices are formally documented in the research and may be well suited for the implementation of empowerment research models.

CHAPTER DISCUSSION QUESTIONS

1. How has history shaped the provision of care to people with disabilities?

2. How do the different disability definitions impact policy for people with disabilities?

3. There are a number of programs and policies that are designed for very young children (e.g., birth to 5 years) and their families. Discuss the impact of early intervention and preschool on program and policies.

4. What unique challenges confront adults and older adults who have disabilities? How have employment opportunities impacted the lives of individuals with disabilities?

5. In what arenas might social work be underutilized, and how might the profession address this challenge?

CASE EXAMPLE AND DISCUSSION QUESTIONS

Case Example 16.2

Sam is 3 years old and was born with cerebral palsy. He struggles with gross and fine motor functions, balance, and coordination. Sam has some difficulty swallowing and feeding himself. Sam has showed signs of speech impairment. His parents started early intervention and therapies to help him, but are nervous about the preschool program and what they should do when he enrolls in it, as well what to do after he comes home from preschool. They explain that the early diagnosis has helped their family qualify for government benefit programs to pay for care, but worry that it is not enough.

Questions for Discussion

1.   As the social worker at the preschool program, how would you engage Sam and his family?

2.   Sam's parents are concerned about how to help him when he gets home at night after preschool. How would you work with them to assess their needs?

REFERENCES

Adair, B., Ullenhag, A., Keen, D., Granlund, M., & Imms, C. (2015). The effect of interventions aimed at improving participation outcomes for children with disabilities: A systematic review. *Developmental Medicine & Child Neurology, 57*(12), 1093–1104. doi:10.1111/dmcn.12809

Americans with Disabilities Act. (1990). Americans with Disabilities Act of 1990. Retrieved from https://www.eeoc.gov/eeoc/history/35th/thelaw/ada.html

Americans with Disabilities Act. (2008). American with Disabilities Act of 1990, as amended. Retrieved from https://www.ada.gov/pubs/adastatute08.htm

Bean, K. F., & Hedgpeth, J. (2014). The effect of social work education and self-esteem on students' social discrimination of people with disabilities. *Social Work Education, 33*(1), 49–60. doi:10.1080/02615479.2012.740454

Black, E. (2003). *War against the weak: Eugenics and America's campaign to create a master race.* Washington, DC: Digit Press.

Centers for Disease Control and Prevention. (2016a, May). *Health, United States, 2015: With special feature on racial and ethnic health disparities.* U.S. Department of Health and Human Services Publication No. 2016-1232. National Center for Health Statistics. Retrieved from https://www.cdc.gov/nchs/data/hus/hus15.pdf#042

Centers for Disease Control and Prevention. (2016b). Key findings: Adults with one or more functional disabilities—United States, 2011–2014. Retrieved from https://www.cdc.gov/ncbddd/disabilityandhealth/features/keyfinding-adults-with-multiple-functional-disabilities.html#disabiltytypes

Chapin, R. K. (2014). *Social policy for effective practice: A strengths approach* (3rd ed.). New York, NY: Routledge.

Cullen, J. M., & Alber-Morgan, S. R. (2015). Technology mediated self-prompting of daily living skills for adolescents and adults with disabilities: A review of the literature. *Education and Training in Autism and Developmental Disabilities, 50*(1), 43–55.

Cummings, S. M., & Kropf, N. P. (2011). Aging with a severe mental illness: Challenges and treatments. *Journal of Gerontological Social Work, 54*(2), 175–188. doi:10.1080/016 34372.2010.538815

DiPipi-Hoy, C., & Jitendra, A. (2004). A parent-delivered intervention to teach purchasing skills to young adults with disabilities. *The Journal of Special Education, 38*(3), 144–157. doi:10.1177/00224669040380030201

Dolgoff, R., & Feldstein, D. (2013). *Understanding social welfare: A search for social justice* (9th ed.). Boston, MA: Pearson.

Dunn, P. A., Hanes, R., Hardie, S., & MacDonald, J. (2006). Creating disability inclusion within schools of social work. *Journal of Social Work in Disability & Rehabilitation, 5*(1), 1–19.

Dunst, C. J. (2002). Family-centered practices: Birth through high school. *The Journal of Special Education, 36*(3), 139–147.

Erickson, W., Lee, C., & von Schrader, S. (2017). *Disability Statistics from the 2015 American Community Survey (ACS)*. Ithaca, NY: Cornell University Employment and Disability Institute (EDI). Retrieved from www.disabilitystatistics.org

Ewen, H. H., Hahn, S. J., Erickson, M., & Krout, J. A. (2014). Aging in place or relocation? Plans of community-dwelling older adults. *Journal of Housing for the Elderly, 28*, 288–309. doi:10.1080/02763893.2014.930366

Gollaher, D. (1995). *Voice for the mad, the life of Dorothea Dix*. New York, NY: Free Press.

Hayward, B., & Schmidt-Davis, H. (2003). *Longitudinal study of the vocational rehabilitation services program*. Final report: VR services and outcomes (ED Contract No. HR92022001). Washington, DC: U.S. Department of Education, Rehabilitation Services Administration.

Hiebert-Murphy, D., Trute, B., & Wright, A. (2008). Patterns of entry to community-based services for families with children with developmental disabilities: Implications for social work practice. *Child & Family Social Work, 13*(4), 423–432. doi:10.1111/j.1365-2206.2008.00572.x

Imms, C., Adair, B., Keen, D., Ullenhag, A., Rosenbaum, P., & Granlund, M. (2016). "Participation": A systematic review of language, definitions, and constructs used in intervention research with children with disabilities. *Developmental Medicine & Child Neurology, 58*(1), 29–38. doi:10.1111/dmcn.12932

Janke, M. C., Payne, L. L., & Van Puymbroeck, M. (2008). The role of informal and formal leisure activities in the disablement process. *The International Journal of Aging and Human Development, 67*(3), 231–257. doi:10.2190/AG.67.3.c

Kraus, L. (2017). *2016 Disability statistics annual report*. Durham, NH: University of New Hampshire.

Lawton, M. P. (1986). *Environment and aging* (2nd ed.). Albany, NY: Center for the Study of Aging.

Mackelprang, R. W., & Salsgiver, R. O. (1996). People with disabilities and social work: Historical and contemporary issues. *Social Work, 41*(1), 7–14.

Mahoney, G., Boyce, G., Fewell, R. R., Spiker, D., & Wheeden, C. A. (1998). The relationship of parent-child interaction to the effectiveness of early intervention services for at-risk children and children with disabilities. *Topics in Early Childhood Special Education, 18*(1), 5–17.

Mathis, J. (2017). The importance of framing mental health policy within a disability rights framework. *Human Rights, 42*(4), 14–16.

Mattila-Holappa, P., Joensuu, M., Ahola, K., Koskinen, A., Tuisku, K., Ervasti, J., & Virtanen, M. (2016). Psychotherapeutic and work-oriented interventions: Employment outcomes among young adults with work disability due to a mental disorder. *International Journal of Mental Health Systems, 10*(1), 68. doi:10.1186/s13033-016-0101-7

Meekosha, H., & Dowse, L. (2007). Integrating critical disability studies into social work education and practice: An Australian perspective. *Practice: Social Work in Action, 19*(3), 169–183. doi:10.1080/09503150701574267

Parker, M., Baker, P. S., & Allman, R. M. (2002). A life-space approach to functional assessment of mobility in the elderly. *Journal of Gerontological Social Work, 35*(4), 35–55. doi:10.1300/J083v35n04_04

Peele, R. (1985). The Willowbrook wars. *The American Journal of Psychiatry, 142*(9), 1111–1112. doi:10.1176/ajp.142.9.1111-a

Singleton, M. M. (2014). The "science" of eugenics: America's moral detour. *Journal of American Physicians and Surgeons, 19*(4), 122–125.

Stern, M. J., & Axinn, J. (2012). *Social welfare: A history of the American response to need* (8th ed.). Boston, MA: Pearson.

Strock-Lynskey, D., & Keller, D. W. (2007). Integrating a family-centered approach into social work practice with families of children and adolescents with disabilities. *Journal of Social Work in Disability & Rehabilitation, 6*(1–2), 111–134. doi:10.1300/J198v06n01_07

Stroul, B., & Blau, G. (Eds.). (2008). *The system of care handbook* (pp. 3–23). Baltimore, MD: Paul Brookes Publisher.

Trattner, W. (1999). *From poor law to welfare state: A history of social welfare in America* (8th ed.). New York, NY: Free Press.

U.S. Department of Education. (2015). Protecting students with disabilities: Frequently asked questions about Section 504 of the Education of Children with Disabilities. Office for Civil Rights. Retrieved from https://www2.ed.gov/about/offices/list/ocr/504faq.html

Van Laarhoven, T., Kraus, E., Karpman, K., Nizzi, R., & Valentino, J. (2010). A comparison of picture and video prompts to teach daily living skills to individuals with autism. *Focus on Autism and Other Developmental Disabilities, 25,* 195–208. doi:10.1177/1088357610380412

Whiteford, H. A., Degenhardt, L., Rehm, J., Baxter, A. J., Ferrari, A. J., Erskine, H. E., . . . Burstein, R. (2013). Global burden of disease attributable to mental and substance use disorders: Findings from the Global Burden of Disease Study 2010. *The Lancet, 382*(9904), 1575–1586. doi:10.1016/S0140-6736(13)61611-6

World Health Organization. (2007). *International Classification of Functioning, Disability, and Health: Children & Youth Version: ICF-CY*. Geneva, Switzerland: Author.

17

Health Care and Serving Veterans

Jose E. Crego and Sharon L. Young

Today, a significant number of veterans who have served in Iraq and Afghanistan suffer some type of traumatic injury sustained through their exposure to the atrocities of battle. A 2015 meta-analysis of 4.9 million post 9/11 veterans found a posttraumatic stress disorder (PTSD) prevalence rate of 23% (Fulton et al., 2015). Since 2000, the number of traumatic brain injury (TBI) incidents in post 9/11 veterans was reported to be 253,330 and amputations in this population totaled 1,753 (Fisher, 2013). Non-suicidal self-injury (NSSI) was found in 14% of a sample of post 9/11 veterans (Kimbrel et al., 2015). NSSI is not uncommon in service members and veterans and may be a marker for likelihood of suicide. In a study of active duty soldiers, 40% of those with a history of NSSI went on to attempt suicide (Bryan, Rudd, Wertenberger, Young-McCaughon, & Peterson, 2015). The suicide data report published by the Department of Veteran Affairs in 2012 reported that 27,062 deaths by suicide were confirmed to be veterans. However, 21 states reporting 34,027 deaths listed unknown veteran status on death certificates. Veterans comprised approximately 22.2% of all suicides reported during the project period. If this prevalence estimate is assumed to be constant across all states, an estimated 22 veterans died from suicide each day in the calendar year 2010 (Kemp & Bossarte, 2012).

Social workers, both in the community and within the Department of Veterans Affairs (VA), provide a comprehensive range of services to a broad demographic of veterans. Service provision for veterans can address a wide range of issues including aging, homelessness, reintegration, sexual assault, physical and psychological war injuries, and substance abuse. Research-informed practice allows social workers to effectively address the special needs of veterans. This chapter discusses the landscape of social work practice with veterans and the interconnectedness of research, policy, and service delivery.

Since World War II, social workers have had an active role in providing mental health and behavioral support for veterans and their families. While much of the work is done by social workers who are employed by the VA, there is an increasing need for social workers in and outside of the VA to be aware of the nuances associated with the veteran as well as his or her family (Jackson, 2013). Social workers should have a working knowledge of military culture, the impact of deployment, subsequent redeployments, reintegration, and adjustment to civilian life. It is essential for social workers to have knowledge about the physical and psychological aspects of trauma, particularly war-related trauma.

PRACTICE

Social workers in the civilian health care sector regularly work with clients who currently serve or have served in the military. They also frequently encounter family members of service members and veterans. Family social work involves working with spouses, partners, children, siblings, and parents, who are in some way affected by the veteran's reaction to his or her service (National Association of Social Workers [NASW], 2012). Through their training, experience, and expertise in assisting individuals and families of varying cultures from across the life span, social workers are in a unique position to assist service members/veterans and their families as they address challenges. Having a basic understanding of military-related challenges enables social workers to better address the needs of service members, veterans, and their families.

Military Culture

All service members undergo an intense initial training often referred to as *boot camp*. This initial training provides for a complete immersion into the military lifestyle and culture (Halvorson, 2010). Recruits, as they are often called, are taught the history of their specific service, military customs and courtesies, and how to properly wear the uniform and understand what each component signifies. They are taught such characteristics as military bearing, military values and ethics, as well as other information that is critical to an individual's success in their respective branch of service.

Military society has been famously described as a "fortress" by Mary Wertsch (1991) who used the term to describe the paradoxical reality lived by those who serve in our military. Those who serve, especially today, are volunteers who guard our American democratic values, yet do not themselves live in a democracy. Our military has a very rigid authoritarian structure. The service member must adhere to the regimentation and conformity that is required within our military system. It is imperative for successful functioning of military society that the individual not become an autocrat (Hall, 2011). Obedience and discipline is required of individuals in order to create a cohesive and focused group. Military life breeds two primary concepts that are embodied by all who serve and have served: honor and sacrifice.

According to Wertsch (1991), honor and sacrifice are best understood by gaining knowledge of the dynamics central to military culture. These dynamics are secrecy, stoicism, and denial. Secrecy is understood as the importance of keeping what goes on within the mission as secret; this is also true for the service member in his or her home life. Stoicism and secrecy serves to keep the veteran from seeking help when needed. This barrier to treatment is exacerbated by stigmatization of mental illness within the military culture.

A crucial element of military culture is the bond that is forged by men and women who serve together, especially in battle. Service members of all branches are expected to conduct themselves in a manner that shows discipline in their actions and words. This includes an expectation of maintaining control of their emotions and their physical selves, always. It is in this environment where they learn that there is no greater bond than the one they share with their fellow serviceman or woman, the ones located all around them in training and combat. For many, this bond of brotherhood/sisterhood is a bond that transcends the military. This bond is highly valued, nurtured, and protected. In life-or-death situations, it is the bond that allows one service member to know that those around him or her "have their back." There is an unspoken understanding that those who will see them through danger or will come for them if they are wounded or killed in combat are those brothers and sisters who are fighting right by their side. This

is embodied in the mantra "leave no one behind" (Halvorson, 2010, p. 9). It is this cama-
raderie (brotherhood/sisterhood) that most men and women of the military continue to
seek long after they no longer wear the uniform.

The Experience of War

The effects of war are known to be long lasting and life changing. The experience of
war often involves death and destruction, and taking part in such an experience can
take years to overcome. These effects are felt by those involved directly or indirectly by
combat operations (Halvorson, 2010). Even within a single military platoon, each service member experiences combat differently. Despite these differences, there are many
common experiences they all share. The combat zone can best be described as intense,
where activity is flourishing in one moment only to drag to a painfully slow pace the next.
"Hurry up and wait" is not just a phrase, but is a reality of life in a war zone (Halvorson,
2010). Soldiers, sailors, and Marines move quickly to prepare for a mission only to find
themselves waiting for minutes or hours as plans change, intelligence is gathered, and
the leadership adjusts its decisions. Adrenal glands are exercised to the maximum as
service members prepare for the mission at hand only to be told to standby and await
further instruction. This constant drain on the adrenals as well as other physiological
aspects of the human body create exhaustion, especially on troops that may already be
sleep deprived (Priebe et al., 2013).

The constant physical strain endured by the troops is further exacerbated by unfamiliar terrain, extreme temperatures, and climate situations as well as the load of the gear
they carry on their backs, often over 150 pounds (Hoge, 2010). There is no such thing
as a simple mission: Each mission is prepared for in its entirety, troops are outfitted in
their protective equipment, including interceptor body armor (IBA), helmet, extra am-
munition, water, weapon(s), and in some cases food (Halvorson, 2010). These stressors
coupled with a near-constant lack of sleep lend to increased levels of stress that have
a significant effect on the troops' ability to function in combat. This daily exposure to
stress and the need to have constant tactical awareness follows the service member into
civilian life, leading to hypervigilance and anxiety (Rubin, Weiss, & Coll, 2013). This
anxiety and hypervigilance can be attributed to the differences of today's battlefield
when compared to those of previous eras. Today, there are no easy demarcation lines,
no front line that marks where the battle begins and where behind it one can rest and
gather supplies and safety. In both World Wars, these demarcation lines were very visible and respected. Behind the lines served as a place of safety, out of reach of enemy
guns and cannons (Wright, 2013). Support personnel remained behind the front lines
numbering in the thousands and worked in support of the troops on the front lines.
Today no clear line exists: All military personnel live and work on posts in the middle of
a terrain that in one moment is peaceful and the next shattered by gunfire. Everyone on
location is at risk of harm or death at any given time from a barrage of munitions such
as mortars that are lobbed over base walls, sniper fire, or improvised explosive devices
(IED) that are used to attack convoys (La Bash, Vogt, King, & King, 2009). Though there
may exist a semblance of safety, there is none, and change can occur without warning.
This knowledge causes those in the situation to maintain a perpetual state of vigilance
and tactical awareness (Hoge, 2010). Consistent awareness at this level of operationality
requires troops to make split-second decisions that involve life and death outcomes.
Troops as young as 21 or 22 have expectations placed on them to make immediate decisions and live with the consequences, something many find nearly impossible to do
after the war (Hall, 2011).

Multiple losses, grief, and guilt are commonplace in battle. Oftentimes the young men and women in combat are not prepared to deal with such matters and fewer still make or have time to adequately process what has occurred before they are back out on the next mission (Halvorson, 2010). Combat has a way of challenging an individual's spiritual and moral fiber through the decisions service members are asked to make. These decisions in the civilian world have clear black-or-white answers but in the fog of battle appear in multiple shades of gray (Hoge, 2010). The act of killing, even when justified by the needs of war, can create dilemmas that affect the service member's spiritual or moral belief code. The impact of this act sits at a deeper level even when the decision to do so is determined by logic or military training. Daily life in combat is filled with confusion, fear, uncertainty, and disruption. This reality for the service member continues for as long as the tour of duty, sometimes 9 or 12 months. Military training and culture have prepared service members to survive this reality. However, the skills and tactical awareness that saw them through combat may continue, maladaptively, into their civilian lives after war. For some veterans, responses born of combat experience, such as hypervigilance and a constant questioning of one's decisions, may never go away (Hoge, 2010).

Readjustment

The period of reintegration that occurs after deployment is perhaps the most challenging of the deployment cycle. Military spouses eagerly await reunion while setting high expectations for what will happen. Romantic evenings are envisioned and a spouse who returns home and is eager to assist in the home chores is wished for and expected. Unfortunately, these expectations are often not fulfilled and this tends to add disappointment to an already tenuous situation (Halvorson, 2010). The reality is that many service members are exhausted both physically and emotionally when they return home and there is an increased need for isolation. This increased need for isolation often leads to withdrawal from family activities as well as being uninterested or incapable of physical intimacy (Jackson, 2013). Some return home and face their own anxieties and uncertainties. Others bring the horrors of war home with them, struggling with PTSD, nightmares, and depression (Moore, 2012). Others may have suffered physical injuries, have lost limbs, or may be suffering with TBI. TBI is a physical injury that often has psychological symptoms including issues with moods, personality, and cognitive abilities (Franulic, Carbonell, Pinto, & Sepulveda, 2009). Readjustment after long separations is challenging for all couples and families; however, the psychological sequelae of combat exacerbate the transition process.

If children are part of the family unit, the service member often finds himself or herself attempting to reconnect with children they have been long separated from. In their absence, the family dynamic has shifted, children have grown, and they are unsure where their role is within the family (Jackson, 2013). There is often a "change of guard" situation and these changes can be tumultuous as resentments may get in the way of resolution. In some cases, the waiting family member who has held down the fort during the deployment may be hesitant to give back this role to the service member who is returning home and thus creating a power struggle. As an example, the husband, before deploying was in charge of household finances, but during the deployment the wife was forced to fulfill that role learning all that is associated with the financial management of a home. Upon return, the husband wants to retake this responsibility and the wife may be reluctant. Another example is the growth of a child from baby to toddler; when the service member left the child barely walked or talked. Upon return, he is confronted with a walking, talking child who has a mind of his or her own and requires a different kind of parenting. These shifting parenting demands create a power struggle as to how things will be done, in contrast to how they have been done (NASW, 2012). A returning parent has to integrate into this new family structure as well as adapt his or her parenting skills and co-parenting skills to meet the changing needs of the children. This task is compounded if the child is the couple's first and the couple lacks fundamental knowledge of child development. Even childless couples struggle at reunification. If the marriage lacked a strong foundation or was not nurtured by communication, honesty, and fidelity during the deployment, there is a greater likelihood of increased stress, which can lead to divorce or abuse (Jackson, 2013).

For Reserve and National Guard members, reintegration is experienced differently than for members of the active duty component. Active duty service members return home to bases that hold their full-time jobs as soldiers, sailors, Marines, or airmen, and to communities that have experience and are familiar with all phases of deployment. In contrast, the Reserve and National Guard components return to the civilian world and to civilian families. This creates some very unique challenges for these service members and their families. A Guard or Reserve member still has the family reintegration challenges previously identified, but these challenges are compounded by trying to find a way to fit back into the civilian world in a community that has little direct experience with the military and less understanding of what they have endured These service members may be excited to return home to friends who are also anxious to hear about their experiences, but the initial excitement quickly wears off as a sense that everything has changed permeates relationships and other personal interactions (Ahern et al., 2015). Everything has changed; the friends and family members who remained behind are different, and the service member has been changed by his or her experiences. There exists an unspoken truth for the veteran that those who stayed behind do not understand what they have been through. Once the excitement has worn off, there is a wish by friends and family to have everything return to the way things were. They want the person back without the effects of the experiences; this is not possible even if the service member wanted it to be so. Veterans express they no longer feel "normal" and wonder if they will ever fit in with civilian friends and family again. Many have a need to reconnect with battle buddies or veterans, but, because of the way the Guard and Reserve are structured, they may not see their fellow service members until they return to training in 30 days or more (Hoge, 2010). National Guard and Reserve members may also feel a loss of mission and purpose, often returning home to jobs and responsibilities that require less skill and authority than they exercised while deployed. While on deployment, they made life and death decisions: now back home veterans are confused by what others see as important. This leads to a feeling of isolation and disconnectedness. Overseas, life had a certain intensity, routine, and pace. Yet back home, out of the military culture, that structure and routine is gone. There is no longer the structure that is so integral in active duty. Many also miss the intensity of combat, with soldiers experiencing an almost constant adrenaline rush as they prepare for each mission. Upon returning home, it feels as if the world has stopped.

In contrast, active duty component members take a couple of weeks' leave and return to life in uniform working side by side with the men and women they served with overseas. They return to their jobs in the military, embedded in military culture, and continue on with their mission. In contrast, Reserve component members take a couple of weeks' leave and go to work side by side with people who are untouched by combat and what is happening several thousand miles away in a distant country. These Reserve component members may have had positions of responsibility in their units—they were decision makers and responsible for the health and well-being of others. In their civilian employment, they may have little or no responsibility, no authority, and thus no feeling of self-worth compared to how they felt in their military position.

Reintegration into a civilian environment with its psychological and social challenges is further complicated when a veteran has war-related injuries. Access to medical care can be a challenge for Reserve and Guard members. While the active component has access to medical and behavioral health care services on base or on post where they are stationed, Reservists and Guardsmen and women may be geographically separated from any military health care facility by several hours. Due to improvements in protective equipment and battlefield medical care, fewer troops are dying from combat-related injuries. As a result, service members, who in previous conflicts would not have survived, are returning home wounded, suffering with severe physical injuries like blindness, amputations, burns, and with debilitating psychological and emotional wounds (Goldberg, 2010). Some are even faced with "poly-trauma" in which they are suffering from multiple and complex combinations of injuries (Clark, Scholten, Walker, & Gironda, 2009).

Medical Considerations and Services

Battle wounds often extend far beyond what the human eye can see. These wounds encompass a full range of issues including, but not limited to, mental health, chronic pain, and addiction and extend far past any time in the war zone. In a recent house hearing, Dr. Stephen Hunt, the national director of the U.S. Department of Veterans Affairs Post-Deployment Care Initiative, stated that individuals "returning from combat have a constellation of health concerns, including physical issues, psychological issues and psychosocial issues concerning things like work and family." He went on to state regarding returning veterans, "this is a population that has unique health care needs that need to be addressed" (U.S. Department of Veterans Affairs, 2017a). Hunt further concedes that this effort must be an integrative system of care including civilian as well as VA resources. His testimony during the Senate hearing led to the discussion of seven common issues with returning combat veterans. These include musculoskeletal injuries and pain, mental health issues, chemical exposure, infectious diseases, noise and vibration exposure, TBI, and urologic injuries (U.S. Department of Veterans Affairs, 2017a).

Treatment for Cognitive and Psychological Wounds

Social workers are involved in the continuum of care offered by the Veterans Health Administration (VHA), which can be in both inpatient and outpatient settings. For those veterans experiencing PTSD, a variety of therapeutic interventions are employed including talk therapies and psychopharmacological treatments; these treatments are often done in conjunction with each other. Medications such as antidepressants, anti-anxiety, and mood stabilizers can address depression and anxiety symptoms, reduce irritability, improve sleep patterns, and help to ease nightmares or intrusive thoughts (NASW, 2012). The talk therapies often associated with PTSD include cognitive behavioral therapy (CBT), acceptance and commitment therapy (ACT), and interpersonal therapy (IPT). These modalities can help affected veterans reduce emotional pain and reestablish positive social relationships. Certain types of therapies—such as cognitive processing therapy (CPT) or prolonged exposure therapy (PE)—may also be used to promote positive thought patterns and behaviors in veterans experiencing mental health issues. Medical guidelines strongly recommend both CBT and PE for the treatment of posttraumatic stress. For cases of severe PTSD, Mental Health Residential Rehabilitation Treatment Programs (MHRRTPs), established by the VA, provide a 24/7 health care setting for veterans with PTSD (U.S. Department of Veterans Affairs, 2017b).

Veterans with TBI may experience a variety of mental health issues. Different therapeutic strategies may be applied, depending on which areas of a person's functioning are affected. Common treatments for TBIs include rehabilitation therapies (e.g., speech-language therapy), medication, assistive devices, and learning strategies to address cognitive, emotional, and behavioral deficits (U.S. Department of Veterans Affairs, 2017c).

Case Example 17.1

Anthony is a 69-year-old Caucasian male who is retired and living with his wife of 23 years (his second marriage). He presents at an outpatient veterans readjustment services center (Vet Center) clinic after referral from his primary care doctor to address a violent reaction to anesthesia and an inability to sleep. Anthony states that the inability to sleep became more pronounced after retirement 3 years ago. He states that sometimes he has dreams that he can't really remember but reports he wakes in a pool of sweat. Anthony also reports that he has been more irritable lately. Regarding the reaction to the anesthesia, he states he does not know what happened but he thought he had been captured by the North Vietnamese and saw the medical staff after his procedure as the enemy. He says he feels silly and bad for the people at the hospital, but it seemed so real to him. He feels he does not need to be at a mental health clinic, and does not understand why he is there. Anthony says he has never needed any help in the past. Anthony reports during the intake that he served 13 months in Vietnam from May 1967 to June 1968. He said he was involved in the Tet offensive, but that was nothing compared to his having to place the remains of fallen soldiers in body bags. He says that those memories often return to him and he tries hard not to remember. Sometimes he can't stop these thoughts and this angers him and makes him sad as well. He says he feels he was the last person to touch those men with dignity and he felt an obligation to them. "At times, I wonder why I was not in one of those bags. That thought is too much for me, so I just have to stop thinking about that!" he states angrily. After the intake, Anthony agrees to return for another counseling session.

While his story is poignant, it is not unique. Anthony lives with the memory of experiences and emotions he cannot fully understand. With his presentation, it is clear that the invisible wounds of his experience are not far from the surface of his day-to-day life. While not common, emergence agitation, the phenomenon which Anthony experienced, is an indicator of the subconscious existence of his posttraumatic stress. Emergence agitation has an overall occurrence of 4.7% in the general population; however, the occurrence in combat veterans is estimated to be 20% (Lovestrand, Phipps, & Lovestrand, 2013).

Anthony's story is characteristic of the diagnostic and stereotypical signs and symptoms of veterans with combat posttraumatic stress. There are four types or clusters of symptoms associated with PTSD; these include reliving the event or re-experiencing, avoiding any situation that may remind the individual of the trauma, negative changes in beliefs and feelings, and lastly feeling on edge or hyperarousal. When he speaks of his memories of the placing of remains of fallen soldiers in body bags, this is a clear example of reliving the event. His reluctance to think about the situation is avoidance; as avoidance does not always have to be in a physical sense. These are just two of the symptoms that are evident in his initial presentation. It is important to note that oftentimes these signs and symptoms are much more subtle in presentation.

POLICY

Veterans Administration

The VA has been on the forefront of the research and policy agenda for veterans since its inception in 1930 (U.S. Department of Veterans Affairs, 2016a). The VA is the largest health care system in the United States serving close to nine million veterans each year (U.S. Department of Veterans Affairs, 2017b). A common misconception about the VA is that it serves all veterans. Eligibility for VA services is determined by duration and type of military service, disability, enrollment periods following military discharge, income, type of discharge, and other factors (U.S. Department of Veterans Affairs, 2017b). After 1990, the military instituted a transition training called TAP that informed exiting service members about VA benefits (Westat, 2010). This education paired with higher use of the Internet by younger veterans has created greater awareness of VA services in younger veterans (see Figure 17.1). This awareness, however, is not reflected in the VA utilization rates of younger veterans. VA usage is determined by a number of factors, including size of military cohort, access to other health care systems, VA eligibility, and socioeconomic factors.

The demand for VA services is a reflection not only on historic fluctuations in troop levels, but also current economic and health care policy factors. The VA or VHA does not provide the sole source of health care for the majority of veterans. For some veterans, for example, the VHA acts as a medical safety net. Veterans will access services at the VHA during times of economic stress or changes in their civilian health care coverage. For example, Yee, Frakt, and Pizer (2016) determined that the passage of the Patient Protection and Affordable Care Act (ACA) with the expansion of Medicaid led to a reduction in VHA use in some states. Shifts in VHA usage will continue as the Vietnam Era veterans age and begin to access civilian care through Medicare (Hynes et al., 2007). As a safety net for some, the VHA must adapt to the changing economic landscape and manage shifts in demand for services.

The historic expansion and retraction of troop strengths has also resulted in changes in the demographics and medical needs of VHA participants. Currently, the largest consumers of VHA services are older veterans. The VHA serves veterans who are older, sicker, poorer, and have a higher level of disability than their non-VHA using peers

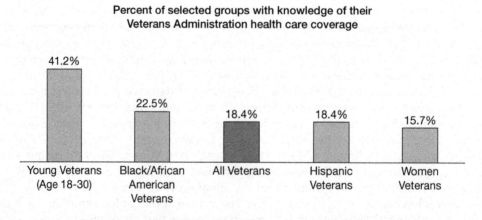

Figure 17.1 Greater knowledge of Veterans Administration health care coverage in younger veterans.

(Hynes et al., 2007). Over half of VHA patients are 65 or older and tend to have more chronic illnesses than veterans who do not use VA health care (Farmer & Hosek, 2016). The graying of veterans can be seen in VHA usage data. In 2014, for example, only 10% of those using VA services were post 9/11 veterans (U.S. Department of Veterans Affairs, 2017a). The 3.9 million post 9/11 veterans represent about one fifth of all veterans in the United States (JEC United States Congress, 2015) but only make up 10% of VHA utilizers.

As the overall number of veterans has been decreasing over the past three decades with the loss of World War II and Korean veterans, the demand for veterans services will eventually decline. However, Farmer and Hosek (2016) have anticipated a short-term increase in demand for VA services until 2019. To manage the fluctuations in usage and the systemic issues surrounding access to VA health care, the Veterans Access, Choice and Accountability Act of 2014 was passed (Farmer & Hosek, 2016). This act was designed to eliminate long wait times for VHA appointments and to allow veterans to access health care in a timely and convenient manner. This is being achieved by allowing eligible veterans to use their VA benefits to access civilian health care and changing administrative processes within the VA to maximize efficiencies. Additionally, the act was designed to provide training, to hire additional VA health care providers, and to improve services for special populations including veterans who experienced military sexual trauma or TBI (Veterans Access, Choice and Accountability Act of 2014). This act allows for the expansion of purchased civilian care for veterans who might live farther than 40 miles from a VA medical facility or have been told they need to wait more than 30 days for a medical appointment (U.S. Department of Veterans Affairs, 2017b). This act further expands the care of veterans into civilian health care systems.

It has been suggested the VA health care policy should continue to shift toward an integrated health care model where the VA is part provider and part payer (Martsolf, Tomoaia-Cotisel, & Tanielian, 2016). This is especially important given the need for expanding services is only predicted until 2019, following which the contracting number of veterans will reduce demand. Purchasing services in the civilian sector will allow greater flexibility for the VA to meet the changing demands for service.

Expanding veterans' health care into the civilian health care system will allow veterans who are dependent on VA for health care better access to timely service. However, this policy has some pitfalls. Veterans have many specialized health care needs related to their military service. Civilian medical professionals may lack an understanding of the medical complications of exposure to chemical toxins from burn pits or Agent Orange. Additionally, non-VA medical staff might be less experienced in treating blast-related TBIs, amputations, and injuries from explosive mechanisms. Social workers not trained or experienced in working with military populations may have difficulty in treating war-related psychological injuries. Although the evidence-based treatments for combat-related PTSD are not dissimilar to civilian methods, social workers treating veterans should have familiarity with the combat experience and an understanding of military culture.

The Civilian Sector

The civilian health care sector plays a vital role in caring for our nation's veterans. Approximately 77% of all veterans receive health care from outside of the VHA (Yee, Frakt, & Pizer, 2016). The reality is medical and clinical social workers encounter veterans in many different community practice settings: hospitals, nursing homes, hospice, mental health clinics, substance abuse treatment centers, and more. Civilian entities such as the NASW have adopted standards for social work practice to help those serving the needs of service members, veterans, and their families.

In September 2012, the NASW adopted standards for practice with service members, veterans, and families (NASW, 2012). These standards were designed to help enhance and maintain the quality of service social workers provide by increasing knowledge of military culture as well as the unique medical challenges of veteran populations. Additionally, the NASW intends to provide the foundation for continuing education, to promote social worker engagement in public policy, and to stress the importance of a profession-wide response to the needs of military and veteran populations. This document looks at the 12 professional standards through a military social work lens.

The professional standards outline how social workers should prepare to work with military and veteran populations through knowledge and training. For example, social workers should have knowledge of military and veteran benefits, services, and resources. Veterans and military members have exclusive access to educational, medical, social support, mental health, and even burial benefits and services. When working with veteran populations, it is vital that the social worker have a basic understanding of these systems and know how clients can access them. The NASW has outlined very specific biopsychosocial knowledge areas essential for those working with this population. These include, but are not limited to, issues related to loss, grief, substance abuse, PTSD, depression, suicidal ideation, intimate partner violence, and TBIs. Further, social workers should understand the nuances of military culture, military justice, and understand how information flows through various military and veteran entities. This includes an understanding of the meaning of different discharge types and the impact this has on the veteran and his or her family. When working with military and veteran families, the NASW recommends social workers understand the deployment cycle and the impact of military life on family members.

The NASW also recommends social workers integrate their understanding of deployment, reintegration, a client's military history, and experiences with Department of Defense and Veteran's Administration services when assessing veterans. Assessment should also take into consideration physical injuries such as TBI, chemical exposure, burn pit exposure, and amputations as well as psychosocial issues such as military sexual trauma, intimate partner violence, suicide, and homelessness. Through the 12 professional standards, the NASW has provided a blueprint for social workers who serve members of the military, veterans, and their families. This framework spans from ethics and values to assessment and intervention to leadership and advocacy. It serves as a guideline for social workers who may be working through Tricare (the Department of Defense–managed care system), at the VA, or in a community setting.

RESEARCH

The Office of Policy and Planning at the U.S. Department of Veterans Affairs (2016b) has set a research agenda to guide VA strategic planning and policy. This Veterans Policy Research Agenda (VPRA) covers four basic areas: benefits and disability compensation, public–private partnerships, families, and reintegration. This research effort was developed by an interdisciplinary team of stakeholders in the veterans community.

The VA administers the second largest disability program in the United States (Agha, Lofgren, Van Ruiswyk, & Layde, 2000). The VA offers compensation based on service-connected disabilities. The degree of compensation is determined by a lengthy and bureaucratic disability claims process. Once a service-connected disability is verified by this process, the claimant is offered a disability rating that will then determine the payment amount as well as priority status at VA health care centers. The number of veterans receiving disability compensation has nearly doubled since 2001 (Shane, 2016). This surge in disability compensation applicants has created a backlog in claims applications and long wait times for applicants. Since 2012, the VA has automated and adjusted some claim systems and devoted additional staff time to reducing the hundreds of thousands of pending claims. Despite these efforts, the VA has failed to eliminate the backlog. The U.S. Government Accountability Office (2017) recommended that the VA further increase staff to work on pending appeals, reform the application and appeals process, and update the IT hardware used to process claims. The VPRA acknowledges these challenges and has called for an examination of the efficiency, modernization, and effectiveness of the current disability benefits system. Rising parallel with disability compensation, demand for VA health care has been steadily rising. Data from the National Center for Veteran Analysis and Statistics (2016) show the number of disabled veterans utilizing VA for health care has increased from 57% in 2005 to 68% in 2014. Also, veterans with the highest disability rating are most likely to use the VA health care system. Almost all (90.5%) veterans with a 100% disability rating are using VA Health Care (National Center for Veterans Analysis and Statistics, 2016). The cost of providing this care has been steeply rising from $37.8 billion in 2006 to $91.2 billion in 2016 (Draper, 2017). In response, the VPRA has added to the policy research agenda to examine technologically advanced treatments that will lead to economic efficiency. The VPRA has also called for research to address the fiscal and systemic challenges of providing disability health care and social protections in relation to other industrialized countries.

Public–Private Partnerships

As the VA moves toward a greater reliance on public–private partnerships, there is a call for research that examines the impact of the design and management of these programs. The VPRA is interested in knowing how to define, monitor, and evaluate public–private partnership programs. The VA has been expanding its purchased care expenditures nearly threefold over the past decade and this will continue to expand with the Veterans Choice Act (Farmer & Hosek, 2016). The VA has successfully integrated private services to support and expand VA services (Moore, 2015). Public–private partnerships can also be an opportunity to provide innovative programs involving veterans services and research. One example of such a partnership is the Veterans Metric Initiative, a collaborative research project that examines the impact of various transition programs on four domains of well-being in veterans (Center for Public-Private Partnerships, 2013).

Families and Reintegration

Reintegration is the process where a service member and perhaps his or her family transition from military to civilian life. Reintegration can occur when a service member returns from a combat deployment, when a military contract ends and a family moves off the military base, or at retirement after a long military career. Reintegration is described by Elnitsky, Fisher, and Blevins (2017) as both a process and an outcome related to the resumption of family, community, and workplace roles following military service. The authors see this multidimensional process being marked by changes in physical and psychological health, identity, financial status, social functioning and engagement, social support, productivity, and community involvement. This change process can be influenced by a variety of factors that can be precipitants or ameliorants to transition difficulties. Precipitants that can exacerbate reintegration, for example, are combat exposure, being wounded, having PTSD, and having multiple or long deployments (Beder, Coe, & Summer, 2011). Ameliorating factors can include: medical and mental health services, employment services, VA benefits, and social support (Bloeser et al., 2014; Nelson et al., 2016; Pietrzak et al., 2010). A contemporary perspective on reintegration uses Bronfenbrenner's Ecological Model to demonstrate this complex system of distal and proximal impacts on the transitioning service member (Elnitsky, Blevins, Fisher, & Magruder, 2017). This research highlights that reintegration is a complex process involving layers of biopsychosocial factors. The VPRA aims to determine how best and how long to measure the process of reintegration. The VPRA has also drawn attention to how reintegration affects families, specifically, how post-military employment of the service member or spouse impacts the family. The opportunities for exploration on the subject of reintegration of veterans and their families are expansive and rich.

As the largest health care system in the United States with millions of pieces of demographic and health data gathered from electronic health records, the U.S. Department of Veterans Affairs is uniquely positioned to be on the forefront of medical, psychological, and social research. An example of this is the Million Veteran Program, an observational cohort study that is using genomic data to track genetic influences on health and disease (Gaziano et al., 2016). Research like this not only contributes to the health care of veterans, but the findings can be used to advance health and medicine around the world.

The latest research findings on veterans can be readily accessed from the research and data clearinghouse websites of the U.S Department of Veterans Affairs: Office of Research and Development, the National Center for Veterans Analysis and Statistics, and the National Center for PTSD. These websites showcase the breadth of medical and psychological research produced by VA researchers, often alongside researchers from government and nongovernment entities. There are also many private research organizations who have a veterans focus. For example, the Rand Corporation, in addition to its Army Research Division, examines veterans' health care and psychosocial issues and publishes accessible and relatable findings. There are also military, veteran, and family research centers at universities across the country supporting and producing research on veterans' issues. Examples of university research centers include the University of Pittsburgh Center for Military Medicine, the National Center for Veterans Studies at the University of Utah, and the Institute for Veterans and Military Families at Syracuse University. These resources provide easy access to the most current research findings and give a glimpse of ongoing research initiatives.

CONCLUSION

This chapter offers an introduction to working with veterans from a practice, policy, and research perspective. When working with veterans, it is essential for social workers to have a basic understanding of military culture and the processes related to deployment, reintegration, and adjustment to civilian life. Although the VA is the largest employer of social workers in the United States (Manske, 2006), private sector social workers are very likely to encounter veterans and their families.

Veterans return to the civilian world carrying their military culture and experiences with them. Military culture values honor, duty, and sacrifice, and a strong sense of collectivism. The majority of veterans are able to successfully integrate these values into their civilian lives. Some returning veterans, however, struggle with the psychological and physical wounds of war. Coping with combat stressors, being responsible for keeping others alive, and constant tactical awareness while deployed creates a skill set that can be maladaptive in the civilian world. Veterans may need support to help their transition and to heal from psychological and physical combat injuries. The Veterans Administration has faced many challenges in meeting the needs of veterans. With continued efforts through research and public–private partnerships, the VA is striving to improve the lives of veterans. Social workers have an important role to play in promoting a policy and research agenda for veterans as well as helping them in clinical settings to successfully reintegrate into the community.

CHAPTER DISCUSSION QUESTIONS

1. What is the relationship between tactical awareness and PTSD symptoms?

2. What socioecological factors make readjustment harder for members of the National Guard when compared to active duty service members?

3. Compare how veterans may experience private sector care versus that which they receive at the Veterans Administration Hospital?

4. Why do you think suicide rates are high in veterans?

5. List several reasons why a service member would have trouble reconnecting to his or her family during readjustment.

6. How would the Veterans Access, Choice, and Accountability Act improve care for veterans?

CASE EXAMPLE AND DISCUSSION QUESTIONS

Case Example 17.2

Vanessa, age 31, was admitted to the hospital for surgery related to a broken leg from a motorcycle accident. She has recently split up with her girlfriend of 5 years and plans to return home following discharge. The medical staff is concerned that she will need assistance with activities of daily living, but she insists that she can do it on her own. Vanessa served in the National Guard for 6 years as a medic and was deployed to both Iraq and Afghanistan. In addition to her injuries from the motorcycle accident, she reports having other medical conditions related to her deployments including chronic back pain, hearing loss, headaches, and knee pain. She also reports that she has had difficulty sleeping since she returned from Afghanistan. She is currently taking medication for anxiety, depression, and sleep. In planning her discharge, Vanessa takes an active role in planning her wound care and rehabilitation. She has a comfort with discussing medical issues, but she appears agitated and jumpy while in the hospital, especially when she hears commotion or instruments dropping outside of her room. She reports she has been diagnosed with PTSD, but has been too busy with school to make time for counseling. She is a sophomore in a nursing program, and has been struggling with concentrating on her studies and memorizing terms. She jokes about the fact that she has trouble hearing through stethoscopes because her ears are always ringing. Vanessa is determined to finish the nursing program and hopes to work in emergency room settings because she likes the excitement.

(continued)

Case Example 17.2 *(continued)*

Questions for Discussion

1. Taking into consideration the NASW ethical standard of self-determination, do you discharge Vanessa home to "do it on her own"?

2. What five elements of her presentation are likely related to her experiences in combat?

3. How do the excitement-seeking behaviors relate to her combat experiences and how would you address them?

4. What benefits and services could the VA and the VHA Hospital system provide to this client?

5. If Vanessa told you she would have to travel at least 50 miles to receive services from the VA and she could not drive there regularly, what options would you explore with her?

REFERENCES

Agha, Z., Lofgren, R. P., Van Ruiswyk, J. V., & Layde, P. M. (2000). Are patients at Veterans Affairs medical centers sicker? A comparative analysis of health status and medical resource use. *Archives of Internal Medicine, 160*(21), 3252–3257. doi:10.1001/archinte.160.21.3252

Ahern, J., Worthen, M., Masters, J., Lippman, S. A., Ozer, E. J., Moos, R., & Bearer, E. L. (2015). The challenges of Afghanistan and Iraq veterans' transition from military to civilian life and approaches to reconnection. *Plos One, 10*(7): e0128599. doi:10.1371/journal.pone.0128599

Beder, J., Coe, R., & Summer, D. (2011). Women and men who have served in Afghanistan/Iraq: Coming home. *Social Work and Health Care, 50*, 515–526. doi:10.1080/00981389.2011.554279

Bloeser, K., McCarron, K. K., Batorsky, B., Reinhard, M. J., Pollack, S. J., & Amdur, R. (2014). Mental health outreach and screening among returning veterans: Are we asking the right questions? *U.S. Army Medical Department Journal, 7*, 109–117.

Bryan, C. J., Rudd, M. D., Wertenberger, E., Young-McCaughon, S., & Peterson, A. (2015). Nonsuicidal self-injury as a prospective predictor of suicide attempts in a clinical sample of military personnel. *Comprehensive Psychiatry, 59*, 1–7. doi:10.1016/j.comppsych.2014.07.009

Center for Public-Private Partnerships. (2013). The veterans metrics initiative. Retrieved from http://www.hjfcp3.org/tvmi

Clark, M. E., Scholten, J. D., Walker, R. L., & Gironda, R. J. (2009). Assessment and treatment of pain associated with combat-related polytrauma. *Pain Medicine, 10*(3), 456–469. doi:10.1111/j.1526-4637.2009.00589.x

Draper, D. (2017) Veterans Health Care: Limited progress made to address concerns that led to high risk designation. U.S. Government Accountability Office Testimony before the

Committee on Veterans Affairs, U.S. Senate. Retrieved from https://www.veterans.senate .gov/imo/media/doc/GAO%20Draper%20testimony%20and%20study%203.15.17.pdf

Elnitsky, C. A., Blevins, C. L., Fisher, M. P., & Magruder, K. (2017). Military service member and veteran reintegration: A critical review and adapted ecological model. *American Journal of Orthopsychiatry, 87*(2), 114–128. doi:10.1037/ort0000244

Elnitsky, C., Fisher, M., & Blevins, C. (2017). Military service member and veteran reintegration: A conceptual analysis, unified definition, and key domains. *Frontiers in Psychology, 8*, 369–379. doi:10.3389/fpsyg.2017.00369

Farmer, C. M., & Hosek, S. D., (2016). Balancing demand and supply for veterans' health care: A summary of three RAND assessments conducted under the Veterans Choice Act. Retrieved from http://www.rand.org/pubs/research_reports/RR1165z4.html

Fisher, H. (2013, October 18). U.S. military casualty statistics: Operation New Dawn, Operation Iraqi Freedom, and Operation Enduring Freedom (congressional research service report). Retrieved from FAS.ORG website: http://www.fas.org/spg/crs/ natsec/RS22452.pdf

Franulic, A., Carbonell, C. G., Pinto, P., & Sepulveda, I. (2009). Psychosocial adjustment and employment outcome 2, 5 and 10 years after TBI. *Brain Injury, 18*(2), 119–129. doi:10.1080/0269905031000149515

Fulton, J. J., Calhoun, P. S., Wagner, H. R., Schry, A. R., Hair, L. P., Feeling, N., . . . Beckham, J. C. (2015). The prevalence of posttraumatic stress disorder in Operation Enduring Freedom/Operation Iraqi Freedom (OEF/OIF) veterans: A meta-analysis. *Journal of Anxiety Disorders, 31*(8), 98–107. doi:10.1016/j.janxdis.2015.02.003

Gaziano, J. M., Concato, J., Brophy, M., Fiore, L., Pyarajan, S., Breeling, J., . . . O'Leary, T. J. (2016). Million Veteran Program: A mega-biobank to study genetic influences on health and disease. *Journal of Clinical Epidemiology, 70*, 214–223. doi:10.1016/j .jclinepi.2015.09.016

Goldberg, M. S. (2010). Death and injury rates of U.S. military personnel in Iraq. *Military Medicine, 175*(4), 220.

Hall, L. K. (2011). The importance of understanding military culture. *Social Work in Health Care, 50*(1), 4–18. doi:10.1080/00981389.2010.513914

Halvorson, A. (2010). *Understanding the military: The institution, the culture, and the people.* Washington, DC: Substance Abuse and Mental Health Service Administration.

Hoge, C. W. (2010). *Once a warrior always a warrior.* Guilford, CT: Lyon Press.

Hynes, D. M., Koelling, K., Stroup, K., Arnold, N., Mallin, K., Sohn M.W., . . . Kock, L. (2007). Veterans' access to and use of Medicare and Veterans Affairs health care. *Medical Care, 45*(3), 214–223. doi:10.1097/01.mlr.0000244657.90074.b7

Jackson, K. (2013). Working with veterans and military families. *Social Work Today*, 12–19.

JEC United States Congress (2015). 10 Key Facts about Veterans of the Post-9/11 Era. Retrieved from https://www.jec.senate.gov/public/index.cfm/democrats/2016/ 11/10-key-facts-about-veterans-of-the-post-9-11-era

Kemp, J., & Bossarte, R. (2012). *Suicide data report 2012.* Washington, DC: Department of Veteran Affairs. Retrieved from https://www.va.gov/opa/docs/suicide-data-report-2012-final.pdf

Kimbrel, N. A., Gratz, K. L., Tull, M. T., Morissette, S. B., Meyer, E. C., DeBeer, B. B., . . . Beckham, J. C. (2015). Non-suicidal self-injury as a predictor of active and passive suicidal ideation among Iraq/Afghanistan war veterans. *Psychiatry Research, 227*, 360–362. doi:10.1016/j.psychres.2015.03.026

La Bash, H., Vogt, D. S., King, L. A., & King, D. W. (2009). Deployment stressors of the Iraq war: Insights from the mainstream media. *Journal of Interpersonal Violence, 24*(2), 231–258. doi:10.1177/0886260508317177

Lovestrand, D., Phipps S., & Lovestrand S. (2013). Posttraumatic stress disorder and anesthesia emergence. *AANA Journal, 81*, 199–203.

Manske, J. E. (2006). Social work in the Department of Veterans Affairs: Lessons learned. *Health & Social Work, 31*(3), 233–238.

Martsolf, G. R., Tomoaia-Cotisel, A., & Tanielian, T. (2016). Behavioral health workforce and private sector solutions to addressing veterans' access to care issues. *JAMA Psychiatry, 73*(12), 1213–1214. doi:10.1001/jamapsychiatry.2016.2456

Moore, B. A. (2012). *Handbook of counseling military couples.* London: Routledge.

Moore, C. D. (2015). Innovation without reputation: How bureaucrats saved the veterans health care system. *Perspectives on Politics, 13*, 327–344. doi:10.1017/S1537592715000067

National Association of Social Workers. (2012). *NASW standards for social work practice with service members, veterans, and their families.* Washington, DC: Author.

National Center for Veterans Analysis and Statistics. (2016). Unique veteran users report FY 2014. United States Department of Veterans Affairs. Retrieved from https://www.va.gov/vetdata/docs/SpecialReports/Profile_of_Unique_Veteran_Users_2014.pdf

Nelson, C. B., Abraham, K. M., Miller, E. M., Kees, M. R., Walters, H. M., Valenstein, M., & Zivin, K. (2016). Veteran mental health and employment: The nexus and beyond. In S. MacDermid Wadsworth & D. Riggs (Eds.), *War and family life* (pp. 239–260). Cham, Switzerland: Springer International Publishing.

Pietrzak, R. H., Johnson, D. C., Goldstein, M. B., Malley, J. C., Rivers, A. J., Morgan, C. A., & Southwick, S. M. (2010). Psychosocial buffers of traumatic stress, depressive symptoms, and psychosocial difficulties in veterans of Operations Enduring Freedom and Iraqi Freedom: The role of resilience, unit support, and postdeployment social support. *Journal of Affective Disorders, 120*, 188–192. doi:10.1016/j.jad.2009.04.015

Priebe, S., Gavrilovic, J. J., Bremner, S., Ajdukovic, Franciskovic, T., Galeazzi, G. M., . . . Bogic, M. (2013). Psychological symptoms as long-term consequences of war experiences. *Psychopathology, 46*(1), 45–54. doi:10.1159/000338640

Rubin, A., Weiss, E., & Coll, J. E. (2013). *Handbook or military social work.* Hoboken, NJ: Wiley.

Shane, L. (2016). VA disability backlog tops 70,000—7 months after it was supposed to be zero. *Military Times.* Retrieved from http://www.militarytimes.com/story/veterans/2016/07/10/va-disability-claims-backlog-veterans-affairs/86862716/

U.S. Department of Veterans Affairs. (2016a). FY Agency Financial Report. Retrieved from https://www.va.gov/finance/docs/afr/2016VAafrFullWeb.pdf

U.S. Department of Veterans Affairs. (2016b). Office of policy and planning veterans policy research agenda. Retrieved from https://www.va.gov/op3/docs/StrategicPlanning/FY_2016_Veterans_Policy_Research_Agenda.pdf

U.S. Department of Veterans Affairs. (2017a). Analysis of VA Health Care Utilization among Operation Enduring Freedom (OEF), Operation Iraqi Freedom (OIF), and Operation New Dawn (OND) veterans. Retrieved from http://www.publichealth.va.gov/docs/epidemiology/health care-utilization-report-fy2015-qtr3.pdf

U.S. Department of Veterans Affairs (2017b). Health benefits. Retrieved from https://www.va.gov/healthbenefits/apply/veterans.asp

U.S. Department of Veterans Affairs. (2017c). Veterans health administration: About VA. Retrieved from https://www.va.gov/health/aboutvha.asp

U.S. Government Accountability Office. (2017). VA disability benefits: Additional planning would enhance efforts to improve the timeliness of appeals decisions. Report to congressional addressees. Retrieved from http://www.gao.gov/assets/690/683637.pdf

Veterans Access, Choice, and Accountability Act of 2014, Pub. L. No. 113–146, § 128 Stat. 1754 (2014).

Wertsch, M. E. (1991). *Military brats: Legacies of childhood inside the fortress.* New York, NY: Brightwell Publishing.

Westat. (2010). *National survey of veterans, active duty service members, demobilized national guard and reserve members, family members, and surviving spouses: Final report, deliverable 27.* Washington, DC: Department of Veterans Affairs.

Wright, J. E. (2013). *Those who have borne the battle: A history of America's wars and those who fought them.* New York, NY: Public Affairs.

Yee, C., Frakt, A., & Pizer, S. (2016). U.S. Department of Veterans Affairs: Economic and policy effects on demand for VA care. Partnered evidence-based resource center policy brief. Retrieved from https://www.queri.research.va.gov/partnered_evaluation/YeeFraktPizer.pdf

Future Directions for Health and Social Work

Lynn Videka and Janna C. Heyman

The future of American health care is being shaped by a number of factors, including efforts toward improving the quality of care, measuring health care outcomes, increasing access to care, reframing the delivery system, containing escalating costs, partisan politics that increasingly reflect fundamental values and ideological divides concerning health care as a societal responsibility, and redistribution of wealth to achieve health equity (Congressional Budget Office [CBO], 2017a; Dzau et al., 2017; Institute of Medicine [IOM], 2015; National Center for Health Statistics, 2016; Roy, 2017). As highlighted throughout this book, social work plays an important role for various facets of the health care system. Social work's distinct contribution to health care in the United States is for analysis AND action to reduce health disparities (Spencer et al, in press).

As detailed in Chapter 1, from the progressive era to today, social work has been in the forefront in taking action to improve the accessibility and quality of health care and in addressing the social and behavioral determinants of health. From the days of the progressive era, health care, especially for those who are excluded from American society, has been a concern of American social workers. Social workers have continued to serve the individuals, families, and communities that are the most vulnerable and affected by social and behavioral influences on health as well as a fragmented health care system.

Social workers are playing an increasingly important role in health care, and this sector is a focal area of growth for the profession. The labor force need for social workers in health care is growing. The projected demand for social workers is expected to increase by 12% between 2014 and 2024, faster than the average rate of all positions, with employment growth estimated due to the demand for health care and social services (U.S. Department of Labor, Bureau of Labor Statistics, Social Workers, 2016). As the national health care landscape is changing (Council on Social Work Education [CSWE], 2014b), the role of social work is also evolving. This chapter summarizes the health care issues raised throughout the book, contemplates factors that will drive future health care policy and practice decisions, and considers the future roles of social workers in health care.

CURRENT AND FUTURE HEALTH CARE IN THE UNITED STATES

Historically, health care in the United States has been characterized by its lack of attention to reducing health disparities and to providing health care to all Americans. The future of health care will be shaped by changing demographics as well as focuses on population health and health disparities. Our nation's health has undergone significant changes with the Patient Protection and Affordable Care Act (ACA), including a decrease in the uninsured population and more financial security for families affected by serious health problems. At the same time, the current proposals to reform the ACA may reverse the gains made in the number of insured individuals (CBO, 2017a). As discussed in Chapter 1, the 2010 ACA led the way for improving access to health care for the uninsured. The ACA "implemented comprehensive reforms designed to improve the accessibility, affordability, and quality of health care" (Obama, 2016, p. 525). After the ACA was enacted, the percentage of uninsured individuals saw a significant decline, from 16.0% in 2010 to 8.9% in the first 6 months of 2016 (Zammitti, Cohen, & Martinez, 2016). Despite the enactment of the ACA, potential barriers remain for the uninsured, including eligibility on immigration status, awareness, and out-of-pocket financial expenses (Obama, 2016; Shartzer, Kenney, Long, & Odu, 2016).

While progress toward universal health insurance has been made, concerns for maintaining and improving access to quality health insurance remains in the forefront. Partisan attacks and opposition to the ACA began with the law's passage on March 23, 2010. There have been over 70 attempts to repeal the ACA, including Supreme Court challenges and the insurance mandate, alternative legislation, and budget strategies (Riotta, 2017). Since President Trump took office, there have been several failed attempts to replace the legislation, with some proposals never reaching House and Senate votes. In the latest action to dismantle the ACA, the Tax Cut and Jobs Act (Public Law 115-97) removes the mandate for individual insurance coverage, but leaves in place the government subsidy for middle income Americans to purchase health insurance and Medicaid expansion.

The likely impact of the discontinuance of the ACA health insurance mandate is that healthier and younger Americans will be less likely to purchase insurance on the insurance exchanges, but the government subsidies will remain in place. If healthier Americans decline to purchase insurance, then the population pools for the insurance exchanges will be older and poorer, leading almost certainly to insurance rate hikes that will make it harder for lower income Americans to afford insurance, and increasing reliance on governmental spending for subsidies. Analysts believe the effects of this law will be to increase the cost of insurance on the exchanges, mostly because the pools will now be comprised of higher risk individuals than with the mandate. The Congressional Budget Office forecasts that the law will also increase the U.S. government deficit, leading the uninsured to seek less health care and to possible downsizing of the health care sector of the economy. This could lead to negative effects for the economy as a hole. The Republican efforts to dismantle the ACA are likely to continue, creating uncertainty for American health policy context, and leading to a less healthy American public (Blumenthal, 2017).

While the gains of the ACA have been described by Obama (2016) and recognized by many other analysts, concerns remain, especially among conservative political points of view, about the cost of the ACA, the hesitance of market-based insurance companies to participate in insurance exchanges, and the costs of providing the additional health care. This is all taking place in the context of American mediocre health outcomes and high costs when compared globally with health care in other developed nations.

WHAT WE KNOW ABOUT SOCIAL NEEDS AND HEALTH OUTCOMES

While there has been progress in the United States with respect to health status, with life expectancy at birth increasing from 76.8 years in 2000 to 78.8 years in 2014 (National Center for Health Statistics, 2016), the United States still ranks 43rd globally on this indicator (IOM, 2014). Similarly, the infant mortality rate has declined from 6.91 per 1,000 live births to 5.82 from 2000 to 2014 (National Center for Health Statistics, 2016). However, as a country, the United States has higher infant mortality rates than most other developed countries (Organisation for Economic Co-operation and Development [OECD], 2017). These poor to mediocre U.S. health performance indicators are driven by health disparities in the United States. People of color and those from low-income households account for the overall lackluster American health outcomes, especially considering that the United States is the world's highest per capita spending nation on health care (Central Intelligence Agency, 2017; World Health Organization, 2012). As one also examines changes in the age-adjusted death rate per 100,000, the United States has decreased from 869.0 to 724.6 between 2000 and 2014 (National Center for Health Statistics, 2016), but, as a nation, the United States has higher death rates than other countries (OECD, 2017), and recent reports show an alarming increase in substance use–related deaths that are lowering the life span for middle-aged men (Case & Deaton, 2015).

There is also a significant shift in the age of the population. In the United States, by 2030, one in every five persons is expected to be in the 65 and over age cohort (Ortman, Velkoff, & Hogan, 2014). Many baby boomers have reached their 65th year, and many are living longer than past over-65 cohorts. According to the National Institutes of Health (2010), life expectancies may be attributed to improved medical treatments, changes in health behaviors, increase in use of assistive technologies, and improvement in education and socioeconomic status. Many older Americans are diagnosed with multiple chronic conditions. These require a coordinated approach to care in order to achieve effective outcomes and efficient care. Palliative and end-of-life care, as discussed in Chapter 9, brings balance and options for people at the end of their life, to make choices concerning aggressive versus palliative or "comfort" care and the degree to which they want their health care driven by technology.

While many of these statistics paint a picture of increasing longevity, it is important to recognize that income, as well as racial and ethnic disparities, still exist today. Individuals in higher income brackets have longer life expectancies compared to those with lower income (Chetty, 2016). With respect to racial and ethnic differences, the National Center for Health Statistics (2016) released *Health, United States, 2015: With Special Feature on Racial and Ethnic Health Disparities*, noting that "Differences in life expectancy, infant mortality, cigarette smoking among women, influenza vaccinations among those aged 65 and over, and health insurance coverage narrowed among the racial and ethnic groups" (p. 21). However, despite progress, there are still racial and ethnic disparities. For example, non-Hispanic Black adults are more likely to have high blood pressure than adults in other racial and ethnic groups. Other indicators, such as age-adjusted obesity rates, highlight these differences, with non-Hispanic Black adults at 48.1% and Hispanics at 42.5%, compared to 34.5% for non-Hispanic White and 11.7% for non-Hispanic Asian adults (Ogden, Carroll, Fryar, & Flegal, 2015).

Persons with a disability, discussed in Chapter 16, often have higher health care needs, and differences by racial and ethnic groups need to be understood. Individuals with disabilities experience limitations in a range of areas, including mobility, hearing, vision, cognition, and emotional or behavioral disorders. Estimates indicate that approximately one in eight working-age adults have some type of disability; with over half (51.0%) having a mobility disability and 38.3% with a cognitive disability (Stevens et al., 2016). Compared with adults who have no disability, adults with any disability were more likely to be age 45 to 64 and more likely to be Black and non-Hispanic (Stevens et al., 2016).

Elizabeth Bradley and her colleagues have conducted a compelling series of cross-sectional, cross-national comparison studies that examine nations' investments in social services and care and health outcomes (Bradley, Elkins, Herrin, & Elbel, 2011). Their findings show that after adjusting for the level of health expenditures and gross domestic product, nations with higher ratios of social expenditures to health expenditures demonstrated better health outcomes in terms of infant mortality, life expectancy, and increased potential life years lost. Bradley et al. (2016) conducted a second study of U.S. state comparisons of the ratio of social (social services and public health) to health (Medicaid + Medicare expenditures) investment on health outcomes. They found that higher social to health spending states showed better health outcomes in seven areas: adult obesity; asthma; mentally unhealthy days; days with activity limitations; and mortality rates for lung cancer, acute myocardial infarction, and type 2 diabetes. These studies point to the importance of investment in social well-being to produce healthy outcomes.

In a recent article that is part of the National Academy of Medicine's Vital Directions for Health and Health Care Initiative, McGinnis et al. (2016) support a social–ecological and life-span model of health that extends beyond the health care system and is highly consistent with social work thinking and practice to improve health behaviors, change health cultures, and to reduce health disparities. The model focuses on people in their environments and makes the point that environmental investments beyond health systems are important to truly improve the health of the nation. This includes investing in public health and education, communities, housing, and in social institutions outside of the health care system, such as schools. Figure 18.1 shows McGinnis et al.'s social–ecological life-span model of health (in

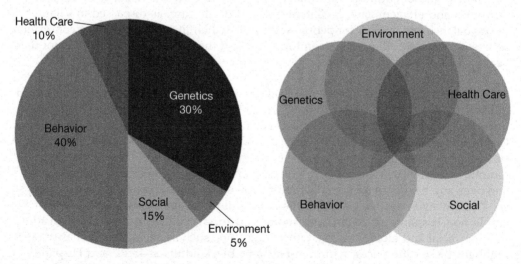

Figure 18.1 Schematics of factors influencing health, their association with premature death, and their intersections.

Source: From McGinnis, J. M., Berwick, D. M., Dascle, T. A., Diaz, A., Fineberg, H. V., Frist, W. H., Gawande, A., Halfon, N., Lavizzo-Mourey, R. (2016). Systems strategies for health throughout the life course. Discussion Paper, Vital Directions for Health and Health Care Series. National Academy of Medicine, Washington, DC. https:// nam.edu/wp-content/uploads/2016/09/systems-strategies-for-health-throughout-the-life-course.pdf. Reprinted with permission.

the right Venn diagram), and the relative influence of each ecological factor on premature death (in the left pie chart). Social and behavioral variables explain 55% of the variance in premature deaths. In contrast, health care explains 10% of the variance in premature deaths. This model demonstrates clearly how important the social and behavioral determinants of health, and of death, are. Social work is the primary profession that addresses these factors in health care, and as such, can directly impact the health of the nation.

SOCIAL WORK ROLES IN RESPONSE TO THE IMPORTANCE OF SOCIAL AND BEHAVIORAL DETERMINANTS OF HEALTH

The importance of social determinants of health has been a central focus of social work and impacts the health and well-being of society. This book considers in depth the social determinants of health (see Chapter 3) and intersectionality, with multiple and cross-cutting identities as creating unique social positions with respect to health care (see Chapter 4). The chapter authors also discuss foci of health care and specific vulnerable populations (see Chapters 8–17) and they emphasize special populations that are prone to health disparities. These chapters also demonstrate that innovative evidence-based policy and practice approaches reduce the gap in health and in health care that the special populations face. These chapters emphasize the importance of educating social workers in understanding how social determinants of health impact practice. This book challenges social workers to see, not just the child that may come into a clinic for a service, but how support can be provided in the context of the child, family, and the community in which they live. An underlying theme across these chapters is that it is important to deliver evidence-based interventions that are built upon understanding clients' social circumstances and their value and preferences, the best research evidence, the practitioners' expertise, and clients' cultural and community preferences. While social workers have been using intersectional (i.e., cross-cutting and overlaying) approaches to understanding the complexities of social identities and their impact on social determinants of health and inequities, further work in evidence-based and culturally relevant approaches is needed. Social workers can also advocate for policy change to work with other professionals to both identify levels of intervention for action related to social determinants of health (Solar & Irwin, 2010).

The Social Work Grand Challenges identifies health equity as an important focus of the social impact for the profession. Rine (2016) suggests that all "forms of health and well-being are social in nature, not only in their etiology, but also by virtue of how they are disparately managed. . . . This broad, holistic, collective, and interdependent understanding of health, well-being, and social problems is evident across these 12 challenges" (p. 143).

Over the past several years, the American Academy of Social Work and Social Welfare (AASWSW) has supported the development and expansion of Grand Challenges for Social Work (AASWSW, 2017). The Grand Challenges aim to set an achievable agenda for social work research and practice that will solve 12 major societal problems over the next generation. "Achieving Health Equity" is the title of the health-focused Grand Challenge. Walters et al. (2016) lay out the agenda for this social work Grand Challenge. Spencer et al. (in press) have expanded the narrative on social work's role in health disparities and lay out a model of practice that includes community and social system interventions as well as individual behavioral interventions. This scholarship calls for social work to address the very fabric of society that produces health inequity, those social and structural factors that are viewed as distal from health problems, but that comprise the predictors of inequality. These include housing, education, financial resources, neighborhood environments, social media access, expanding community assets including access to nutritionally rich food. It is consistent with the framework advanced by McGinnis et al. (2016) calling for community and social structural changes that reduce health inequalities, as well as continued attention to evidence-based individual and family-level interventions that are culturally relevant and acceptable to specific populations to improve health outcomes. These are especially important to address for children so that the protective and nurturing environments allow the child to develop healthily, and to be protected from trauma. A nurturing and protective environment will launch children into a lifetime of good health, physical and behavioral.

Spencer et al. (in press) identify several frameworks and strategies for addressing health equities. One approach deploys an ecological framework, similar to the one developed by McGinnis et al. (2016); another deploys a translational science approach, moving from "social laboratory" to "natural environment." The various methods have some common characteristics including community-based decision making and participation, respect for community beliefs norms and traditions, attention to physical and social environments, collaborative problem-solving approaches, a deep knowledge of and interaction with the community, and multi-sector approaches that include working with the community, families, government, and social and health institutions in order to achieve desired equity goals.

Social workers are already the dominant behavioral health workforce, with most direct care, especially for low-income people, being delivered by social workers. These skills are increasingly important to health care today. But social workers should also seize the opportunity to lead the development of community and larger system changes by developing evidence-based community-targeted models of health in the future.

INTEGRATED ROLES FOR SOCIAL WORK IN HEALTH CARE

Social workers in health care cannot view themselves as practicing in a silo; they need to have the competency to " integrate and apply social work knowledge, values, and skills to practice situations in a purposeful, intentional, and professional manner to promote human and community well-being" (CSWE, 2015, p. 6). They must function at all levels of intervention in the health care system. Social workers need to be leaders that integrate practice, policy, and research in shaping the future of health care. Figure 18.2 illustrates future roles that social workers will have in health promotion, prevention, and health service delivery.

Prevention

Since enactment of the ACA in the United States, access to health care for uninsured people has increased and there is a renewed focus on prevention. However, as the ACA is challenged, it begs the question, will the United States be able to continue to encourage models that have prevention as their core focus? Rishel (2015) calls upon social workers to "be able to implement a prevention-focused integrative approach to practice in order to effectively function and provide leadership in the new era of health care" (p. 125).

Research conducted by Ruth and colleagues (2015) found that topics within social work prevention, such as substance abuse, violence, aging, and disease, although still a minority focus as compared with treatment or intervention approaches, have increased in the social work professional literature between 2000 and 2010. This increased attention

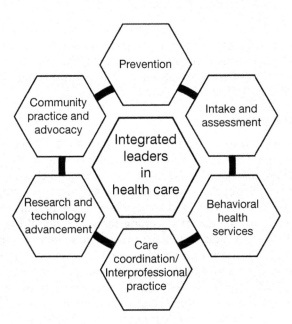

Figure 18.2 Social work roles in future health care.

to prevention-based practice is important not only for social work in services to children and youth, before the onset of most health morbidities, but throughout the life cycle and the illness cycle.

Social workers contribute to improving health care and reducing health disparities through health promotion. Examples include media campaigns on prenatal care and infant development, or on recognizing the signs of depression and advertising depression screening days.

Universal prevention includes interventions delivered to entire populations. Examples include health education classes and substance abuse prevention education for middle school students to reduce the arc of risk over the adolescent years and through condom distribution (see Chapter 14 on HIV prevention) to prevent HIV and other sexually transmitted infections.

Selective prevention includes interventions to high-risk populations. Many states have home visiting–based prevention programs such as "Healthy Families America," or the "Nurse Family Partnership" for high-risk families. These programs are designed to promote healthy child development and nurturing parent–child interactions from the prenatal period through school entry.

Indicated prevention includes services to high-risk populations who have early signs of morbidity, such as diabetes education programs to persons with borderline blood sugar levels or motivational interventions to help reduce substance use in adolescents with a first driving under the influence arrest.

Prevention approaches include evidence-based treatment and case identification (e.g., for sexual partners of HIV-positive persons).

Prevention also extends into rehabilitation and maintenance after treatment for an acute condition. Examples include harm reduction models such as needle exchanges for drug-using populations, psychiatric or physical rehabilitation, and "booster treatment" or follow-up sessions for a variety of conditions. The prevention model is a framework that integrates health throughout the life span and uses interventions much broader in scope and approach than those thought of as "clinical treatments." Social workers must be competent in the range of evidence-based prevention approaches in health care today.

Intake and Assessment

Screening and assessment for behavioral health problems is becoming routine in primary care and in people with multiple chronic health conditions (Claiborne et al., 2010; Videka, Ohta, Blackburn, Luce, & Morton, in press). Several chapters in this book illustrate the increasing number of evidence-based screening and assessment tools that social workers are using in primary, acute, and tertiary health care practice. Every social worker should be competent with the use of screening tools, and should be mindful to ensure evidence-based follow-up strategies when a positive assessment is made.

Claiborne et al. (2010) show that problem alcohol use screening is routinely completed in a medical center, and that the electronic medical record with prompts helps support screening. The same study showed that follow-through with post assessment positive results was much more lax due to cultural factors in the health care system. Social workers can play a critical role as the team behavioral health specialist, to ensure that evidence-based follow-up methods such as Screening, Brief Intervention, Referral, and Treatment (SBIRT), or referral methods are correctly implemented.

Behavioral Health Services

Social workers are typically the health team member with specialized skills in delivering behavioral health services. With the increasing recognition that this domain is an important driver of overall health care and medical treatment adherence, social workers should educate other health professionals about the role of behavioral health in the overall health of a person. As several chapters in this volume illustrate, there is a growing number of evidence-based and short-term interventions that help people improve their health and to manage self-care and wellness. Social workers have a professional responsibility to provide the most effective services available and to help the interprofessional team identify when these services are needed.

Interprofessional Practice and Team Work

Social workers are valuable members of the interprofessional team, which typically includes physicians, nurses, pharmacists, and other health care professionals. Now more than ever, in their behavioral health care specialist roles, social workers provide behavioral health services in interprofessional primary care settings. While the evidence for the health outcomes contributions of interprofessional health services is just beginning to be studied, there is evidence that interprofessional education leads to better team functioning, and that for some conditions, produce better patient health outcomes (Reeves, Perrier, Goldman, Freeth, & Zwarenstein, 2013; Renders et al., 2000).

Social workers should be leading the research focus on interprofessional care. These studies will demonstrate the positive effects that social work services produce. They are vital to working with the individual and family members to listen, respect, and collaborate on shared decision making. In interprofessional, integrated care teams, social workers have the knowledge and skills to be able to engage, assess, facilitate, communicate, and provide care coordination/case management and connection to resources.

Research and Technology Advancement

Dzau et al. (2017) state, "The rise of digital health technology has opened the door to enhanced health care and provider access, greater patient engagement, as well as data and tools to support more personalized and tailored health care" (p. 4). Social workers need to be in the ready to be part of the digital health technology (see Chapter 5). It plays a vital role in communication methods, today in the use of medical records and in the future, it will continue to be a part of communication. As part of the Centers for Disease Control and Prevention, the National Center for Health Statistics (2017) is also working to improve the technology infrastructure in the United States, moving from paper-based systems to an integrated web-based system, including efforts to improve electronic health records and public health information systems. These advances are essential to improve data sources for the health care system to address prevention, disease, future research, and policy. Social workers need to be a part of these advances.

Whatever health care policy changes will occur, it is likely that newer models of evidence-based interprofessional, coordinated care will continue to meet the needs of people with multiple chronic conditions and limited social resources and health behavioral repertoires. Furthermore, with the high rates of comorbid behavioral health conditions in primary care and in many chronic health conditions, social work practice will need to adapt its methods to fit the fast-paced world of primary care. This will require a change in the mind-set of social work primary health behavioral care intervention—from long-term to consulting, single-episode approaches that may include annual or more frequent follow-up. The new single-episode (with follow-up as needed and requested) approaches hold great promise for reaching the majority of people with behavioral health needs who never seek specialty mental health or addictions care. More and more primary care services, especially the federally qualified health centers (FQHCs) that provide care to the populations that have faced health disparities, employ social workers in primary care clinics and deploy short-term interventions for behavioral health problems on a consulting, rather than specialty care, basis. It is especially important for behavioral health care to be available to more young and middle-aged adults, with the highest rates of mental health and substance use problems, and with a specialized help seeking rate for these problems at less than 10%, as described in Chapter 8. Given the long-term health risks that mental health and substance use patterns of behavior pose, response and short-term, evidence-based interventions such as motivational interviewing and SBIRT should be readily available for every youth and adult in the United States.

Community Practice and Advocacy

McGinnis et al. (2016) and Spencer et al. (in press) provide compelling cases for health advancement strategies that take environments seriously and intervene at the community level to create health-supporting environments. One example of this approach is the increasing community planning and engagement emphasis of *Communities that Care* (www.communitiesthatcare.net), a community intervention strategy that aims to create health environments that support youth development. In this model, a community planning process engages community leaders to work together to identify culturally acceptable strategies to increase safety and healthy recreational alternatives for youth. Another Detroit-based program, Midnight Golf (www.midnightgolf.org), supports youth evening golf leagues to provide healthy evening activities for youth. Spencer et al. (2011) created a community-wide, community health-worker–led diabetes prevention program in an inner city. The intervention demonstrated lower A1c levels community-wide. Another program being established in urban communities with vacant lots is the community garden program. Community Centers and Settlement Houses across the nation are banding together to provide better and affordable health food environments for their communities (George, Rovniak, Kraschnewski, Hanson, & Sciamanna, 2015). More of these types of interventions are needed. Social workers are in just the right position to create them in partnership with the communities themselves.

SPECIAL POPULATIONS AND HEALTH CARE

In Health Promotion and Public Health (Chapter 6), we are reminded that public health and social work share the perspective that caring for the health and social needs of the population, especially the most vulnerable subpopulations, helps to benefit society as a whole. Much of the content of this book focuses on the special needs and circumstances and special interventions for these special populations who are at risk of health disparities. The settlement house movement's work emphasized public health and prevention as a central focus in social work history. Today, there needs to be a continued emphasis on understanding the person in the environment and commitment to work in communities utilizing public health approaches (Ruth, Marshall, & Velásquez, 2013). These efforts need to empower social workers to advocate for change in the community and globally. Rishel (2015) captures this thinking well in stating, "It is important to note that the need for prevention-focused integrative services goes beyond the health care system. Other service systems, including the child welfare system, juvenile justice system, and education system, also have a need for and will benefit from this type of approach to service delivery and practice" (Rishel, 2015, p. 126). This view corresponds to McGinnis, Williams-Russa, and Knickman's (2002) work that challenged readers to remember that U.S. health policy and health spending is often focused on payment for medical treatment. However, "The fact that many of the conditions driving the need for treatment are preventable ought to draw attention to policy opportunities for promoting health" (p. 78). Social workers need to be educated about the importance of prevention.

The Integrative Behavioral Health chapter highlights the goals of the "Triple Aim" in health care, including: (a) improving the health of the population; (b) reducing the per capita cost; and (c) enhancing the patient experience (Berwick, Nolan, & Whittington, 2008). As behavioral health needs increase, social workers play a vital role. Social workers focusing on the patient-centered needs of individuals are trained in screening and conducting biopsychosocial assessment, which plays a critical role in working with individuals, their families, and the health care team on shared decision making. They are involved in addressing patients' attitudes toward their treatment plan, adherence, and barriers to care. In integrated care, social workers are core members of the interprofessional team. The diverse knowledge and skills of social workers can help to strengthen the behavioral health workforce. Given the health vulnerability that substance use behaviors create, social worker's role as behavioral health providers contributes substantially toward improving the health of our nation.

Social workers are also integral members of palliative and end-of-life care teams. Chapter 9 expands on the changes in palliative care. When faced with a life-threatening illness at any stage, palliative care focuses on improving the quality of life of individuals and their loved ones. Palliative care can touch the lives of individuals at any age and this approach has pioneered interprofessional approaches to health care service delivery. As palliative care has developed across different settings, social workers are in the forefront helping to communicate with individuals and families and playing a crucial role in interprofessional teams. This may include working with advance care planning, which involves planning to ensure that the patient's/individual's wishes are followed when the patient is no longer able to communicate them. The future role for social workers should continue to focus on assessment, communication, and family engagement.

IMPLICATIONS FOR SOCIAL WORK EDUCATION AND PRACTICE

The dramatic changes needed to truly deliver effective and efficient health care and to reduce the substantial health disparities in our nation call for a very different social work education than prevails today. The CSWE Commission on Accreditation and the Commission on Educational Policy (COEP) established the 2015 Educational Policy and Accreditation Standards (EPAS) for accrediting baccalaureate and master's degree programs in social work education. CSWE's 2015 EPAS is guided by "a person-in-environment framework, global perspective, respect for human diversity, and knowledge based on scientific inquiry, the purpose of social work is actualized through its quest for social and economic justice, the prevention of conditions that limit human rights, the elimination of poverty, and the enhancement of the quality of life for all persons, locally and globally" (p. 5). While the EPAS is not specifically developed for social work and health care, it lays the foundation for the breadth and depth of the knowledge, skills, and values critical for future social work and health care professionals. The holistic view of competency addresses both performance and judgment in regard to practice (CSWE, 2015). CSWE has also included prevention in its 2015 EPAS.

The National Association of Social Workers (NASW) Code of Ethics addresses the core values of the profession, addressing human dignity and worth and the pursuit of social justice. NASW has integrated prevention into its practice standards for social workers in health care.

Competencies that focus on cultural competence, collaborative practice, short-term, evidence-based intervention skills, and the ability to work effectively in organizations and to deliver clinical assessment, treatment, and evaluation services with individuals, families, groups, and communities are important. Understanding and competency to work in health care organizations is important. But there are several competencies for today's and tomorrow's public health–focused practice that need more attention in the social work curriculum. These include interprofessional practice, the use of technology in delivering social work care, and organizational leadership.

In 2013, a survey of CSWE-accredited MSW programs showed that 71% of incoming social work students chose a "clinical" or direct intervention track for their social work studies, and that 18% of students were enrolled in generalist practice tracks (CSWE, 2014a). Only 11% of all social work students were enrolled in larger social system–emphasis tracks. This demonstrates the trend toward clinical practice in the profession and raises concern about preparation of the future workforce who will have the interest in and the competency to lead community and social system change efforts that sustain the health of marginalized populations. Furthermore, only 14% of all social work students reported that year enrolled in a health-focused curriculum track, suggesting that not enough social workers are being educated to competently manage the huge knowledge base of health care along and to integrate this knowledge with social work principles and competencies.

The best available knowledge today suggests that in order for social workers to play an important role in reducing health disparities and contributing to better health for all Americans, they need to understand how to intervene at multiple social system levels, and particularly to address the gaps in maximizing the role of social disparities and environments on health. Therefore, based on the data presented, there is a gap between the micro-focused practitioners of today and the macro environmental needs our nation has to improve the health of our population. This reasoning suggests that social work education should reorient itself to address the structural and environmental determinants of health inequality as well as the behavioral aspects that view the individual as the agent of self-change.

With 45% of the social work workforce employed in health or behavioral health settings, and with this sector being the fastest growing sector of the profession through 2025, the emphasis on public health and prevention efforts as well as community and social structural interventions must grow (U.S. Department of Labor, Bureau of Labor Statistics, Social Workers, 2016). To contribute to better health, every social worker must know how to lead community assessment and change. Every social worker must be knowledgeable about social policy (which the current CSWE competencies address), and must also know how to influence the adoption of progressive policies and how to use his or her discretion in practice to deliver the most progressive services possible under insurance plan stipulations and government policies.

Social work today and in the future will be highly interprofessional. Social work students must have competencies in understanding and articulating their roles and contributions in health care. With paraprofessional providers such as home health aides, community health workers, peer providers, and patient navigators, the fastest growing sector of the health care workforce interprofessional practice must include working collaboratively and effectively with paraprofessionals in health care. Paraprofessional workers are those who are typically most culturally similar to the recipients of health care, who often have the "lived experience," that is similar life experiences, as the health recipient, who inhabit the social systems of the health recipient, and have the best linguistic and cultural competence of their neighborhoods and communities. All social work students need to understand health disparities, how they work, and how they are dismantled, in order to clearly understand and articulate their contributions to the quality of health of the health care recipient. Social workers need to be able to communicate their contribution with confidence and poise.

CONCLUSION

Social work services will grow in the next 20 years with the aging of the population and the growing disparities in income and in health in our society. In order to be prepared to play an integral role in the health care of the future, social workers need education that equips them with competence and confidence. They need to understand and be able to articulate what they can contribute to interprofessional care of the complex and sometimes disenfranchised health care recipient. They need to be able to motivate those seeking care and those giving care to aspire to the best actions that will advance health. They need to always carry a prevention focus, which is entirely consistent with the optimistic "strengths" perspective that is a hallmark of our field. They need to lead the health care team in understanding and respecting the diversity of clients and cultures and communities. They need to advocate for health care recipients and they need to be able to intervene with larger social systems—communities, social institutions including the health care system, and the policy arena—to deliver the best possible health care for all Americans.

This is a moment of opportunity for social work. It is up to our profession to advance the potential of universal and quality health care for all Americans.

REFERENCES

American Academy of Social Work and Social Welfare. (2017). Grand challenges for social work. Retrieved from http://aaswsw.org/grand-challenges-initiative/

Berwick, D. M., Nolan, T. W., & Whittington, J. (2008). The Triple Aim: Care, health, and cost. *Health Affairs, 27*(3), 759–769. doi:10.1377/hlthaff.27.3.759

Bradley, E. H., Canavan, M., Rogan, E., Talbert-Slagle, K., Ndumele, C., Taylor, L., & Curry, L. A. (2016). Variation in health outcomes: The role of spending on social services, public health, and health care. *Health Affairs, 35*(5), 760–768. doi:10.1377/hlthaff.2015.0814

Bradley, E. H., Elkins, B. R., Herrin, J., & Elbel, B. (2011). Health and social services expenditures: Associations with health outcomes. *British Medical Journal: Quality and Safety, 20*(10), 826–831. doi:10.1136/bmjqs.2010.048363

Case, A., & Denton, A. (2015). Rising morbidity and mortality in midlife among white non-Hispanic Americans in the 21st century. *Proceedings of the National Academy of the Sciences of the United States of America, 112*(49). doi:10.1073/pnas.1518393112

Central Intelligence Agency. (2017). The world factbook. Country comparison: Health expenditures. Retrieved from https://www.cia.gov/library/publications/the-world-factbook/rankorder/2225rank.html

Chetty, R., Stepner, M., Abraham, S., Lin, S., Scuderi, B., Turner, N., Bergeron, A., & Cutler, D. (2016). The association between income and life expectancy in the United States, 2001-2014. *Journal of the American Medical Association, 315*(16), 1750-1766.

Claiborne, N., Videka, L., Postiglione, P., Finkelstein, A., McDonnell, P., & Krause, R. D. (2010). Alcohol screening, evaluation, and referral for veterans. *Journal of Social Work Practice in the Addictions, 10*(3), 308–326. doi:10.1080/1533256X.2010.500963

Council on Social Work Education (2014a). *Survey of social work programs: 2013 research brief.* Alexandria, VA: Author. Retrieved from https://www.cswe.org/CMSPages/GetFile.aspx?guid=19672b43-fab2-42b0-8a91-8ed7771e95d5

Council on Social Work Education. (2014b). *The role of social work in the changing health care landscape: Principles for public policy.* Alexandria, VA: Author.

Council on Social Work Education. (2015). *Educational policy and accreditation standards.* Alexandria, VA: Author.

Dzau, V. D., McClellan, M., Burke, S., Coye, M. J., Daschle, T. A., Diaz, A., . . . Zerhouni, E. (2017). Vital directions for health and health care: Priorities from a National Academy of Medicine initiative. Report prepared for the National Academy of Medicine. Retrieved from https://nam.edu/wp-content/uploads/2017/03/Vital-Directions-for-Health-Health-Care-Priorities-from-a-National-Academy-of-Medicine-Initiative.pdf

George, D. R., Rovniak, L. S., Kraschnewski, J. L., Hanson, R., & Sciamanna, C. N. (2015). A growing opportunity: Community gardens affiliated with US hospitals and academic health centers. *Preventive Medicine Reports, (2)*, 35–39. doi:10.1016/j.pmedr.2014.12.003

Institute of Medicine. (2014). *U.S. health in international perspective: Shorter lives, poorer health.* Washington, DC: National Academies Press.

Institute of Medicine. (2015). *Vital signs: Core metrics for health and health care progress.* Washington, DC: National Academies Press.

McGinnis, J. M., Berwick, D. M., Dascle, T. A., Diaz, A., Fineberg, H. V., Frist, W. H., . . . Lavizzo-Mourey, R. (2016). Systems strategies for health throughout the life course (Discussion Paper). In *Vital Directions for Health and Health Care Series.* Washington,

DC: National Academy of Medicine. Retrieved from https://nam.edu/wp-content/uploads/2016/09/Systems-Strategies-for-Better-Health-Throughout-the-Life-Course.pdf

McGinnis, J. M., Williams-Russo, P., & Knickman, J. R. (2002). The case for more active policy attention to health promotion. *Health Affairs, 21*(2), 78–93. doi:10.1377/hlthaff.21.2.78

National Center for Health Statistics. (2016). *Health, United States, 2015: With Special Feature on Racial and Ethnic Health Disparities*. Hyattsville, MD: Author.

National Center for Health Statistics. (2017). National vital statistics system. Retrieved from https://www.cdc.gov/nchs/data/factsheets/nvss_fact_sheet.pdf

National Institutes of Health. (2010). Disability in older adults. Retrieved from https://report.nih.gov/NIHfactsheets/Pdfs/DisabilityinOlderAdults(NIA).pdf

Obama, B. (2016). United States health care reform: Progress to date and next steps. *Journal of the American Medical Association, 316*(5), 525–532. doi:10.1001/jama.2016.9797

Ogden, C. L., Carroll, M. D., Fryar, C. D., & Flegal, K. M. (2015). *Prevalence of obesity among adults and youth: United States, 2011–2014*. NCHS Data Brief, No. 219. Hyattsville, MD: National Center for Health Statistics.

Organisation for Economic Co-operation and Development. (2017). Infant mortality rates (indicator). Retrieved from https://data.oecd.org/healthstat/infant-mortality-rates.htm

Ortman, J., Velkoff, V., & Hogan, H. (2014). *An aging nation: The older population in the United States*. Current Population Reports, P25-1140. Washington, DC: U.S. Census Bureau.

Reeves, S., Perrier, L., Goldman, J., Freeth, D., & Zwarenstein, M. (2013). Interprofessional education: Effects on professional practice and health care outcomes (update). *Cochrane Database of Systematic Reviews, 3*. doi:10.1002/14651858.CD002213.pub3

Renders, C. M., Valk, G. D., Griffin, S. J., Wagner, E., van Eijk, J. T., & Assendelft, W. J. J. (2000). Interventions to improve the management of diabetes mellitus in primary care, outpatient and community settings. *Cochrane Database of Systematic Reviews, 4*, CD001481. doi:10.1002/14651858.CD001481

Rine, C. M. (2016). Social determinants of health: Grand challenges in social work's future. *Health & Social Work, 41*(3), 143–145. doi:10.1093/hsw/hlw028

Riotta, C. (2017). GOP aims to kill Obamacare again after failing 70 times. *Newsweek*, July 29, 2017. Retrieved from http://www.newsweek.com/gop-health-care-bill-repeal-and-replace-70-failed-attempts-643832

Rishel, C. (2015). Establishing a prevention-focused integrative approach to social work practice. *Families in Society: The Journal of Contemporary Social Services, 96*(2), 125–132. doi:10.1606/1044-3894.2015.96.15

Roy, A. (2017). The new Senate Republican bill will transform American health care. *Forbes: The Apothecary*. June 23, 2017. Retrieved from https://www.forbes.com/sites/theapothecary/2017/06/23/the-new-senate-republican-bill-will-transform-american-health-care/#562a4d284318

Ruth, B. J., Marshall, J. W., & Velásquez, E. M. (2013). Prevention in social work scholarship: A content analysis of *Families in Society* 2000–2010. *Families in Society, 94*(3), 182–185. doi:10.1606/1044-3894.4304

Ruth, B. J., Velásquez, E. M., Marshall, J. W., & Ziperstein, D. (2015). Shaping the future of prevention in social work: An analysis of the professional literature from 2000 through 2010. *Social Work, 60*(2), 126–134. doi:10.1093/sw/swu060

Shartzer, A., Kenney, G. M., Long, S. K., & Odu, Y. (2016). A look at remaining uninsured adults as of March 2015. Retrieved from Urban Institute website: http://hrms.urban.org/briefs/remaining_uninsured_march_2015.pdf

Solar, O., & Irwin, A. (2010). A conceptual framework for action on the social determinants of health. Social Determinants of Health Discussion Paper 2 (Policy and
Practice). Retrieved from the World Health Organization website: http://www.who
.int/sdhconference/resources/ConceptualframeworkforactiononSDH_eng.pdf?ua=1

Spencer, M.S., Rosland, A., Kieffer, E., Sinco, B., Vlaerio, M., Palmisano, G., … Heisler, M.
(2011). Effectiveness of a community health worker intervention among African American
and Latino adults with Type 2 diabetes: A randomized control trial. *American Journal
of Public Health, 101*(12), 2253–2260. doi:10.2105/AJPH.2010.300106

Stevens, A. C., Carroll, D. D., Courtney-Long, E. A., Zhang, Q. C., Sloan, M. L.,
Griffin-Blake, S., & Peacock, G. (2016). Adults with one or more functional disabilities—United States, 2011–2014. *Morbidity and Mortality Weekly Report (MMWR), 65*,
1021–1025. doi:10.15585/mmwr.mm6538a1

U.S. Department of Labor, Bureau of Labor Statistics, Social Workers. (2016). Occupational
Outlook Handbook, 2016–17 Edition. Retrieved from https://www.bls.gov/ooh/
community-and-social-service/social-workers.htm

U.S. Senate. (2017). Better Care Reconciliation Act of 2017. Retrieved from https://assets
.documentcloud.org/documents/3872487/SenateHCBill.pdf

Videka, L., Ohta, B., Blackburn, A., Luce, V., & Morton, P. (in press). Integrated health
care roles for social workers. In V. Stanhope, & S. L. Straussner (Eds.), *Social work and
integrated health care: From policy to practice and back*. New York, NY: Oxford University
Press.

Walters, K., Spencer, M., Smukler, M., Allen, H. L., Andrews, C., Browne, T., … Uehara, E.
(2016) Health equity: Eradicating health inequalities for future generations. Grand
challenges for social work initiative, Working Paper # 19. American Academy of
Social Work and Social Welfare. Retrieved from http://aaswsw.org/wp-content/
uploads/2016/01/WP19-with-cover2.pdf

World Health Organization. (2012). *Spending on health: A global overview*. Fact Sheet No. 319.
April 2012. Geneva, Switzerland: Author.

Zammitti, E. P., Cohen, R. A., & Martinez, M. E. (2016). Health insurance coverage:
Early release of estimated from the National Health Interview Survey, January–June
2016. Report prepared for the National Center for Health Statistics. Hyattsville, MD:
National Center for Health Statistics. Retrieved from https://www.cdc.gov/nchs/
data/nhis/earlyrelease/insur201611.pdf

Index